Craniofacial Distraction

Joseph G. McCarthy
Editor

Craniofacial Distraction

Springer

Editor
Joseph G. McCarthy, M.D.
Wyss Department of Plastic Surgery
NYU Langone Medical Center
New York, NY
USA

ISBN 978-3-319-52562-4 ISBN 978-3-319-52564-8 (eBook)
DOI 10.1007/978-3-319-52564-8

Library of Congress Control Number: 2017941723

Printed on acid-free paper

This Springer imprint is published by Springer Nature
The registered company is Springer International Publishing AG
The registered company address is: Gewerbestrasse 11, 6330 Cham, Switzerland

Foreword

A revision may require an introduction for, as an example, taking the position of a ship at sea. But an original work is self-sufficient; it can stand by itself. It does not need a foreword, which is embarrassing for one to write who is ignorant in the matter.

New ideas—some often ridiculous—are daily occurrences in surgery, but successful clinical applications of them are rare. Moreover, when the applications of a new surgical concept extend rapidly to several areas, the fact deserves to be sharply emphasized. This is presently the case for Distraction Osteogenesis, called the "D.O.G." system by the writer. From the basic principles to animal experiments to quantitative evaluations and the wide spectrum of clinical applications, "D.O.G." is splendidly illustrated and its therapeutic appeals made convincing in this book.

Memories

Ilizarov's concept (1952) for limb reconstruction was born in remote, deep-frozen Siberia. Then Snyder experimented (1973) with the canine mandible, but his work escaped the facial surgeon's vigilance. However, Joe McCarthy made subsequent canine experiments and presented the first applications on the human in Florence in 1989; the "D.O.G." method then exploded within only 6 years. The fact is so much more remarkable when one considers that, in general, it takes *one generation* from the infant's first steps to easy jogging; other examples are the transitions from Medawar's tissue compatibility to current kidney transplantation and from chips to personal computers and the development of safety in lens or total hip replacements.

Paleoconcepts

It also took *one generation* for interceptive craniofacial surgery to be applied to the corrections of the deformities resulting from Crouzon syndrome, Apert syndrome, plagiocephaly, Franceschetti syndrome, hemifacial microsomia, "rare" facial clefts, and hypertelorbitism through the intracranial route. One generation of painful effort for all specialties, but only 6 years for McCarthy's performance in attracting facial and cranial surgical leaders.

Jubilation

The writer of this foreword feels the situation so much more ironic because several of the surgical steps mentioned above have been dramatically short-circuited by a simple "jackscrew" device skillfully used. A mandibular endless screw has opened an unlimited adventure. This is a revolution that has spread to the maxilla in Mexico; then the midface and calvarium in France, Germany, and the United States; and so on.

Panoramic Perspectives

Will an endless screw put an end to interceptive facial and cranial surgical procedures, which can still stand as landmarks and references for treatment goals? The D.O.G. system has been elaborated by Joe McCarthy for the child's mandible, which has a high potential for generating new bone. But D.O.G. has rapidly expanded to other young bones, and the method will probably remain a privilege for children. However, the principles have been already applied to nongrowing bones, such as those in craniosynostosis, and also to older posttraumatic mandibular deformities by the process of "bone transport," which might avoid the need for intraoral soft tissue transfers in adults.

Is it not amazing that the D.O.G. method has already attracted the orthodontists? Is it not encouraging that another gate of hope is now opened to the hopeless microphthalmic patients?

Further applications in the human will no longer be "human experiments," but sound applications of investigative surgeons who had either surrendered or had overwhelmed the problems by other means or other tools at different age groups.

Thank You

For the surgery of the human face, the year 1987 was a fabulous milestone. When Joe McCarthy uncorked the first bottle of "D.O.G." in Florence in 1989, he was continuing a half-century NYU tradition for innovation and education.

Paris, France Paul Tessier

Reproduced from the 1999 book

Preface

I suspect every author, contemplating writing a textbook, asks himself the obvious question: Why? Is there a need? Will it be worth the effort? For me, the answer is an unequivocal yes.

First of all, craniofacial distraction has been a personal odyssey beginning with our initial canine experiments in 1986. As our experience with the technique increased, both at New York University and other worldwide centers, I recognized the need to collect the relevant material and make it available to interested clinicians. The first effort was a workshop, probably the first ever on the subject, held at the NYU Medical Center in 1994. It was a small, but spirited, meeting with no more than 50 participants from around the world. We shared ideas and learned from each other. At the conclusion of the meeting, we recognized that craniofacial distraction, with many of the techniques first developed in animal models, had a sound research/clinical foundation and had resulted in significant advances in craniofacial surgical treatment.

Ten years after the first mandibular distraction, the first textbook, the forerunner of the current book, was published with multiple authors writing on laboratory research, as well as the clinical experience in mandibular and midface distraction. While there have been many meetings on the subject in the subsequent interval, I now believe, almost two decades later, that a new edition is indicated because of significantly new developments and findings in research and clinical distraction.

In organizing the book outline, I have arranged it according to the anatomic components of the craniofacial skeleton. Following the Introduction, there is a chapter entitled the "Biomechanical and Biomolecular Aspects of Distraction," detailing classic research that harks back to the historic work of Gavriil Ilizarov of Russia. Future research advances, beyond those chronicled in this chapter, will have profound effects on the practice of craniofacial distraction.

The chapter on mandibular distraction mainly reflects the experience and clinical protocols of the NYU team. However, there is a complete review of the international literature and the contributions of other teams are also discussed in the chapter.

I was fortunate to work closely with my NYU orthodontic colleague, Barry Grayson, right from the beginning of the craniofacial distraction project. We worked as a team and I learned a great deal from him. He excelled at preoperative planning, data collection and long-term outcome analysis. I should also note he is the father of craniofacial orthodontics, now recognized as a subspecialty of the American

Dental Association. He and Dr. Pradip Shetye have contributed a chapter entitled "Orthodontic Aspects of Mandibular Distraction" in which the critical role of the orthodontist in the clinical protocol is emphasized, followed by a chapter on midface/monobloc distraction.

I have recruited contributing authors from those areas of craniofacial distraction where they have made innovative contributions and have acquired a large clinical experience. Dr. Cesar Guerrero has a unique experience in intraoral mandibular distraction and has demonstrated inventive skills in the design of devices used to replace traditional orthognathic mandibular procedures.

My former trainee, James Bradley, recognized that cleft palate patients, while they may have a satisfactory occlusal relationship, often lack adequate midface projection or contour; hence, his promotion of Le Fort I level distraction before craniofacial maturity is attained.

Working with my former trainee and current NYU faculty member, Roberto Flores, I have outlined the NYU protocol and practices for midface and monobloc distraction. Our experience is predominantly based on the application of the RED or halo devices. We have shared follow-up outcome data extending out to 20 years postoperative.

David Dunaway and Aina Greig of London have a remarkable bipartition distraction experience in which they simultaneously correct orbital hypertelorism and midface hypoplasia. I have also recruited Jesse Taylor of Philadelphia who has developed new applications of the distraction method to expand the cranial vault in pediatric patients with craniosynostosis.

In my over 40 years at the Institute of Reconstructive Plastic Surgery at the NYU Langone Medical Center, I was fortunate to be a member of a remarkable clinical/research team with many of my colleagues drawn from basic science and clinical disciplines outside the specialty of plastic surgery. They have been collegial and we have spent many enjoyable hours together both in and outside the clinical setting. They have challenged me and also exchanged ideas and suggestions. Candor and hard work in such an environment are the key ingredients for clinical innovation and progress.

I wish to acknowledge those team colleagues and NYU fellows/residents who have been involved in the craniofacial distraction journey with me (and apologize to those inadvertently omitted): Joseph Bernstein, Sean Boutros, James Bradley, Lawrence Brecht, E.J. Caterson, Court Cutting, Wojciech Dec, Roberto Flores, Dale Franks, Scott Glasberg, Paul Glat, Arun Gosain, Barry Grayson, Aina Greig, Geoffrey Gurtner, David Hirsch, Craig Hobar, William Hoffman, Larry Hollier, Richard Hopper, Jordan Jacobs, John Jensen, Hitesh Kapadia, Nolan Karp, Tim Katzen, Jamie Levine, Michael Longaker, Richard Mackool, Susan McCormick, Babak Mehrara, Parit Patel, Norman Rowe, Doug Roth, Pierre Saadeh, John Schreiber, Pradip Shetye, John Siebert, Pedro Santiago, Jason Spector, David Staffenberg, Doug Steinbrech, Eric Stelnicki, Oren Tepper, Charles Thorne, Bruno Vendittelli, Stephen Warren, Katie Weichman, Robert Wood and Barry Zide.

I am also indebted to my colleagues beyond NYU, especially Drs. Fernando Ortiz-Monasterio and Fernando Molina of Mexico City. They early recognized the potential of craniofacial distraction and collected a large clinical series confirming the efficacy of the technique. Likewise, Drs. John Polley and Alvaro Figueroa of Chicago introduced the halo frame for midface distraction, a device whose reliability greatly influenced me. I must also acknowledge Drs. Diner and Vasquez who organized several meetings in Paris that did so much to disseminate the worldwide clinical experiences with this new technique. The biannual meeting of the International Society of Craniofacial Surgery (ISCFS), likewise, highlighted this subject in their programs.

My patients and their families have been my true heroes. Their spirit and courage continue to inspire and energize me. Their optimism and gritty determination were so impressive as they committed to new surgical procedures and the compilation of long-term clinical data. I must pay special attention to Pat Chibbaro, nurse clinician par excellence, who never lost sight of all details of a large clinical program and, yet, remained so devoted to the interests and needs of our patients and their families. Mary Spano, outstanding medical photographer, made sure our photographic records were of the highest quality to ensure important clinical data gathering. Her work is apparent to all who look at the illustrations in this book. Margy Maroutsis, working with Drs. Grayson and Shetye, saw to it that orthodontic visits with cephalograms and ICAT scans were coordinated.

Sandra Cummings, my executive secretary, was ever loyal and capable. Her organizational and computer skills were critical in this new era of electronic publishing. She has managed to keep my professional life on track, always with elegance and good humor.

Unlike the 1999 edition when I worked with a Springer publishing team working less than 15 city blocks away in New York, this book was developed and processed electronically continents apart. Yet, despite initial misgivings, I quickly realized I was working with highly skilled professionals whose help and cooperation I wish to acknowledge:

Ms. Wilma McHugh, production contact; Ms. Tanja Maihoefer from editorial team; Ms. Mahalakshmi Sathishbabu, project coordinator; and Mr. Rajesh Sekar, project manager

I dedicate this book to three departed mentors—all giants of the world of craniofacial surgery. They had endless energy, passion for surgery, intellectual curiosity and unquenchable commitment to surgical problem solving. Colleagues and friends, we shared many happy and warm times together.

John M. Converse—New York
Paul Tessier—Paris
Fernando Ortiz-Monasterio—Mexico City

My successor, Eduardo Rodriguez, in the Wyss Department of Plastic Surgery has graciously allowed me to continue some of my academic work. I am proud that Dr. Rodriguez is at the helm of NYU Plastic Surgery six decades after its founding.

Roberto Flores, my former resident and fellow, has fortunately been recruited back to the NYU Craniofacial Surgery Center. He has been involved in these chapters and has provided many important insights and ideas.

Most of all, I owe so much to Karlan, my wife of almost 55 years. She shared this distraction journey with me—and a "distraction" in our personal lives it could be. She, however, encouraged me and made it all possible, overseeing so many parts of my personal and family life. She tolerated a work schedule, often too fast paced. I will always be grateful for the joy, love and laughter she brings to my life.

New York, NY, USA
2017

Joseph G. McCarthy, M.D.

Contents

Craniofacial Distraction: A Personal Odyssey

1

Joseph G. McCarthy

By the mid-1980s, approximately 20 years after Tessier reported remarkable achievements in the reconstruction of the craniofacial skeleton with radically new surgical techniques, successful massive en bloc skeletal movements were routinely employed to improve craniofacial function and appearance. Moreover, CT imaging and rigid skeletal fixation systems had been developed, allowing even more complex craniofacial surgical reconstructions. Nevertheless, there remained unsolved problems. The surgical procedures were invasive, and the operations and hospitalizations were lengthy. There was often the need for bone graft harvest, and extensive blood replacement was necessary. Soft tissue problems were often not addressed, and many of the procedures represented what I call "bone carpentry." The relapse rate for many procedures was relatively high because of the acute intraoperative advancement of skeletal segments against restrictive and deficient soft tissue.

It had been my custom, as chief, to make plastic surgery rounds at Bellevue Hospital on Wednesday mornings. In 1986, at the completion of rounds, the residents suggested that I accompany them to the orthopedic surgery floor to see "something interesting." On arrival, we visited a bedside where there was a male patient lying in bed with Ilizarov distraction devices on his lower extremities for lengthening purposes. Prior to this visit, I was unaware of the concept of distraction osteogenesis. Immediately, I recognized that this novel technique of augmenting bone should be considered for reconstruction of the craniofacial skeleton. It was my Eureka moment!

We had been working in the laboratory to lengthen bone, and I must admit we were singularly unsuccessful. We had developed a canine mandible model in which the bone was osteotomized at the angle, and specially constructed skin expanders were inserted after the gap had been enlarged, the plan being to expand the expander

J.G. Mccarthy, M.D.
Wyss Department of Plastic Surgery, NYU Langone Medical Center, New York, NY, USA
e-mail: Joseph.mccarthy@nyumc.org

J.G. McCarthy (ed.), *Craniofacial Distraction*,
DOI 10.1007/978-3-319-52564-8_1

with serial saline injections. Regrettably, we had an excessively high infection rate and abandoned the experiment.

Following my visit to the orthopedic service, I knew it was time to return to the laboratory. I had always felt that translational research began on the clinical service where a problem was recognized and a solution sought. The laboratory should be used to develop a solution, which was then "translated" back to the clinical setting, in reality, a two way path. At that time, Nolan Karp was my research fellow and Charles Thorne the craniofacial surgery fellow. They were the first of many fellows and residents who were key members of the NYU craniofacial distraction team, working both in the laboratory and clinic setting. For the distraction experiment, we used a similar canine mandible model, and the Howmedica Corporation modified an existing finger distraction device. We followed the Ilizarov protocol as published (translated by my son who read and spoke Russian).

We made the osteotomy behind the last molar and secured the distraction device with two bicortical pins on either side of the osteotomy. As recommended by Ilizarov, we observed a latency period of 5 days and activated the device at the rate of 1 mm per day for 20 days. We maintained the device in consolidation for 8 weeks.

After euthanasia and stripping of the soft tissue, we were stunned to see robust and solid bone at the distraction zone. I was also struck at the three-dimensional expansion of the mandible. This series of mandibular distraction experiments was submitted to the journal, Plastic and Reconstructive Surgery. It was rejected but subsequently published in another journal [1]. Its rejection is ironic because this publication became the second-most cited paper in the plastic surgery literature.

In a follow-up study [2], the same NYU team reported a serial histologic study to ascertain the biologic events in the distraction zone:

1. An initial fibrous central zone with laying down of collagen in parallel bundles in the direction of the distraction forces
2. A transition zone characterized by the deposition of osteoid on the collagen matrix
3. A remodeling zone with the appearance of osteoblasts and osteoclasts
4. A mature bone zone

After extensive canine laboratory experience, I was convinced distraction of the mandible was ready for human application. I thought the ideal candidate would be a young child because I had recognized in my clinical work that the younger patient was a "bone factory" in its ability to produce bone. I was also looking for a patient with severe deficiency and an associated marked craniofacial dysmorphism. I believed that the mandible was the ideal bone for initial clinical distraction, especially since the teeth and radiographs/cephalograms would allow us to document the progress and result of the distraction. Moreover, unilateral mandibular distraction allowed the contralateral side to serve somewhat as a control.

I selected an 18-month-old boy with right-sided craniofacial microsomia. The parents and I had multiple conversations about the clinical problem, the novelty of the recommended surgical technique, and also the extensive laboratory experience supporting the use of a distraction device. The first craniofacial distraction procedure was performed in May 1989. I have followed the patient for 27 years, and his mother at one time was the president of our family support group. We subsequently operated on other children, and in our first clinical paper, we reported a series of patients with unilateral craniofacial microsomia [3].

Throughout this odyssey, my orthodontist colleague, Barry Grayson, was of invaluable assistance in documenting and advising me in terms of the three-dimensional change in mandibular morphology and the effects on the occlusion. I was always impressed with his creative ideas and his focus on the effects of surgical intervention on craniofacial growth and development in the younger patient.

It quickly became apparent that in patients with bilateral mandibular deficiency and obstructive sleep apnea, distraction was a major clinical breakthrough or milestone in the treatment of neonatal sleep apnea due to mandibular deficiency and glossoptosis. Many times, it precluded the need for a tracheotomy, a challenging therapeutic decision in the young child. The role of the pediatric otolaryngologist and the pediatric anesthesiologist was critical, and I learned a great deal from them on safely managing a dangerous airway.

In a series of patients with previous bone graft mandibular reconstructions, we learned that adequate bone volume was critical for distraction success [4]. Distraction of narrow caliber rib grafts led only to fibrous union. In the growing or young patient, we reported the value of removal of tooth follicles with a delay of several months before mandibular distraction in order to increase bone volume for the osteotomy and device application [5].

The next logical step was to develop an intraoral mandibular distraction device, and after the device had been fabricated, we demonstrated in the canine model that there was not an increase in the infection rate and there was bone of adequate volume and strength, even though the surgical wound had been exposed to the oral flora [6].

As I lectured around the world about this new technique, a common question, especially from oral maxillofacial surgeons, was what was the effect of mandibular distraction on the TMJ. Our team, with Susan McCormack leading, demonstrated in the laboratory and clinical setting that mandibular distraction had little negative effect on the normal TMJ [7, 8]. There was slight, but temporary, flattening of the condylar cartilage with no effect on the glenoid fossa. These findings were also borne out with the absence of temporomandibular joint problems in our clinical series. However, it was noted that with vertical vectors, there could be discomfort in the TMJ, and, on occasion, we would unload the joint by an orthodontically constructed occlusal splint.

These studies also led to a new surgical approach to the correction of TMJ ankylosis [9]. In the clinical setting, an L-shaped osteotomy was made, and transport distraction was performed after a gap arthroplasty to release the ankylosis. It is noteworthy that the leading edge of the transport segment had a fibrocartilaginous cover, simulating the condylar cartilage.

By this time, we recognized that distraction osteogenesis has a more global effect than simply lengthening or augmenting the affected bone. This led to the concept of "distraction histogenesis" or enlargement of not only the bone but also the associated soft tissue, i.e., the muscles of mastication and nerves [10].

I must acknowledge my gratitude for the early support and recognition of craniofacial distraction by the late Fernando Ortiz Monasterio and his young and dynamic colleague, Fernando Molina, of Mexico City. They embraced the technique and published an impressive large series of patients with successful mandibular distraction. Moreover, the father of craniofacial surgery, Paul Tessier of Paris, visited our canine laboratory at NYU, and I demonstrated one of our animals who had undergone unilateral mandibular distraction. I happened to remark that the name of the animal was Florence, as we were preparing to report the experiment at the biannual meeting of the International Society of Craniofacial Surgeons to be held in Florence in 1988. Tessier always spoke about his recognition of the impact of this new technique when he met "the patient Florence in New York." He also wrote a gracious preface to the first edition of this book in 1999 [11].

At the New York University Medical Center in 1994, we hosted the first ever conference on craniofacial distraction, and it was heartwarming to greet my colleagues from around the world who reported on their experience. We all learned a great deal from each other at this conference. It was the first of many worldwide stimulating craniofacial distraction conferences over the next two decades.

After success with mandibular distraction in the laboratory and clinical setting, the next logical step was to apply the technique to other components of the craniofacial skeleton. Along with other groups around the world, we were one of the first to demonstrate successful midface distraction osteogenesis in a canine model [12], and we also developed a model for multidimensional distraction of the canine zygoma [13]. This was later followed by laboratory demonstration of transport distraction in the rabbit calvaria [14]. The combined laboratory studies confirmed that all components of the craniofacial skeleton were amenable to successful distraction.

The development of midface or subcranial Le Fort III distraction had an enormous impact. Buried and external (halo) devices were developed, but we preferred the latter. The experience in midface distraction showed that it was safer in the younger child as manifest by reduced operating times and reduced hospital stays. The technique also allowed greater advancement or overcorrection in the growing child. Moreover, in monobloc distraction, the infection problem, previously associated with acute monobloc advancement and the resulting retrofrontal dead space, had been significantly reduced.

Our team also had other associated midface distraction projects including a canine model demonstrating an endoscopic Le Fort III osteotomy [15]. In a serial CT clinical study, we demonstrated the sites of bone deposition following midface distraction [16]. For example, more bone was generated when the osteotomy was made through the body of the zygoma rather than the thinner arch.

As our clinical experience with mandibular distraction progressed, we initiated a combined laboratory and clinical study of multiplanar distraction or "molding of the generate." We reported a three-part series of papers: (1) Development of Multiplanar

Device [17], (2) Laboratory Study of Sagittal and Vertical Movements [18], and (3) Sagittal and Horizontal Movements [19]. This was followed by a report of our clinical experience with multiplanar mandibular distraction or molding of the generate [20].

Long-term clinical research of distraction osteogenesis continued under Dr. Grayson's leadership with follow-up of patients who had undergone mandibular distraction to document the presence or absence of mandibular growth on the operative and nonoperative sides. These studies confirmed that in the growing child, there was growth on the operative side, albeit at a slower rate than the contralateral side [21, 22]. Long-term studies extending well into completion of craniofacial growth documented that there were two groups of patients: one which achieved satisfactory craniofacial form without additional surgery and another group that would require two-jaw surgery [23].

In our continuing clinical study, the NYU team further refined surgical planning by introducing the concept of the vector of mandibular distraction and outlining three vectors (vertical, oblique, and horizontal) based on the relationship of the distraction device to the maxillary occlusal plane [24]. In this way, it was demonstrated that surgeons can work with the orthodontists preoperatively in planning a mandibular distraction, whether bilateral [25] or unilateral [26], just as one would also plan traditional orthognathic surgery.

Our team at NYU was also able to conduct long-term clinical studies following the course of patients who underwent midface distraction. Dr. Pradip Shetye, an orthodontist working with Dr. Grayson, compared three groups of midface advancement patients followed over three decades: (1) acute Le Fort III advancement with intermaxillary fixation and wire fixation and bone grafts, (2) another group with acute advancement but with rigid skeletal fixation, and (3) the group with midface distraction [27]. Comparison of the three groups showed that with midface distraction, a much greater advancement could be obtained at orbitale and point A; the length of the operation and hospital stay were greatly reduced, as was the complication rate. In addition, a subsequent study showed the associated change in soft tissue contour in relation to the change in skeletal advancement [28]. Subsequent midterm follow-up studies [29] were extended to 5 years [30]. Another study documented the quantitative increase in airway volume [31].

A significant advance was the development of a rigid occlusal platform to prevent posterior descent of the Le Fort III segment [32] and to plan control and vector of the distracted midface segment [33].

Simultaneous with the clinical research, a team of laboratory researchers was developed to study the role of extracellular matrix proteins and the biomolecular mechanisms in the distraction zone in smaller animal models. We were particularly interested in developing methods of accelerating the activation phase and reducing the length of the consolidation phase in mandibular distraction. This resulted in a three-part publication. In part one, the rat mandibular distraction model was outlined along with histologic and radiographic analysis [34]. In the second report, there was a molecular analysis of TGF Beta-1 and osteocalcin gene [35]. It was demonstrated, for example, at what times in the biology of the distraction process VEGF, TGFB, and osteocalcin were uploaded. In another report, a device was outlined to deliver bioactive agents to the bone during distraction osteogenesis [36].

After all of the studies, I became convinced that Ilizarov had worked on the wrong bones of the human skeleton! In reality the bones of the craniofacial skeleton were much more amenable to distraction. They were thinner (membranous) and had a better blood supply. Moreover, they were capable of multidimensional molding and tolerated wider subperiosteal dissection for ease of device application, and we could also employ a faster activation rate than could Ilizarov. Finally, the accessibility of the teeth and cephalograms facilitated the study of the dynamic changes occurring during and after the distraction process.

As this book is being published, one must look to the future. I have no doubt that there will be substantial improvements in the distraction technique in the future. The goal remains to reduce the length of treatment by accelerating the activation rate and shortening the period of consolidation. Ideally, one hopes for a "spot weld" of the newly generated bone. I think in the future endoscopic techniques and miniaturized devices will be developed to reduce the extent of surgical exposure and make the surgical procedure less invasive. Resorbable distraction devices may preclude the need for a second surgical procedure; however, rigid fixation is an *absolute* requirement during the activation and consolidation phases. In the infant, there may be successful osteotomy-free distraction across suture sites. Distraction procedures in the future may become multidimensionally more complex, not unlike contemporary two-jaw surgery. There could be simultaneous multisegment distraction, including the midface and mandible with multivector plans combined. It could be entitled "combined orthognathic distraction."

As a prelude to the future, our research team reported several promising studies of gene therapy manipulation of the distraction zone [37]. A mandibular osteotomy was made and VEGF adenovirus injected in the distraction zone, and, after 10 days of activation, the BMP-2 adenovirus was injected. The studies showed earlier ossification in the gene-manipulated animal group as compared to the control group. This finding portends a future of shorter consolidation periods. There is also the potential of using adult stem cells (endothelial progenitor cells) to augment blood vessel formation and to transport to the distraction zone mesenchymal stem cells to promote more rapid bone generation [38]. In so many ways, craniofacial distraction osteogenesis represents the union of plastic surgery and tissue engineering. The opportunities for research and clinical innovation are endless.

The Biomedical Research of Today Is the Clinical Medicine of Tomorrow. Without It the Clinical Medicine of Tomorrow Will Be the Clinical Medicine of Today

James C. Thompson

In closing, I want to emphasize that by choice my summary is deliberately personal and relates the contributions to the emerging field of craniofacial distraction by our clinical and research teams at New York University. I thank them and I salute them. I must also acknowledge the significant contributions by similar teams around the world. Their work has contributed greatly to progress in the field and I have learned so much from my colleagues who have challenged and inspired me. Their contributions are documented in the bibliographies at the conclusion of the individual chapters of this book.

I am honored and grateful that several colleagues have authored chapters with subjects in which they have demonstrated unique expertise. It has been especially heartwarming for me to watch other workers in the craniofacial surgical world adopt the technique of distraction osteogenesis for addressing unresolved problems in craniofacial surgery, a discipline celebrating its fiftieth anniversary at the time of the publication of this book.

Glossary

Activation phase Often erroneously termed "distraction," the period of active device lengthening during distraction osteogenesis.

Appendicular skeleton Comprised of bones of the four limbs, pectoral girdle, and pelvic girdle.

Axial skeleton Comprised of bones of the face, skull, chest wall, and vertebrae.

Bifocal distraction Distraction osteogenesis to fill a central bony defect, by distracting one flanking transport segment toward the center. One osteotomy is made.

Consolidation phase The period following activation, during which the bony generate undergoes remodeling.

Distraction device Hardware that facilitates movement of bones during distraction. May be categorized as internal or external, based upon relation to soft tissue surrounding the bone. Not to be referred to as "distractor."

Distraction osteogenesis The generation of bone between vascularized bone surfaces which are separated by gradual distraction.

Endochondral bone Bone that forms via a cartilaginous intermediate.

Fibrous interzone (FIZ) Within the distraction gap, a physis-like organization of osteogenic cells.

Intramembranous bone Bone that forms directly from mesenchymal precursor cells, without a cartilaginous intermediate.

Latency phase The time following the osteotomy when initial fracture healing bridges the cut bone surfaces prior to initiating activation.

Molding of the generate Closed reduction maneuver of the generate, performed prior to or during the consolidation phase. Usually accomplished by manipulation of the distraction device or the application of interdental wire-rubber forces. Typically performed to improve the dental relationship following mandibular distraction.

Primary mineralization front (PMF) Within the distraction gap, a dense line of proliferating osteoblasts flanking the FIZ, that is actively undergoing mineralization.

Rate The number of millimeters per day at which bone surfaces are distracted.

Rhythm The number of device activations per day, usually in equally divided increments to total the rate.

Trans-osteotomy Refers to distraction osteogenesis performed across an osteotomy site.

Trans-sutural Refers to distraction osteogenesis performed across an interosseous suture, without an osteotomy.

Transchondroid bone A histologic finding exclusive to the distraction gap, marked by chondrocyte-appearing cells but without cartilage formation.

Transport distraction The generation of intercalary bone.

Transport segment The segment(s) of bone actively distracted during bifocal or trifocal transport distraction osteogenesis.

Trifocal distraction Distraction osteogenesis to fill a central bony defect, by distracting flanking transport segments toward the center. Involves two osteotomies.

Unifocal distraction Distraction osteogenesis to achieve simple bone lengthening, using a single osteotomy.

Vector The trajectory of applied distractive forces. With respect to the mandible, for example, often characterized as horizontal, vertical, or oblique.

Zone of microcolumn formation (MCF) Columns of ossifying bone forming within the distraction gap, surrounding the blood vessels that extend to the PMF.

References

1. Karp NS, Thorne CHM, McCarthy JG, Sissons HA. Bone lengthening in the craniofacial skeleton. Ann Plast Surg. 1990;24:231.
2. Karp NS, McCarthy JG, Schreiber JS, Sissons HA, Thorne CHM. Membranous bone lengthening: a serial histologic study. Ann Plast Surg. 1992;29:2.
3. McCarthy JG, Schreiber J, Karp N, Thorne CH, Grayson BH. Lengthening the human mandible by gradual distraction. Plast Reconstr Surg. 1992;89(1):1–8; discussion 9–10.
4. Stelnicki EJ, Hollier L, Lee C, Lin WY, Grayson B, McCarthy JG. Distraction osteogenesis of costochondral bone grafts in the mandible. Plast Reconstr Surg Mar 2002;109(3):925–33; discussion 934–5.
5. Regev E, Jensen JN, McCarthy JG, Grayson BH, Eski M. Removal of mandibular tooth follicles before distraction osteogenesis. Plast Reconstr Surg. 2004;113(7):1910–5.
6. McCarthy JG, Staffenberg DA, Wood RJ, Cutting CB, Grayson BG, Thorne CH. The introduction of an intraoral bone lengthening device. Plast Reconstr Surg. 1995;96:978.
7. McCormick SV, McCarthy JG, Grayson BH, Staffenberg DA, McCormick SA. The effect of gradual distraction of the mandible on the temporomandibular joint: part I, experimental canine study. J Craniofac Surg. 1995;6:358.
8. McCormick SV, Grayson BH, McCarthy JG, Staffenberg DA. The effect of gradual distraction of the mandible on the temporomandibular joint: part II, clinical study. J Craniofac Surg. 1995;6:364.
9. Stucki-McCormick SU, Fox RM, Mizrahi RD. Reconstruction of a neocondyle using transport distraction osteogenesis. Semin Orthod. 1999;5(1):59–63.
10. Mackool RJ, Hopper RA, Grayson BH, Holliday R, McCarthy JG. Volumetric change of the medial pterygoid following distraction osteogenesis of the mandible: an example of the associated soft-tissue changes. Plast Reconstr Surg. 2003;111(6):1804–7.
11. McCarthy JG. Distraction of the craniofacial skeleton. New York: Springer; 1999.
12. Staffenberg DA, Wood RJ, McCarthy JG, Grayson BH, Glasberg SB. Midface distraction advancement in the canine without osteotomies. Ann Plast Surg. 1995;34(5):512–7.

13. Glat PM, Staffenberg DA, Karp NS, Holliday RA, McCarthy JG. Multidimensional distraction osteogenesis: the canine zygoma. Plast Reconstr Surg. 1994;94:753.
14. Bouletreau PJ, Warren SM, Paccione MF, Spector JA, McCarthy JG, Longaker MT. Transport distraction osteotomies: a new method to heal calvarial defects. Plast Reconstr Surg. 2002;109:1074.
15. Levine JP, Rowe NM, Bradley JP, Williams JK, Mackool RJ, Longaker MT, McCarthy JG. The combination of endoscopy and distraction osteogenesis in the development of a canine mid-face advancement model. J Craniofac Surg. 1998;9:423.
16. Jensen JN, McCarthy JG, Grayson BH, Nussbaum AO, Eski M. Bone deposition/generation with Le Fort III (midface) distraction. Plast Reconstr Surg. 2007;119(1):298–307.
17. McCarthy JG, Williams JK, Grayson BH, Crombie JS. Controlled multiplanar distraction of the mandible: part I device development and clinical application. J Craniofac Surg. 1998;9:323.
18. Williams JK, Rowe NM, Mackool RJ, Levine JP, Hollier LH, Longaker MT, Cutting CB, Grayson BH, McCarthy JG. Controlled multiplanar distraction of the mandible part II: laboratory studies of sagittal (anteroposterior) and vertical (superoinferior) movements. J Craniofac Surg. 1998;9:504.
19. Hollier LH, Rowe NM, Mackool RJ, Williams JK, Kim JH, Longaker MT, Grayson BH, McCarthy JG. Controlled multiplanar distraction of the mandible part III: laboratory studies of sagittal and horizontal movements. J Craniofac Surg. 2000;11:83.
20. McCarthy JG, Hopper RA, Hollier Jr LH, Peltomaki T, Katzen T, Grayson BH. Molding of the regenerate in mandibular distraction: clinical experience. Plast Reconstr Surg. 2003;112(5):1239–46.
21. Hollier LH, Kim JK, Grayson BH, McCarthy JG. Mandibular growth after distraction in patients under 48 months of age. Plast Reconstr Surg. 1999;103:1361.
22. Shetye PR, Grayson BH, Mackool RJ, McCarthy JG. Long-term stability and growth following unilateral mandibular distraction in growing children with craniofacial microsomia. Plast Reconstr Surg. 2006;118(4):985–95.
23. Weichman K, Jacobs JMS, Patel PA, Shetye PR, Grayson BH, McCarthy JG. Early distraction for mild to moderate unilateral craniofacial microsomia (UCFM): long-term follow-up outcomes and recommendations. Plast Reconstr Surg. 2017.
24. Grayson BH, McCormick S, Santiago PE, McCarthy JG. Vector of device placement and trajectory of mandibular distraction. J Craniofac Surg. 1997;8(6):473–80; discussion 461–2.
25. Vendittelli BL, Dec W, Warren SM, Garfinkle JS, Grayson BH, McCarthy JG. The importance of vector selection in preoperative planning of bilateral mandibular distraction. Plast Reconstr Surg. 2008;122(4):1144–53.
26. Dec W, Peltomaki T, Warren SM, Garfinkle JS, Grayson BH, McCarthy JG. The importance of vector selection in preoperative planning of unilateral mandibular distraction. Plast Reconstr Surg. 2008;121(6):2084–92; discussion 2093–4.
27. Shetye PR, Davidson EH, Sorkin M, Grayson BH, McCarthy JG. Evaluation of three surgical techniques for advancement of the midface in growing children with syndromic craniosynostosis. Plast Reconstr Surg. 2010;126(3):982–94.
28. Shetye PR, Caterson EJ, Grayson BH, McCarthy JG. Soft-tissue profile changes following early Le Fort III distraction in growing children with syndromic craniosynostosis. Plast Reconstr Surg. 2013;132(4):945–54.
29. Shetye PR, Boutros S, Grayson BH, McCarthy JG. Midterm follow-up of midface distraction for syndromic craniosynostosis: a clinical and cephalometric study. Plast Reconstr Surg. 2007;120(6):1621–32.
30. Patel PA, Shetye PR, Warren SM, Grayson BH, McCarthy JG. Five year follow-up of midface distraction in growing children with syndromic craniosynostosis. Plast Reconstr Surg. 2016.
31. Flores RL, Shetye PR, Zeitler D, Bernstein J, Wang E, Grayson BH, McCarthy JG. Airway changes following Le Fort III distraction osteogenesis for syndromic craniosynostosis: a clinical and cephalometric study. Plast Reconstr Surg. 2009;124(2):590–601.
32. Shetye PR, Grayson BH, McCarthy JG. Le Fort III distraction: controlling position and path of the osteotomized midface segment on a rigid platform. J Craniofac Surg. 2010;21(4):1118–21.

33. Shetye PR, Giannoutsos E, Grayson BH, McCarthy JGL. Fort III distraction: part I. Controlling position and vectors of the midface segment. Plast Reconstr Surg. 2009;124(3):871–8.
34. Rowe NM, Mehrara BJ, Dudziak ME, Steinbreck DS, Mackool RJ, Gittes G, McCarthy JG, Longaker MT. Rat mandibular distraction osteogenesis, Part I. Histologic and radiographic analysis. Plast Reconstr Surg. 1998;102:2022.
35. Mehrara BJ, Rowe NM, Steinbrech DS, Dudziak ME, Saadeh PB, McCarthy JG, Gittes GK, Longaker MK. Rat mandibular distraction osteogenesis: part II. Molecular analysis of transforming growth factor beta-1 and osteocalcin gene expression. Plast Reconstr Surg. 1999;103:536.
36. Grayson BH, Rowe NM, Hollier Jr LH, Williams JK, McCormick S, Longaker MT, McCarthy JG. The development of a device for the delivery of agents to bone during distraction osteogenesis. J Craniofac Surg. 2001;12:19.
37. Ashinoff RL, Cetrulo Jr CL, Galiano RD, Dobryansky M, Bhatt KA, Ceradini DJ, Michaels VJ, McCarthy JG, Gurtner GC. Bone morphogenic protein-2 gene therapy for mandibular distraction osteogenesis. Ann Plast Surg. 2004;52:585.
38. Cetrulo Jr CL, Knox KR, Brown DL, Ashinoff RL, Dobryansky M, Chang EI, Bhatt KA, McCarthy JG, Gurtner GC. Stem cells and distraction osteogenesis: endothelial progenitor cells selectively home to the regenerate during activation and consolidation. Plast Reconstr Surg. 2005;116:1053.

Distraction Osteogenesis: Biologic and Biomechanical Principles

2

Christopher M. Runyan, Roberto L. Flores, and Joseph G. McCarthy

2.1 A Brief History

Distraction osteogenesis (DO) is a bone-regenerative process in which an osteotomy is followed by gradual distraction of the surrounding vascularized bone segments, with formation of new bone within the distraction gap. This process was first described by Alessandro Codivilla at the turn of the twentieth century [1, 2]. Codivilla demonstrated the ability to lengthen the chronically deformed femur or tibia 3–8 cm following an oblique osteotomy. He did this by applying a 25–30 kg distractive force across a full extremity plaster cast, which was serially and circumferentially cut near the level of deformity. Application of traction occurred only at the time of cast adjustment, causing a gap to form, which was then filled with additional plaster. This frequently resulted in pressure necrosis due to rubbing of the cast against the soft tissues of the leg.

Early limb lengthening attempts were met with complication and poor predictability and thus were not generally accepted before the work of Gavriil Ilizarov in the 1950s and 1960s. An orthopedist in Russia, Ilizarov conducted a series of experiments using the canine tibia to optimize distraction osteogenesis using a multi-pin circumferential external fixator. His advances included determination of optimal pin stability within the fixator, minimization of soft tissue disruption including periosteum preservation to maintain blood supply, demonstration of feasibility of corticotomies rather than osteotomies, determination of ideal latency and activation periods, and a rigorous histologic assessment of the distraction site, including description of the *neo-physis* [3, 4]. Ilizarov applied his findings to limb lengthening operations in over 15,000 patients, but his clinical work was unknown to the Western world until 1980. That year he operated on the Italian explorer, Carlo Mauri, who had a 10-year-old tibial deformity from a skiing accident deemed uncorrectable.

C.M. Runyan, M.D., Ph.D. • R.L. Flores, M.D. (✉) • J.G. McCarthy, M.D.
Wyss Department of Plastic Surgery, NYU Langone Medical Center, New York, NY, USA
e-mail: roberto.flores@gmail.com; Joseph.mccarthy@nyumc.org

J.G. McCarthy (ed.), *Craniofacial Distraction*,
DOI 10.1007/978-3-319-52564-8_2

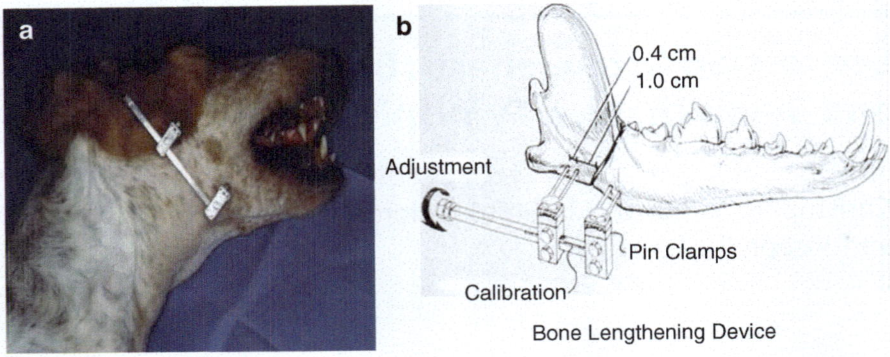

Fig. 2.1 (**a**) Canine with NYU extraoral distraction device. (**b**) Drawing of NYU canine model with osteotomy site and extraoral distraction device

Ilizarov corrected this deformity and pseudoarthrosis using his technique, and upon Mauri's return, Ilizarov was promptly invited to present his work at a conference in Bellagio in 1981. This was the first time Ilizarov spoke outside the Iron Curtain. His technique then spread rapidly throughout Europe and to the US by the late 1980s.

Within the craniofacial skeleton, distraction osteogenesis was first attempted experimentally in 1972 by Snyder [5]. His group surgically shortened one side of a canine mandible and then corrected the resultant crossbite using an external screw-driven distractor device. It was, however, the work of McCarthy and his colleagues at New York University who conducted a series of canine experiments [6, 7] (Fig. 2.1) that resulted in the first human application in 1989, when the mandibular body and ramus were lengthened in four young patients with congenital micrognathia [8]. This report ushered in the era of craniofacial distraction osteogenesis. Subsequent experiments in animal models further demonstrated the utility of distraction osteogenesis for lengthening or expanding the midface [9, 10], zygoma/glat [11], and cranial vault [12, 13]. Based on these studies and others, the use of distraction has since expanded to treat a wide range of congenital anomalies and acquired deformities throughout the craniofacial skeleton.

2.2 Classification of Distraction Osteogenesis

Distraction osteogenesis may be classified based on treatment goal, type of distraction device, anatomic location, or operative approach. When considering the goals of treatment, there are three modalities: (1) pure lengthening procedures, (2) bone segment transportation for correction of defects without lengthening, (3) and corrective distraction osteotomies. Bone lengthening is the most common application and requires a single osteotomy or corticotomy followed by application of distractive forces (Fig. 2.2, *top panel*). Bone transport osteogenesis is used to fill bony defects by advancing adjacent bone or "transport segment" into the gap. One or two transportation segments may be used, depending upon defect size and

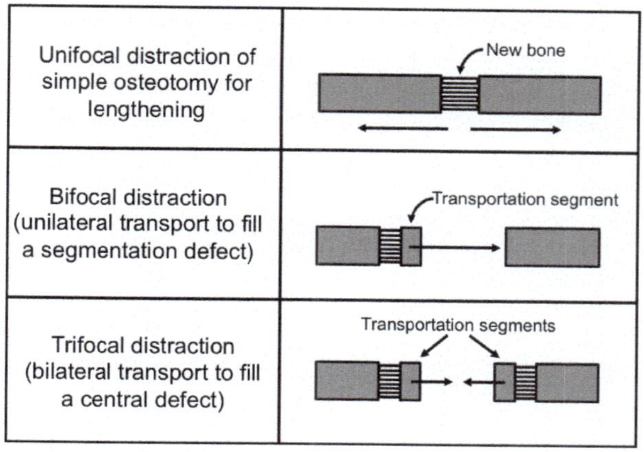

Fig. 2.2 Modalities of distraction osteogenesis

surgeon preference (Fig. 2.2, *middle and bottom panels*). Corrective distraction osteotomies combine bone lengthening with additional movements to correct shortened limbs with varus/valgus or rotational deformities. Both lengthening procedures and bone segment transport modalities are used within the craniofacial skeleton.

Distraction osteogenesis devices may also be classified as either external or internal. Both classic limb lengthening and early mandible distraction utilized external distraction devices. These devices generally have threaded drive shafts, which interface with the osteotomized bone by pin fixation. More recently internal devices have gained in popularity for use in craniofacial applications, particularly for the mandible and cranial vault. These are typically directly applied to the bone via screw fixation in a subperiosteal plane. Internal devices have the advantage of increased rigidity and absence of cumbersome external hardware, but may decrease bone blood supply, as they require greater periosteal dissection and require a separate procedure for device removal. Internal distraction for limb lengthening is now possible using periosteum-sparing telescoping intramedullary nails [14].

Anatomic location is another means of classifying distraction osteogenesis. Within the appendicular skeleton, the procedure is most commonly described within the long bones of the lower extremity (Table 2.1). Within the craniofacial skeleton, distraction osteogenesis was initially applied to the mandible; however, its use has increasing popularity within the maxilla (particularly the alveolus), the midface, and the cranial vault.

A final classification consideration is whether a *trans-sutural* (closed) or *trans-osteotomy* (open) operative approach is used. It is arguable whether closed approaches actually constitute distraction osteogenesis, as no osteotomies are performed; however, they do utilize an activation and consolidation period. A closed approach within the appendicular skeleton is called "distraction epiphysiolysis." This utilizes an external ring distractor to apply tension across an open growth plate, with external pins placed across the epiphysis and metaphysis. Its use is associated with risk of damage to the growth plate resulting in growth reduction [15] and therefore is often reserved

Table 2.1 Relative popularity of anatomic sites of distraction osteogenesis, based on the number of references obtained from a PubMed query (01/2016) using the search terms "distraction osteogenesis" and the "operative sites/indications"

Appendicular skeleton		Craniofacial skeleton	
Search term	# References	Search term	# References
Tibia	558	Mandible	1529
Femur	243	Maxilla	742
Radius	74	Alveolus	588
Metatarsal	58	Palate	476
Metacarpal	39	LeFort	420
Humerus	32	Craniosynostosis	287
Pelvis	9	Monobloc	80

for adolescents nearing closure of the growth plates. The membranous bones of the craniofacial skeleton lack growth plates, but during childhood individual bones may be distracted across interosteal suture lines. Palatal expansion is a well-known example of this trans-sutural approach. Recent studies suggest this approach may also be applied to the maxilla for midface advancement [16–18]. Without an osteotomy there is limited control of the bone using this method, and its value will require a future assessment of relapse and long-term outcomes.

2.3 Phases of Distraction Osteogenesis

Distraction osteogenesis may be divided into three dynamic or temporal phases: *latency*, *activation*, and *consolidation*. The period of delay following the osteotomy and prior to activation of the distraction device is known as the latency period. Short latency periods are generally associated with decreased volume of callus and inadequate osteogenesis, whereas long latency periods may lead to premature consolidation [4]. However, latency duration for the craniofacial skeleton (0–4 days) is by necessity much shorter than that for the appendicular skeleton (5–10 days), because of more rapid bone healing of the thin, membranous bones. Also, the majority of craniofacial distraction is performed in children, whose skeleton is actively growing, and who heal facial fracture rapidly at baseline. Some have even advocated for eliminating the latency phase in craniofacial applications. Slack et al. found that, although there are decreases in osteogenic activity at the cellular and molecular level when latency is eliminated, clinically there is no difference in the distracted mandible receiving a 48 h latency versus no latency period [19]. Other human [20] and animal models of mandibular distraction [21, 22] similarly found no clinical difference when the latency period was eliminated. Given these data and our clinical experience, a determination of appropriate latency period in craniofacial applications should be optimized to avoid premature consolidation. In neonates the latency period can be reduced to 1 day.

The *activation phase* follows latency. Its duration is determined by the clinical goal for bone production. Two variables during activation are the *rate* (or distance) the device is advanced each day and the *rhythm* (or frequency) of device activation. In his canine tibial distraction model, Ilizarov found that an activation rate of 0.5 mm/day frequently resulted in premature consolidation, but 2.0 mm/day may result in nonunion [4]. McCarthy and the NYU group also reported that 1.0 mm/day had the best outcomes and that increased frequency of device activation resulted in fewer complications [23, 24]. From this many have cited a rate of 1.0 mm/day as the optimal rate for craniofacial device activation [21, 25, 26]. Mathematical [27] and computational [28] models seem to support this clinical finding. However, as with latency, neonates or young children with high healing proclivity may require faster distraction rates, up to 2.0 mm/day, to avoid premature consolidation [20].

Distraction *rhythm* refers to the frequency of activation. Using his canine tibial model, Ilizarov found increased quality and quantity in bone formed by distraction osteogenesis, when activating the distractor 60 times per day compared to only once per day, although both received a total of 1 mm advancement [4]. Histochemical analysis shows increased expression of osteoblastic markers (alkaline phosphatase and adenosine triphosphatase) in the tissues distracted with greater frequency [4]. A direct comparison between continuous and discontinuous distraction protocols further demonstrated improved vascularization and more rapid bone formation in the continuously activated protocol [29]. These findings have led to development of automated continuous distraction devices currently in preclinical testing stages [30]. It is important to note that the rhythm of distraction is not as important as the rate, and a rhythm of twice a day has become the accepted clinical model.

Following activation, the *consolidation phase* ensues during which time mineralization of the new osteoid matrix occurs. For membranous bones and prior to consolidation, it is possible to manipulate the distracted segment, a maneuver known as "molding the regenerate." Reports of this maneuver are largely limited to small case series, which demonstrate that in certain instances it may serve as a useful added step in the distraction protocol to help optimize the generated bone position, particularly to improve dental relationships [31–33]. Compared to the other stages of distraction osteogenesis, little research or controversy surrounds the length of this phase, and yet, this is the longest phase, especially for the patient. Upon completion of activation, the devices are kept in place until radiographic evidence of mineralization is present. In the craniofacial skeleton, the accepted period is at least twice the length of the activation phase, or approximately 8 weeks [34–36]. Inadequate time allowed for consolidation may lead to greater relapse of the regenerate.

2.4 Biology of Bone Formation, Fracture Healing, and Distraction Osteogenesis

Clinical use of distraction osteogenesis is essentially a form of bone tissue engineering. Tissue engineering requires three primary components: a progenitor or stem cell to produce the desired tissue, growth factors to provide the necessary inductive signals to the progenitor cells, and a scaffold to guide appropriate three-dimensional configuration of the growing tissue. During distraction osteogenesis the bone-anchored distraction device provides the rigidity and necessary space that would normally be provided by a scaffold. Progenitor cells and growth factors are conveniently provided by the niche surrounding the distraction site. To the reconstructive surgeon hoping to generate new, vascularized bone, however, these cellular and molecular interactions may be a black box. Bone is unique among all tissues in the body, as it is the only tissue to heal or regenerate without scar formation and to regain its full premorbid strength and function. The complex molecular interactions of healing bone reflect how they formed during development [37, 38]. An understanding of the molecular biology and physiology of bone formation and fracture healing will provide insights into how bone is produced during distraction osteogenesis.

2.4.1 Pathways of Bone Development

During embryonic development, bone forms by one of two pathways: *endochondral* or *intramembranous* ossification (reviewed in [39]). The former requires a cartilaginous intermediate and is responsible for formation of the entire appendicular (limbs and pelvis) and much of the axial skeleton, including the ribs, scapulae, and skull base. *Endochondral bone* forms either from paraxial mesoderm (axial skeleton) or from lateral plate mesoderm, which contributes to the limb buds (appendicular skeleton). *Intramembranous ossification* does not involve a cartilaginous intermediate but instead relies on direct differentiation of mesenchymal precursor or neural crest cells into osteoblasts. It is the mechanism for development of most of the craniofacial skeleton. Intramembranous bones within the craniofacial skeleton (Fig. 2.3) are derived either from neural crest cells for the more cephalad structures and facial bones or from paraxial mesoderm for the more caudal structures and skull base [41]. Some of the caudal-most bones of the skull (occipital, ethmoid, petrous portion of the temporal, and portions of the sphenoid bones) develop by endochondral ossification.

Endochondral and intramembranous bone are first identified as clusters of undifferentiated cells known as mesenchymal condensations, which through an unknown mechanism coalesce in the areas of future skeletal development [39, 42]. Neural crest cells are derived from neuroectoderm of the developing neural tube, but undergo an epithelial-to-mesenchymal transition followed by delamination and ventral migration into craniofacial structures within the developing embryo. As with mesoderm-derived cells within mesenchymal condensations, neural crest cells similarly may lead to bone production via either intramembranous or endochondral ossification [43, 44], although the craniofacial skeleton is predominately formed from neural crest cells via intramembranous ossification (Fig. 2.4). The progression and differentiation of these cells are guided by signaling pathways, many of which are also relevant for fracture healing.

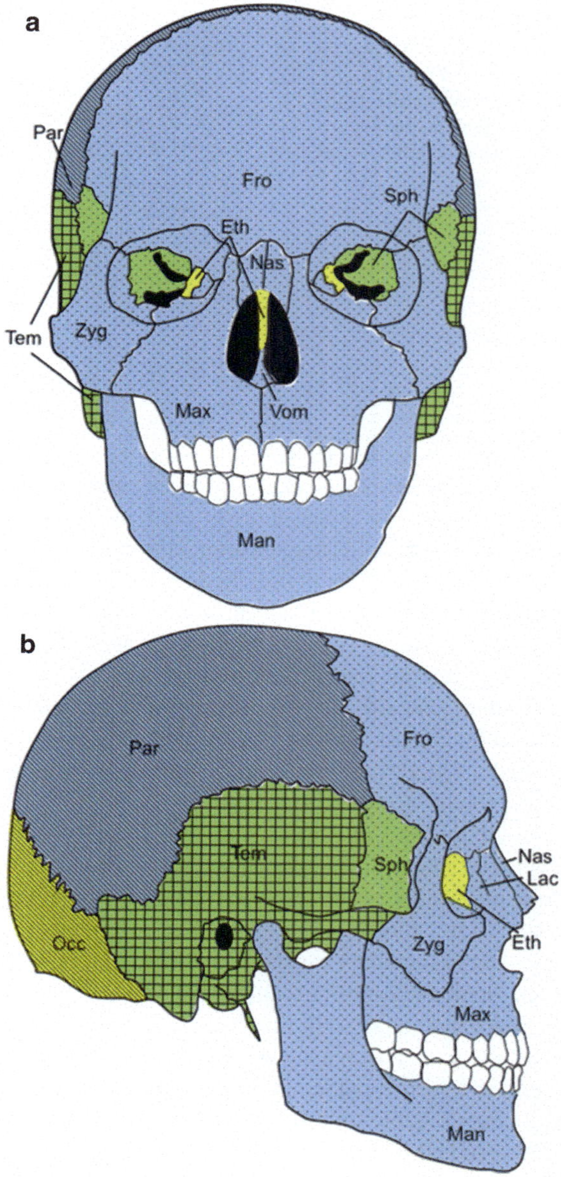

Fig. 2.3 Derivation of bones of the calvarium (adapted from [40], Craniofacial Embryogenetics and Development). (**a**, **b**) Two views of the human craniofacial skeleton, including (**a**) frontal and (**b**) lateral depicting both the cell source and the mechanism of bone formation. *Blue*—intramembranous ossification. *Yellow*—endochondral ossification. *Green*—both intramembranous and endochondral ossification. *Dotted*—neural crest cell derived. *Diagonal lines*—paraxial mesoderm derived. *Crosshatched*—both neural crest and paraxial mesoderm derived. *Eth* ethmoid, *Fro* frontal, *Lac* lacrimal, *Man* mandible, *Max* maxilla, *Nas* nasal, *Occ* occipital, *Par* parietal, *Sph* sphenoid, *Tem* temporal, *Vom* vomer, *Zyg* zygoma

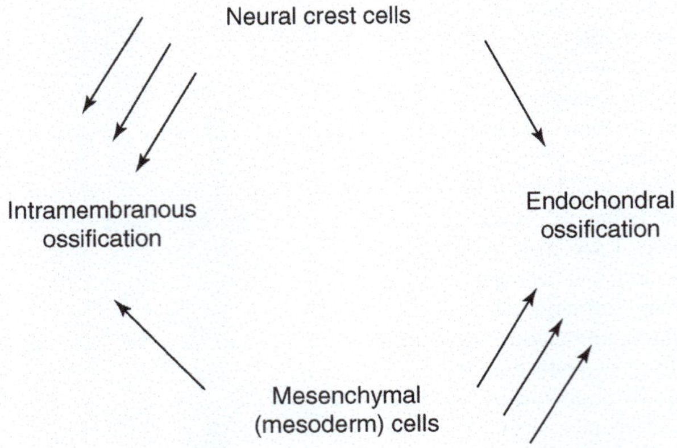

Fig. 2.4 Relative contributions of neural crest cells and paraxial mesoderm cells to the two types of bone within the craniofacial skeleton

Figure 2.5 depicts the possible fates of cells within the mesenchymal condensations. In the craniofacial skeleton, these cells may undergo intramembranous ossification, producing bone directly without a cartilaginous intermediate. In the remainder of the axial and appendicular skeleton, mesenchymal precursor cells give rise to an intermediate tissue, the immature cartilage. From immature cartilage two additional types of cartilage may develop: persistent and replacement cartilages. Persistent cartilage remains relatively avascular and eventually forms the cartilages of the nose, ear, intervertebral discs, and ribs. In contrast, replacement cartilage undergoes chondrocyte hypertrophy and vascularization allowing progression to endochondral ossification. During this process, chondrocytes enter a tightly controlled program of proliferation, pre-hypertrophy, hypertrophy, apoptosis, and replacement by osteoblasts [45].

Many of the signal transduction pathways regulating the progression of mesenchymal condensations to bone and cartilage are understood and are recapitulated in fracture healing. The pro-osteogenic factor runt-related transcription factor 2 (Runx2) is expressed among both pre-osteoblasts in mesenchymal condensations and later in immature cartilage [46]. Mice deficient in both alleles of Runx2 form no bone demonstrating its requirement for both intramembranous and endochondral bone formation [47–49]. Further, a mutation in one copy of Runx2 in humans leads to cleidocranial dysplasia which is marked by hypoplastic clavicles, supernumerary teeth, enlarged fontanelles, and eventual osteoporosis [48]. A similarly important pro-chondrogenic transcription factor, Sox9 [SRY (sex-determining region Y)-related HMG box gene 9], is essential for cartilage development. The absence of Sox9 in mice results in a complete absence of cartilage formation [50–52], and partial loss in humans leads to campomelic dysplasia [53–55], which is marked by craniofacial defects, bowing, and angulation of the long bones, and tracheobronchial hypoplasia which frequently leads to perinatal respiratory distress and lethality. Together Runx2 and Sox9 are master regulatory transcription factors for osteogenic and chondrogenic specification, respectively.

Sox9 promotes expression of essential cartilage-related collagen genes including Coll II [56], Coll IX [57], and Coll XI [58], which together help generate an

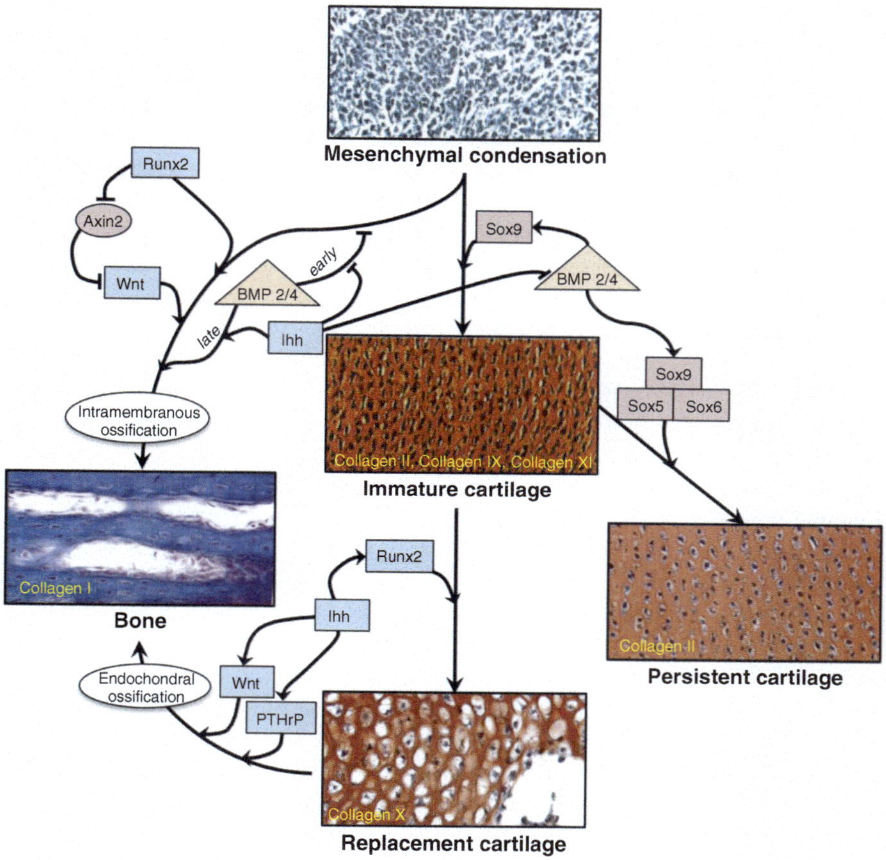

Fig. 2.5 Pathways for bone formation. Modified from Eames and Helms [37]

extracellular collagen matrix. Within immature cartilage chondrocytes rapidly divide and remain undifferentiated. Key factors in stimulating chondrocyte proliferation and Sox9 activity are bone morphogenetic proteins 2 (BMP-2) and BMP-4 [43]. This is perhaps counterintuitive because exogenous BMP-2 is clinically utilized as a powerful morphogen for bone formation. In contrast the transition of immature to replacement cartilage involves chondrocyte maturation through distinct pre-hypertrophic and hypertrophic stages, as well as vascular invasion and activation of bone markers. This requires additional signaling pathways, the most important of which is Hedgehog (reviewed in [59]).

The Hedgehog (Hg) gene is evolutionarily conserved, and mammalian homologues include Sonic (Shh), Desert (Dhh), and Indian (Ihh) hedgehogs. It is expressed by pre-hypertrophic chondrocytes within replacement cartilage and accelerates their hypertrophy and promotes osteoblast differentiation. Ihh does this by activating Runx2, which then activates Osterix (Osx) [60]; without either of these transcription factors, no bone can form. Ihh also decreases BMP-2 activity, which leads to downregulation of Sox5, Sox6, Sox9, and Coll II [61]. Recent experiments performed in a bone organ culture system demonstrated that although BMP-2 has potent pro-osteoblast properties, Hh signaling is required; without the presence of Hh activity, BMP-2 promotes ectopic chondrogenesis within the perichondrium [62]. Ihh also stimulates expression of the hypertrophic cartilage marker, type-X collagen. Perhaps the best understood Ihh-mediated pathway in developing bone is that of parathyroid hormone-related peptide (PTHrP). Within growth plates of endochondral bone, Ihh and PTHrP participate in a feedback loop, regulating the rate of chondrocyte proliferation and differentiation into pre-hypertrophic and hypertrophic chondrocytes.

Development of calvarial bones by intramembranous ossification occurs as presumptive bone cells proliferate and migrate outward from mesenchymal condensations [63]. Instead of growth plates, intramembranous bone relies upon ossification centers that add bone in a radial fashion. Many of the pro-osteogenic molecular pathways essential for endochondral bone formation are essential for intramembranous bone formation, including Runx2, Wnt, Ihh, and BMP. A lack of BMP signaling within the cranial mesenchymal condensations is permissive for osteoblast formation, whereas at later stages BMP signaling is essential for neural crest-derived calvarial bone formation [41, 43]. Ihh also has an important role; it is expressed at the leading edge of growing cranial bones, promoting bone formation by BMP-2- and BMP-4-mediated direct osteogenic differentiation rather than proliferation [64]. Its loss results in significantly decreased calvarial bone formation [43]. Deletion of repressors of Hh signaling (Gli3 and Rab23) results in high Hh activity with associated increased ossification of calvarial bones and craniosynostosis [65, 66]. Runx2 is expressed within calvarial osteoblasts during the process and promotes osteogenesis. Loss of one allele of Runx2 is associated with delayed suture closure and persistent fontanels [67]. The pro-osteogenic effects of Runx2 in intramembranous bone are mediated through Wnt signaling. Activation of the Wnt pathway promotes specification of the osteogenic lineage and represses the chondrogenic lineage within calvarial mesenchyme [41]. TGF-β signaling is also important as it promotes calvarial osteocyte proliferation. Nearly all studies of intramembranous bone development examine the frontal or parietal bones, and relatively little is understood of the process within intramembranous bones of the facial skeleton [68].

2.4.2 Pathways of Appendicular Bone Fracture Healing

Fractures of bones of the appendicular skeleton heal by both intramembranous and endochondral ossification. Endochondral bone formation predominates, occurring outside the periosteum in mechanically unstable regions and immediately adjacent to the fracture site. Intramembranous bone formation occurs subperiosteally at the proximal and distal edges of the callus and forms hard callus [69]. Bridging of the hard callus across the fracture gap provides initial stabilization and leads to restoration of biomechanical function [70]. As endochondral ossification is the mechanism of bone formation in the appendicular skeleton, it is also the mechanism primarily responsible for appendicular skeletal repair.

Four overlapping phases of fracture healing may be evident histologically (reviewed in [71]):

1) *Immediate inflammatory response*. This occurs over the initial 24–48 h post fracture and is marked by hematoma formation, hemostasis, inflammation, and recruitment of mesenchymal stem cells (MSCs).
2) *Cartilage formation with early endochondral ossification and periosteal response*. During this period mesenchymal stem cells differentiate into chondrocytes, which then produce a cartilaginous callus rich in collagen and proteoglycans [72, 73]. The soft, cartilaginous callus grows inversely proportional to the stability of the fracture and does so asymmetrically within the fracture. For example, femur fractures produce larger distal calluses and tibial fractures and larger proximal calluses, suggesting a recapitulation of bone development with the calluses forming nearest the growth plates [70, 74]. The soft callus growth peaks between 7 and 9 days following the fracture [73]. The periosteal response results in early intramembranous ossification and is associated with cell proliferation and early vascular ingrowth and neo-angiogenesis.
3) *Cartilage resorption and primary bone formation*. During this phase chondrocytes proliferate, mature, become hypertrophic, and increase synthesis of collagen, which accumulates within the extracellular matrix. As the chondrocytes then begin to undergo apoptosis, additional mesenchymal progenitor cells are recruited and differentiate into osteoblasts. This leads to callus mineralization, as osteoblasts use the soft callus as a template to deposit woven bone in place of the mineralized cartilage. This is initially manifest as a thin shell of bone around the periphery of the callus. Neo-angiogenesis also continues during this phase.
4) *Secondary bone formation and remodeling*. During this final phase, the bony callus grows and is reshaped by osteoclastic resorption and osteoblastic bone formation, resulting in regeneration of the original cortical and trabecular arrangement with a marrow-containing medullary cavity.

The molecular physiology of these four phases of fracture healing is well understood and shares many molecular similarities with endochondral bone development. A comprehensive description of these factors is beyond the scope of this chapter; however, an updated, concise summary is presented in Table 2.2. Of the many cytokines and growth factors involved, three groups have complex, well-defined overlapping roles during the four stages of bone healing: pro-inflammatory cytokines, TGF-β superfamily members (including the BMPs), and angiogenic factors. A number of other pathways are implicated in the healing process as their loss results in significant perturbations in the ability to heal, although their specific roles in the four phases of bone healing are not well defined. These include the Hedgehog [85] and Wnt signaling pathways ([86–88]; Minear 2010).

In the absence of rigid fixation, fracture healing of the appendicular skeleton occurs through formation of a cartilage scaffold, which is gradually replaced with

Table 2.2 Molecular pathway activation during endochondral bone fracture healing (adapted from [71])

Stage of fracture repair	Biologic process	Signaling molecule activation and proposed functions
Inflammation	Hematoma	IL-1, IL-6, and TNF-α release by circulating granulocytes and lymphocytes recruits inflammatory cells, enhances extracellular matrix synthesis, and stimulates angiogenesis [75]
	Inflammation and recruitment of progenitor cells	TGF-β, PDGF, and BMP-2 expression promote extracellular matrix formation and initial callus formation ([76], [77]). MMP-9 regulates the distribution of inflammatory cells [78]
Cartilage formation	Collagen deposition	Collagens type II and type III accumulate shortly after inflammation, produced by chondrocytes in the cartilaginous callus and periosteal osteoblasts
	Chondrogenesis and endochondral ossification	TGF-β2 and TGF-β3 stimulate chondrogenesis, corresponding with collagen type II synthesis [79]. BMP-2 promotes chondrocyte differentiation [80]. PTH also promotes cartilaginous and bony callus formation, whereas OPG prevents chondroclastogenesis by inhibiting RANKL
	Vascular ingrowth	MMP-9 promotes vascular invasion of hypertrophic cartilage, by promoting VEGF bioavailability [81]. VEGF directly stimulates angiogenesis and is maximally expressed when resorption is initiated [71]
Primary bone formation	Chondrocyte apoptosis and cartilage resorption	TNF-α stimulates mineralized chondrocyte apoptosis and cartilage resorption and helps recruit osteoprogenitor cells ([70, 82]; [83]). RANKL activity increases while OPG decreases, stimulating chondroclastogenesis
	Changes in collagen expression	Collagens type II and type III are removed as cartilage callus resorbs. Collagen type I accumulates as bony trabeculae develop. Collagen type X expression by hypertrophic chondrocytes provides a template for bone formation
	Mesenchymal cell differentiation to osteoblasts	Stimulated by BMP-2, BMP-6, and BMP-9 [84]
	Osteoblast recruitment and maturation	Stimulated by BMP-3, BMP-4, BMP-7, and BMP-8 ([79], [84])
	Neo-angiogenesis	VEGF and PDGF expression continue to promote angiogenesis
Secondary bone formation	Bone remodeling	TNF-α, IL-1, and RANKL activity promote bone remodeling by osteoclast remodeling of woven bone for lamellar bone formation

bone. This healing closely resembles the steps of embryonic endochondral ossification [38]. Mesenchymal precursors coalesce in the shape and location of the bone to be formed both for endochondral ossification and fracture healing. Both processes also involve mesenchymal cell proliferation and differentiation and hypertrophy along a cartilaginous or osteogenic pathway. An obvious difference between the processes is the presence of the inflammatory step in fracture healing that facilitates recruitment of the mesenchymal stem cells. However, once these cells are present, some of the same signaling pathways are involved including Ihh, VEGF, and MMP [38]. It is perhaps the preservation of many of these embryonic pathways that allow fractured bone to avoid forming scar, but to heal through a truly regenerative process.

2.4.3 Pathways of Craniofacial Skeletal Fracture Healing

An early rabbit mandible fracture model demonstrated that in the absence of rigid fixation, mandible fracture healing has some histologic similarities with long bone fractures [89]. Within 2 weeks of fracture, a large subperiosteal callus develops containing chondroid and immature osteoid. Within the subsequent 2 weeks, this callus is gradually replaced with trabecular bone and is completely bridged with new neovascular channels and Haversian systems. Paccione et al. similarly observed in their mouse mandible fracture model that the sequential presence of islands of rudimentary cartilage matrix formation, vascular ingrowth, osteoblast activation, mineralization, and lamellar bone formation resembled secondary bone endochondral bone healing [90]. They suggest that the contribution of a cartilage intermediate in their mandible fracture model (and that of others) was simply due to bony instability. Indeed the presence of instability in long bone fractures results in increased motion at the fracture site, which promotes cartilaginous callus formation during the primary bone healing phase.

Rigorous animal studies have not been performed to examine the histologic and molecular changes of facial bone fractures treated with rigid fixation. There are a number of reasons for this. The small size of rodent facial bones precludes plate fixation. Microplates were not available when bone healing studies were commonly performed. The lack of a straight marrow cavity precludes the use of intramedullary stabilization. Despite this, clinical experience provides overwhelming evidence that bones that develop by intramembranous ossification heal by the same mechanisms, and generally not through a cartilaginous intermediate. Skull fractures illustrate this principle. The scalp provides a tight soft tissue envelope to promote calvarial fracture reduction, while the convexity of the calvarium forms a sturdy keystone arch, which provides natural rigid fixation. Most of the bones of the facial skeleton similarly have a stabilizing periosteum and soft tissue envelope and are not subject to repeated forces. In contrast the mandible is subject to cyclic mechanical loading associated with mastication. However, with immobilization or rigid load-bearing or load-sharing fixation, the mandible heals by direct ossification.

Hasegawa et al. [91] provide experimental evidence opposing a role for chondrogenesis in membranous bone healing. They initially identified multipotent mesenchymal progenitor cells within fracture hematomas of long bones and demonstrated their ability to differentiate into osteocytes, adipocytes, and chondrocytes in vitro [92]. They subsequently cultured human *mandible* fracture hematoma cells and found that although these cells had a similar mesenchymal cell surface expression profile and had good osteogenic and adipogenic potential, they had a significantly reduced ability to differentiate into chondrocytes when compared to progenitors isolated from long bone fracture hematomas.

Compared with long bone fractures, our knowledge of the molecular physiology of healing craniofacial fractures is extremely sparse. Experiments in a rat model of mandible fracture healing implicate TGF-β superfamily members, including TGF-β1, BMP-2, BMP-4, and BMP-7, in osteoblast migration, differentiation, and proliferation [93, 94].

2.4.4 Physiologic Aspects of Distraction Osteogenesis on Bone Healing

Bones undergoing distraction osteogenesis share similar histologic characteristics of healing, regardless of whether they are within the craniofacial or appendicular skeleton [6, 95, 96]. However, there are significant histologic differences between distraction osteogenesis and fracture healing. The latency period of distraction resembles early fracture healing with hematoma formation and recruitment of inflammatory cells and mesenchymal stem cells [24, 71]. Endochondral bone formation may be observed during latency and early during distractor activation, although the endochondral bone is not found within the distraction gap but is limited to areas adjacent to the periosteum. Jazrawi [97] proposed that this observation suggests that the distraction environment may suppress cartilage development, but that a lack of device stability may be responsible for cartilage formation.

Rather than form a cartilaginous callus within the distraction gap, a physis-like structure of cells organizes into a fibrovascular bridge oriented in the direction of distraction called the *fibrous interzone*, or FIZ (see Fig. 2.6, [6, 34, 98]). The FIZ is rich in chondrocyte-like cells, fibroblasts, and oval cells, which are morphologically intermediates between fibroblasts and chondrocytes [6, 34, 98, 99]. As the distraction gap increases, the FIZ remains 4 mm thick, and at the conclusion of the process, the FIZ is the last region to ossify. Adjacent to the FIZ on either side is the *primary mineralization front* (PMF), which contains a high density of proliferating osteoblasts. These osteoblasts undergo primary mineralization in regions of newly formed capillaries and vascular sinuses, leading to formation of columns of bone resembling stalagmites and stalactites, known as the *zone of microcolumn formation* (MCF). When distraction ends, the PMF advances from each end toward the center, bridging the FIZ. Sequential mineralization of osteoid occurs during the activation and especially during the consolidation phase, starting within the surrounding MCF, which then proceeds to bridge the FIZ. During the consolidation period,

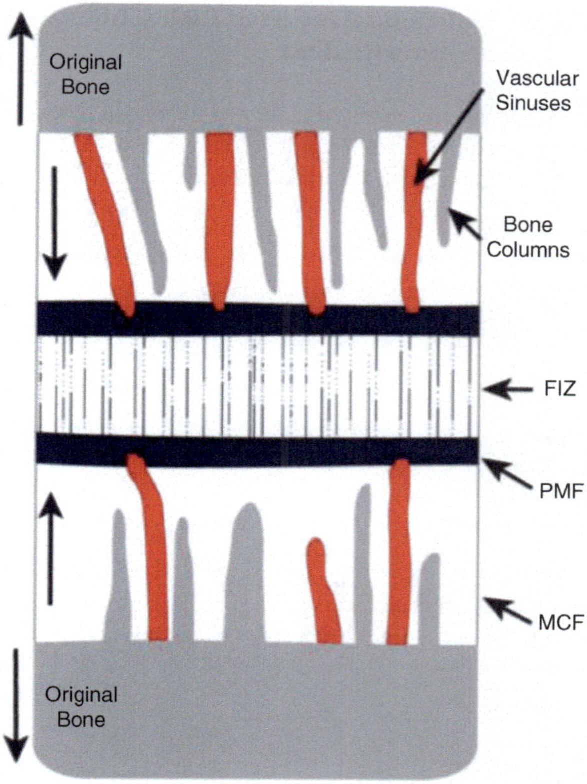

Fig. 2.6 Neo-physis of bone healing with distraction osteogenesis. See text for description. Reproduced, with permission, from [40]

mineralization of new bone is completed, and bony remodeling occurs resulting in formation of mature, lamellar bone with marrow.

The predominant mechanisms of bone formation within this niche are twofold. First, Yasui [100] observed that the FIZ of distracted rat femurs contained chondrocyte-appearing cells within a bony matrix, but without capillary ingrowth as is found in endochondral ossification. Similar to chondrocytes, these chondroid cells expressed type II collagen. However, they transition to type I collagen expression, suggestive of direct transformation of the chondrocyte-like cells into osteoblasts [101]. Yasui named this phenomenon "transchondroid bone formation" and proposed that it represents a new type of bone formation. However, both Yasui and others [3, 4, 6, 102] observed that the predominant mechanism of bone formation during distraction osteogenesis is intramembranous ossification, which may be distinguished from the other mechanisms by the histologic absence of cartilage and the expression of only type I collagen. At the ultrastructural level, disorganized bundles of type I collagen are found at the end of the latency period [103]. As activation begins, these bundles increase in size and become oriented in a plane parallel with the distraction force [6, 102, 104]. Osteoid is then deposited along the collagen bundles by osteoblasts located at corticotomy/osteotomy edges and within the distraction gap [104].

2.4.5 Molecular Aspects of Distraction Osteogenesis on Bone Healing

Distraction osteogenesis is initiated by an osteotomy. The molecular profile during the immediate post-osteotomy (latency) phase thus resembles that of fracture healing (Table 2.3). Pro-inflammatory cytokines IL-1 and IL-6 are upregulated in

Table 2.3 Differential expression of signaling molecules during distraction osteogenesis (adapted from [71])

Signaling molecules	Latency		Activation		Consolidation	
	Early	Late	Early	Late	Early	Late
Cytokines						
IL-1[a]	+++					
IL-6[b]	+++		+++	+++		
TNF-α[a]						+++
RANKL/OPG ratio[a]		++	+++	+++	+	
TGF-β superfamily						
BMP-2[c]	++		+++	+++	+	
BMP-4[c]	++		+++	+++	+	
BMP-6[c] (at endochond)		+++	++	+		
TGF-β[c, d, j]	+	++	+++	+++	+	
Angiogenic factors						
VEGF-A[e]			+++	+++	+	
VEGF-B[e]			+	+	+	
VEGF-C[e]	++		+	+	+	
VEGF-D[e]		++	++	+		
Angiopoietin 1[e]		++	+	+		
Angiopoietin 2[e]			++	+		
HIF-1α[f]			+++	+++		
Other osteogenic factors						
FGF-2 (bFGF)[c]			++	++	+	+
IGF[c]			++	++		
Collagen I[d]	−−−	−−	−		+	+++
Osteocalcin[d, g, h]	−−−	−−	−	+	+	+
Osteopontin[i, g]			−/+++[i]	+++	?	?
Osteonectin[g, h]			−	+++	?	?

"+" indicates gene upregulation, whereas "−" indicates gene downregulation. Empty squares indicate a lack of data or lack of differential gene expression beyond baseline

[a] Ai-Aql et al. [71]

[b] IL-6—Cho et al. [105]

[c] BMP-2, BMP-4, BMP-6, BMP-7, GDF-5—Sato et al. [109], Nuntanaranont et al. [112] (BMP-2, BMP-4), Khanal et al. [113] (BMP-2, BMP-4)

[d] TGF-b, collagen I, osteocalcin—Mehrara and Longaker [114], Nuntanaranont et al. [112] (TGF-β)

[e] VEGFs and angiopoietin—Pacicca et al. [115]

[f] VEGFs and HIFα—Carvalho et al. [116]

[g] Opn, Oc, osteonectin, collagen I—Sato et al. [99]

[h] Osteonectin, osteocalcin—Meyer…Joos

[i] Opn—Perrien (2002) (varies by cell type)

[j] TGF-β superfamily—Choi et al. [117]

the initial period, promoting extracellular matrix synthesis and inflammatory cell recruitment [71, 105]. Osteogenic and chondrogenic differentiation of these progenitors is similarly stimulated by early BMP-2 expression. A separate pro-inflammatory marker, TNF-α, is not expressed during latency, likely because its induction requires a greater traumatic insult than a simple osteotomy [105].

With device activation the molecular expression profile significantly deviates from that of fracture healing. IL-6 is upregulated a second time when activation begins and mechanical strain is applied to the callus. At this time its expression is high in osteoblasts, chondrocytes, and oval cells within the FIZ where tensile strains are the highest. IL-6 upregulation is thought to contribute to intramembranous ossification by enhancing osteogenic differentiation, and IL-6 has an anabolic effect on distraction osteogenesis and catabolic effect in fracture repair [105].

The TGF-β superfamily members are also upregulated during device activation. TGF-β was increased in distracted mandibles compared to those with non-distracted osteotomies [24], and a direct correlation between an increasing rate of mandibular distraction and TGF-β expression has been observed [106]. During activation TGF-β promotes osteoblast proliferation while suppressing their maturation, effectively delaying their differentiation and thus promoting new bone formation [107, 108]. BMP-2 and BMP-4 expression are both expressed immediately following the osteotomy, are downregulated, and then are highly reexpressed during device activation [109]. These BMPs are upregulated specifically within chondrogenic cells at the PMF and within oval cells within the FIZ, in response to the application of mechanical strain [109, 110]. They are maintained throughout activation, but then gradually disappear during consolidation, further implying a role in proliferation of cells required for completion of bone healing. Consistent with this, the addition of exogenous BMP-2 shortens treatment time during DO by accelerating bone formation during the consolidation phase [111]. In contrast to other factors, BMP-6 expression, limited to chondrocytes within the FIZ, begins during the latency phase and declines during the activation phase. BMP-6 downregulation occurs as the primary mode of ossification transitions from endochondral to intramembranous, reflecting its contributions to endochondral bone formation [109].

Two additional growth factors have been identified which are responsive to the increased mechanical strain found during device activation. Insulin-derived growth factor-1 (IGF-1) and fibroblast growth factor-2 (FGF-2, or basic FGF) are both highly expressed around the PMF and may promote osteoblast differentiation before subsequent downregulation during consolidation [22, 106].

As with fracture healing, osteoclastogenesis is necessary to help bone formed by distraction osteogenesis to remodel and form mature, lamellar bone. The RANKL/OPG system is thought to be the key regulator for balanced bone turnover [118]. As with fracture healing, a high RANKL/OPG expression ratio promotes osteoclastogenesis. The RANKL/OPG ratio increases late during latency and peaks within the consolidation phase, with the greatest turnover occurring at 3–4 weeks of consolidation [118, 119]. Activation of osteoclasts by TNF-α occurs throughout fracture healing; however, it is not expressed until later during consolidation, suggesting that RANKL/OPG plays the primary role for bone turnover and maturation [82].

Osteocalcin is expressed by mature osteoblasts and promotes mineralization. Its expression is significantly decreased compared with normal bone during the latency period. Osteocalcin levels gradually increase early during distraction, until reaching normal levels toward the end of consolidation [99, 114]. In contrast, osteocalcin in acutely lengthened mandibles does not significantly increase 6 weeks post distraction. This suggests deficiencies in osseous regeneration in acutely lengthened specimens are due to disturbances in mineralization/bone turnover in addition to decreased bone scaffold production.

2.4.6 Angiogenesis in Distraction Osteogenesis

Angiogenesis is an essential process for distraction osteogenesis. When angiogenesis is chemically inhibited, a lack of ossified bone and blood vessels occurs between the two cut ends of bone, with a resulting fibrous nonunion [120]. Mechanical distraction induces much greater angiogenic response than fracture healing [71]. Blood flow during activation increases up to 10 times the normal blood flow, as measured by quantitative technetium scintigraphy [34, 121]. Histologically, periosteal and endosteal vessels form columns alongside newly developing bone, toward the FIZ [79]. Within the FIZ capillaries are formed by both sinusoidal and transport capillary angiogenesis. During consolidation the periosteal and medullary vascular networks connect at the distraction site, including the FIZ [79]. Although new vessel formation begins during activation, maximal vessel volume increase occurs during consolidation, suggesting a link between angiogenesis and bone formation [122–124].

Among VEGF family members, only VEGF-A and neuropilin (a VEGF receptor) are significantly upregulated during the activation phase [116]. VEGF-D is upregulated briefly during the latency period but is diminished thereafter [116]. VEGF-A is expressed in maturing osteoblasts within the PMF and within osteoclasts in the MCF zone, directing angiogenesis in this region of the distraction gap [117]. Partial blockade of VEGF signaling in a tibial model of DO results in blockade of intramembranous ossification but allows for chondrogenesis, whereas complete VEGF blockade inhibits both osteogenesis and chondrogenesis [125]. The primary source of VEGF-A during DO is mesenchymal cells within the surrounding muscle. These blood vessels then synthesize morphogens (e.g., BMP-2) that promote bone formation in distracted bone [123]. An upstream activator of VEGF-A, HIF-1α, is significantly upregulated in bone undergoing distraction compared with fracture healing [115], suggesting that many of the downstream genes that are targets of HIF-1α (e.g., VEGF-A) play a major role in promoting new bone formation during DO. Deferoxamine enhancement of MDO is thought to be by upregulation of HIF-1α activity [126, 127]. Morgan [124] found that (1) the phase of activation is characterized primarily by arteriogenesis in surrounding muscle; (2) during consolidation, angiogenesis predominates in the intraosteal region; and (3) vessel formation proceeds from the surrounding muscle into the regenerate. Periods of intense osteogenesis are concurrent with those of angiogenesis.

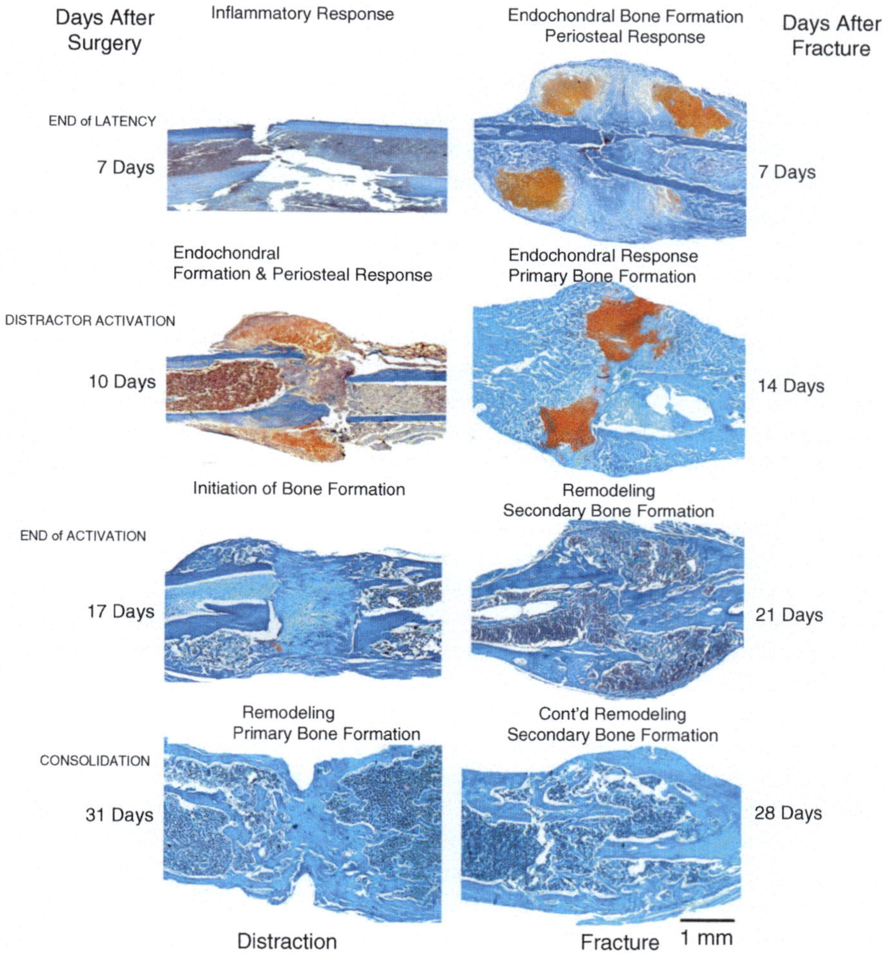

Fig. 2.7 Comparison of the progression of healing in fractures and distraction osteogenesis. Murine femur fracture calluses and tibial distraction gap tissues were prepared at the indicated time points, using Safranin-O/fast *green* staining. Cartilage is identified with *bright red* stain. The scale bar indicates 1 mm for all panels. Used with permission from [71]. The presence of cartilage during distractor activation may indicate some device instability

2.4.7 Contrasting Bone Formation by Fracture Healing and Distraction Osteogenesis

Distraction osteogenesis shares aspects of some of the physiologic pathways of fracture healing, but is clearly a distinct biologic process. This can be easily appreciated by comparing the two processes histologically (Fig. 2.7, [71]). Shortly after fracture of the appendicular skeleton, a robust cartilage callus forms outside the bone, stabilizing the fracture. In distraction osteogenesis, much less cartilage is formed, and its presence is temporally restricted to the early periods after activation is initiated, after which it is rapidly resorbed. Distracted bone also has large amounts of unmineralized osteoid in the central region of the distraction gap, whereas the fracture callus of endochondral bone calcifies rapidly as it undergoes primary bone healing. Bragdon [122] speculates that the lack of cartilage formation during distraction is due to the population of precursor cells that reside within the endosteum. Endosteal cells are restricted to the osteogenic lineage, whereas the periosteum, which contributes to both fracture healing and distraction osteogenesis, has precursor cells capable of differentiating into both chondrocytes and osteoblasts [128].

Angiogenesis is critical for both fracture healing and distraction osteogenesis. VEGFs are expressed during both processes but have higher relative expression during fracture healing. VEGF receptor knockout studies showed that both angiogenesis and osteogenesis during distraction osteogenesis were dependent on activity of both VEGF receptors 1 and 2 [125]. Also, inhibition of VEGF in a fracture-healing model showed delayed healing and failure to progress from a cartilaginous to bony callus. In fracture healing, angiogenesis begins between days 7 and 14 as chondrogenic tissues undergo resorption [71]. However, during distraction osteogenesis, angiogenesis is initiated only after activation has begun and is thought to be driven by the distraction process rather than by signals elaborated from chondrocytes [71, 122]. The observation that the majority of new vessels occur within the medullary space of the distraction regenerate supports this theory [115, 125]. This is in contrast to fracture healing, wherein new vessel formation occurs within the external callus and is associated with the cartilage-to-bone transition.

In certain respects, distraction osteogenesis more closely resembles embryonic bone development than fracture healing. The rate of bone formation during distraction osteogenesis is 200–400 μM/day, which is 4–8× faster than the fastest physeal growth in adolescence, and is equivalent to that of the fetal femur [95, 96, 117]. There is also circumstantial evidence that pathways that are important for bone development are differentially regulated during distraction osteogenesis. Shibazaki reported increased PTHrP activity within distracted mandibular condyles [129]. Kasaai found significant increases in Wnt signaling factors in a mouse tibial distraction model [130]. Hedgehog signaling is also altered in a rabbit model of calvarial distraction [131]. However, there is not enough understanding of DO to determine whether it is a physiologic recapitulation of embryonic bone development. This is certainly an area for future study.

2.5 Biomechanics of Distraction Osteogenesis

Simply stated, biomechanics refers to the effects that mechanical forces have on biologic processes. The distraction process translates mechanical forces to a predictable biologic endpoint. At the distraction site, the mechanical factors that influence the environment include the applied tensile distractive forces, the rigidity of the fixation device, the amount of physiologic loading (muscle action), and the properties of the

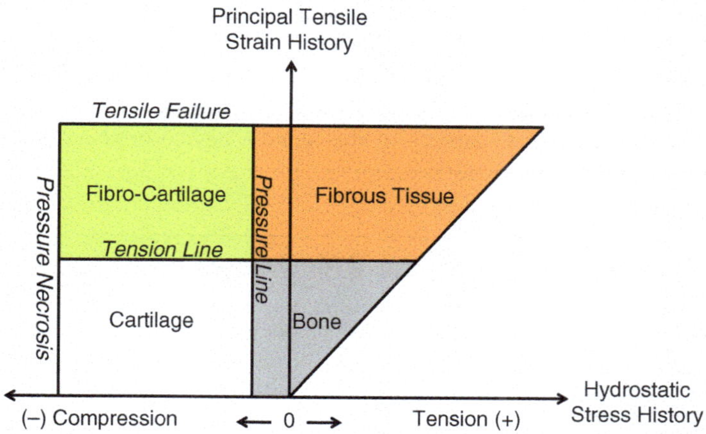

Fig. 2.8 Phase diagram of tissue differentiation concept relating mechanical loading history of multipotent mesenchymal tissue to skeletal tissue formation. Tensile failure line marks cutoff region beyond which failure of tissue occurs and new mesenchymal tissue forms in response to tissue trauma [134, 135]. Adapted with permission from [135]

surrounding soft tissues and regenerate. As distraction proceeds, one would expect tensile forces to increase. This has been confirmed in studies of human limb lengthening, with tensile forces increasing from 2.5 N/kg at initiation of activation and leveling off at 9.5 N/kg at completion [132]. This increase is likely caused by a combination of increasing resistance from the soft tissues and growing bony regenerate. During consolidation the ratio of force carried by the fixator versus the distracted limb can be measured. Increasing mineralization of the regenerate results in an increase in axial stiffness and a decrease in this ratio. For the appendicular skeleton, the regenerate's load-bearing capacity at the beginning of consolidation is 45% and, at least 4 months of consolidation, is typically required to improve to 90% [132, 133].

The type and intensity of the applied forces directly influence bone formation. Finite element modeling of mouse tibial fracture healing and distraction osteogenesis has led to characterization of these influences (Fig. 2.8, [134, 135]):

(1) Intermittent loading in regenerating bone heals by direct intramembranous bone formation in areas of low stress and strain.
(2) Low to moderate magnitudes of tensile strain and hydrostatic tensile stress also stimulate intramembranous ossification.
(3) Poor vascularity can promote chondrogenesis in an otherwise osteogenic environment.
(4) Hydrostatic compressive stresses stimulate chondrogenesis.
(5) High tensile strain stimulates production of fibrous tissue.
(6) Tensile strain with superimposed hydrostatic compressive stress stimulates development of fibrocartilage.
(7) Low shear stress favors cartilage and high shear stress results in fibrous tissue formation.

These principles have been validated in the craniofacial skeleton using a rat mandibular model of the latency and activation phases of distraction osteogenesis [135, 136]. Ultimately, for successful intramembranous bone formation by distraction osteogenesis, a low to moderate magnitude of tensile force (up to 13% reported by Loboa [135]) is required. Instability of the fixation device or shear stresses will favor endochondral bone formation.

2.6 Mechanotransduction and Mechanocoupling

Mechanotransduction is the translation of mechanical loading to cellular signal transduction pathway activation. Bone cells sense the applied tensile forces during distraction and transform these stimuli into biochemical signals into the cellular responses leading to appropriate changes in the architecture of the healing bone [137]. Mechanotransduction consists of the following steps: (1) mechanocoupling, (2) signal transmission, and (3) the effector cell response [138]. Mechanocoupling is the initial detection of a mechanical force with an associated signal pathway activation. The cell within bone responsible for initially sensing and responding to these forces is thought to be the osteocyte [139]. This is because osteocytes are regularly distributed throughout cortical and trabecular bone, because they are connected and communicate through long cellular processes and because they are unlikely to be effector cells due to being trapped within bone [140, 141]. The protein or structure within osteocytes responsible for mechanocoupling during distraction osteogenesis has not been identified, but there are a number of candidates [139]. The cells' cytoskeletons may directly sense changes in cell shape associated with the tensile forces. This "substrate deformation" may act directly on the actin cytoskeletons of the long osteocyte processes or the cell body itself [142, 143]. Alternatively, changes in the lacunocanalicular flow between osteocytes may provide the signals [144]. This may involve activation of stretch- or voltage-activated ion channels, G-protein-coupled receptors, and nodal cilia [140, 145]. Likely, multiple of these mechanisms are involved in sensing the distraction tensile forces.

Following mechanocoupling of the tensile force to the osteocyte, a series of secondary biochemical signaling events occurs, including changes in gene expression, protein and lipid modifications, protein degradation, alteration in cell shape/size, and the release of secreted factors. Collectively these events allow signal propagation within the osteocyte and activation of effector cells, namely, osteoblasts and osteoclasts. A number of signaling pathways have been identified that, when inactivated, inhibit the response of bone to a loading stress, including cyclooxygenase-2/prostaglandins [146], Wnt/LRP-5/β-catenin [147], IGF-1 [148, 149], and nitric oxide [150] pathways. Effector cell responses are manifest in protein expression by osteoblasts and osteoclasts, as new bone is produced. For example, alkaline phosphatase, type I collagen, osteopontin, osteocalcin, Runx2, and Osterix are all upregulated in response to mechanical loading of bone. Specific to distraction osteogenesis, Table 2.3 listed many of the other factors involved in both the signal transmission and effector cell phases of mechanotransduction.

2.7 Advances of Distraction Osteogenesis in the Craniofacial Skeleton

Because this chapter has introduced the foundation of bone healing physiology and biomechanics, a significant focus has been placed upon the historic development of distraction osteogenesis within long bones. Limb lengthening will continue to be a useful tool to the orthopedist, but the frontiers in distraction osteogenesis seem to lie in craniofacial applications (as supported by Table 2.1). As proposed by Dr. McCarthy in his prologue to the initial edition of this text, the craniofacial skeleton is more suited to surgical distraction than the long bones for the following reasons: superior blood supply, easier surgical accessibility, decreased associated pain, shorter required distraction/consolidation period, greater ease of measuring outcomes (dental measurements and cephalograms), and relatively lesser morbidity with wide, subperiosteal dissection.

This speculation has been borne out by the expanded clinical use of distraction osteogenesis within the craniofacial skeleton and the development of a larger literature. Initially described to improve mandibular asymmetry in patients with craniofacial microsomia, craniofacial distraction osteogenesis today is more commonly used to correct severe functional deficits. For example, distraction of the mandible is frequently used to correct tongue-based airway obstruction in neonates with micrognathia or in adults with severe obstructive sleep apnea. Midface distraction has supplanted the traditional or acute advancement technique, especially in the growing child. Posterior cranial vault distraction is used to delay the need for major cranial remodeling by reducing high intracranial pressure in patients with syndromic craniosynostosis, until a time that major surgery can more safely be performed. Distraction osteogenesis will continue to be an important tool in the craniofacial surgeon's armamentarium for treatment of difficult orthognathic or reconstructive cases.

The miniaturization and internalization of external distraction devices have been particularly beneficial to craniofacial applications. Frequently used bilaterally, internal or semi-buried devices have less failure, increased rigidity and stability, and greater convenience for patients and their families compared to the large, conspicuous external devices. External devices are thought to provide greater control over midface distraction vectors and permit molding of the generate during the activation and consolidation phases. Internal devices require a second operation for device removal and require greater periosteal undermining for placement.

Another advance in craniofacial distraction is the growing potential for adjuvant therapies to accelerate and improve the process. Preclinical animal models demonstrate improved bone formation during mandibular distraction osteogenesis (reviewed in [151]) with the addition of growth factors (BMP-2, BMP-4, BMP-7, IGF-1, VEGF, growth hormone, adiponectin, erythropoietin), osteoclast-suppressive medications (alendronate, zoledronic acid), mesenchymal stem cells, hyperbaric oxygen, and a number of mechanical stimuli (low-intensity shock wave therapy, low-intensity pulsed ultrasound). These models are predicated upon an understanding of the basic biomechanics and molecular physiology of bone healing and distraction osteogenesis. These basic principles provide a vast opportunity for both optimizing distraction osteogenesis and reducing the length of the clinical therapeutic process.

Buchman at the University of Michigan developed a high-throughput, reproducible model of rat mandibular distraction (REFs), permitting investigation of adjuvants and new applications for distraction osteogenesis [152]. The pro-angiogenic factor HIF-1α is one such factor [116]. Given its significant upregulation during the activation phase of distraction osteogenesis, it was hypothesized that increasing HIF-1α activity by deferoxamine administration would enhance bone formation during distraction osteogenesis. They demonstrated that deferoxamine increased HIF-1α levels in their model, resulting in enhanced vascular formation [126], more rapid consolidation of the regenerate (Donneys 2013), and greater bone production [127, 153]. Buchman has also examined the effects of radiation on distraction osteogenesis. Osteoradionecrosis of the mandible, a difficult reconstructive challenge, frequently requires autologous bone flaps. It was found that, in response to radiation, bone produced by distraction had significantly reduced osteocyte numbers, decreased bone mineralization, decreased vascularity, and a lower breaking load compared to control hemi-mandibles [154–157]. They also demonstrated that concomitant treatment with a number of factors had a protective effect from radiation damage, including parathyroid hormone [158, 159], amifostine [153, 160], and stem cells [154].

Pearls and Pitfalls

- Classification methods of distraction osteogenesis include treatment goal, distraction device type, anatomic location, and operative approach.
- Phases of distraction osteogenesis include latency, activation, and consolidation. Variables during the activation phase include the rate and rhythm of device activation.
- An understanding of embryonic bone formation and fracture healing helps one understand the physiology and biology of distraction osteogenesis.
- Bone generated by distraction osteogenesis does so predominately by intramembranous ossification, regardless of anatomic location. This is also the same mechanism of bone formation of developing craniofacial bone and fracture healing.
- The type and intensity of applied forces during distraction influence the types of tissue created.

References

1. Codivilla A. On the means of lengthening, in the lower limbs, the muscles and tissues which are shortened through deformity. Am J Orthop Surg. 1905;(4):353–69. http://jbjs.org/content/s2-2/4/353.abstract
2. Jordan CJ, Goldstein RY, Mclaurin TM, Grant A. The evolution of the Ilizarov technique: part 1: the history of limb lengthening. Bull NYU Hosp Jt Dis. 2013;71(1):89–95.
3. Ilizarov GA. The tension-stress effect on the genesis and growth of tissues. Part II. Clin Othop Relat Res. 1989a;(239):263–85.
4. Ilizarov GA. The tension-stress effect on the genesis and growth of tisues. Part I. Clin Orthop Relat Res. 1989b;(239):263–85.
5. Snyder CC, Levine GA, Swanson HM, Browne EZ. Mandibular lengthening by gradual distraction. Plast Reconstr Surg. 1973;51(5):506–8.
6. Karp NS, McCarthy JG, Schreiber JS, Sissons HA, Thorne CHM. Membranous bone lengthening: a serial histological study. Ann Plast Surg. 1992;29(1):2–7.
7. Karp NS, Thorne CHM, McCarthy JG, Sissons HA. Bone lengthening in the craniofacial skeleton. Ann Plast Surg. 1990;24(3):231–7.
8. McCarthy JG, Schreiber JS, Karp NS, Thorne CHM, Grayson BH. Lengthening the human mandible by gradual distraction. Plast Reconstr Surg. 1992;89(1):1–8.
9. Rachmiel A, Potparic Z, Jackson IT, Sugihara T, Clayman L, Topf JS, Forté RA. Midface advancement by gradual distraction. Br J Plast Surg. 1993;46(3):201–7. http://www.ncbi.nlm.nih.gov/pubmed/8490698
10. Staffenberg DA, Wood RJ, McCarthy JG, Grayson BH, Glasberg SB. Midface distraction advancement in the canine without osteotomies. Ann Plast Surg. 1995;34(5):512–7.
11. Glat PM, Staffenberg DA, Karp NS, Holliday RA, Steiner G, McCarthy JG. Multidimensional distraction osteogenesis: the canine zygoma. Plast Reconstr Surg. 1994;94(6):753–8.
12. Bouletreau PJ, Warren SM, Paccione MF, Spector JA, McCarthy JG, Longaker MT. Transport distraction osteogenesis: a new method to heal adult calvarial defects. Plast Reconstr Surg. 2002b;109(3):1074–84. http://www.ncbi.nlm.nih.gov/pubmed/11884839
13. Losken HW, Mooney MP, Zoldos J, Tschakaloff A, Burrows AM, Smith TD, et al. Internal calvarial bone distraction in rabbits with delayed-onset coronal suture synostosis. Plast Reconstr Surg. 1998;102(4):1109–19; discussion 1120–1. http://www.ncbi.nlm.nih.gov/pubmed/9734430
14. Guichet J-M, Deromedis B, Donnan LT, Peretti G, Lascombes P, Bado F. Gradual femoral lengthening with the Albizzia intramedullary nail. J Bone Joint Surg Am. 2003;85-A(5):838–48. http://www.ncbi.nlm.nih.gov/pubmed/12728034
15. Synder M, Niedzielski K, Borowski A. Complication, difficulties and problems in the application of distraction epiphysiolysis. Ortop Traumatol Rehabil. 2002;4(4):464–8. http://www.ncbi.nlm.nih.gov/pubmed/17679880
16. Coeugniet E, Dhellemmes P, Vinchon M, Wolber A, Pellerin P. Midfacial distraction without osteotomy using a transfacial pin and external devices. J Craniofac Surg. 2012;23(1):184–9. doi:10.1097/SCS.0b013e3182418f80.
17. Tong H, Gao F, Yin J, Shi Z, Song T, Li H, et al. Three-dimensional quantitative evaluation of midfacial skeletal changes after trans-sutural distraction osteogenesis for midfacial hypoplasia in growing patients with cleft lip and palate. J Craniomaxillofac Surg. 2015a;43(9):1749–57. doi:10.1016/j.jcms.2015.08.027.
18. Tong H, Wang X, Song T, Gao F, Yin J, Li H, et al. Trans-sutural distraction osteogenesis for midfacial hypoplasia in growing patients with cleft lip and palate: clinical outcomes and analysis of skeletal changes. Plast Reconstr Surg. 2015b;136(1):144–55. doi:10.1097/PRS.0000000000001375.

19. Slack GC, Fan KL, Tabit C, Andrews B, Hindin DI, Kawamoto HK, Bradley JP. Necessity of latency period in craniofacial distraction: investigations with in vitro microdistractor and clinical outcomes. J Plast Reconstr Aesthet Surg. 2015;68(9):1206–14. doi:10.1016/j.bjps.2015.04.012.
20. Hollier LH, Higuera S, Stal S, Taylor TD. Distraction rate and latency: factors in the outcome of pediatric mandibular distraction. Plast Reconstr Surg. 2006;117(7):2333–6. doi:10.1097/01.prs.0000219354.16549.c9.
21. Glowacki J, Shusterman EM, Troulis M, Holmes R, Perrott D, Kaban LB. Distraction osteogenesis of the porcine mandible: histomorphometric evaluation of bone. Plast Reconstr Surg. 2004;113(2):566–73. doi:10.1097/01.PRS.0000101061.99577.09.
22. Tavakoli K, Yu Y, Shahidi S, Bonar F, Walsh WR, Poole MD. Expression of growth factors in the mandibular distraction zone: a sheep study. Br J Plast Surg. 1999;52(6):434–9. doi:10.1054/bjps.1999.3157.
23. McCarthy JG, Stelnicki EJ, Grayson BH. Distraction osteogenesis of the mandible: a ten-year experience. Semin Orthod. 1999;5(1):3–8.
24. McCarthy JG, Stelnicki EJ, Mehrara BJ, Longaker MT. Distraction osteogenesis of the craniofacial skeleton. Plast Reconstr Surg. 2001;107(7):1812–27.
25. Farhadieh RD, Gianoutsos MP, Dickinson R, Walsh WR. Effect of distraction rate on biomechanical, mineralization, and histologic properties of an ovine mandible model. Plast Reconstr Surg. 2000;105(3):889–95. doi:10.1097/00006534-200003000-00010.
26. Mofid MM, Manson PN, Robertson BC, Tufaro AP, Elias JJ, Vander Kolk CA. Craniofacial distraction osteogenesis: a review of 3278 cases. Plast Reconstr Surg. 2001;108(5):1103–14; discussion 1115–7. http://www.ncbi.nlm.nih.gov/pubmed/11604605
27. Schendel SA, Heegaard JH. A mathematical model for mandibular distraction osteogenesis. J Craniofac Surg. 1996;7(6):465–8.
28. Boccaccio A, Pappalettere C, Kelly DJ. The influence of expansion rates on mandibular distraction osteogenesis: a computational analysis. Ann Biomed Eng. 2007;35(11):1940–60. doi:10.1007/s10439-007-9367-x.
29. Djasim UM, Mathot BJ, Wolvius EB, van Neck JW, van der Wal KGH. Histomorphometric comparison between continuous and discontinuous distraction osteogenesis. J Craniomaxillofac Surg. 2009;37(7):398–404. doi:10.1016/j.jcms.2009.03.006.
30. Peacock ZS, Tricomi ÃBJ, Faquin WC, Magill JC, Murphy BA, Kaban LB, Troulis MJ. Bilateral continuous automated distraction osteogenesis: proof of principle. J Craniofac Surg. 2015;26(8):2320–4. doi:10.1097/SCS.0000000000001996.
31. Luchs JS, Stelnicki EJ, Rowe NM, Naijher NS, Grayson BH, McCarthy JG. Molding of the regenerate in mandibular distraction: part 1: laboratory study. J Craniofac Surg. 2002;13(2):205–11. doi:10.1097/00001665-200203000-00004.
32. McCarthy JG, Hopper RA, Hollier LH, Peltomaki T, Katzen T, Grayson BH. Molding of the regenerate in mandibular distraction: clinical experience. Plast Reconstr Surg. 2003;112(5):1239–46. doi:10.1097/01.PRS.0000080726.50460.3E.
33. Pensler JM, Goldberg DP, Lindell B, Carroll NC. Skeletal distraction of the hypoplastic mandible. Ann Plast Surg. 1995;134(2):130–6.
34. Aronson J. Experimental and clinical experience with distraction osteogenesis. Cleft Palate Craniofac J. 1994b;31(6):473–81. doi:10.1597/1545-1569(1994)031<0473:EACEWD>2.3.CO;2.
35. Hopper RA, Altug AT, Grayson BH, Barillas I, Sato Y, Cutting CB, McCarthy JG. Cephalometric analysis of the consolidation phase following bilateral pediatric mandibular distraction. Cleft Palate Craniofac J. 2003;40(3):233–40. doi:10.1597/1545-1569(2003)040<0233:CAOTCP>2.0.CO;2.
36. Polley JW, Figueroa AA. Rigid external distraction: its application in cleft maxillary deformities. Plast Reconstr Surg. 1998;102(5):1360–72.
37. Eames BF, De la Fuente L, Helms J a. Molecular ontogeny of the skeleton. Birth Defects Res C Embryo Today Rev. 2003;69(2):93–101. doi:10.1002/bdrc.10016.

38. Ferguson C, Alpern E, Miclau T, Helms JA. Does adult fracture repair recapitulate embryonic skeletal formation? Mech Dev. 1999;87(1–2):57–66. doi:10.1016/S0925-4773(99)00142-2.
39. Karaplis A. Embryonic Development of Bone and the Molecular Regulation of Intramembranous and Endochondral Bone Formation. In: Bilezikian J, Raisz L, Martin TJ, Editors. Principles of Bone Biology Vol. 1. 2008, ISBN: 9780123738844.
40. Percival CJ, Richtsmeier JT. Angiogenesis and intramembranous osteogenesis. Dev Dyn. 2013;242(8):909–22. doi:10.1016/j.biotechadv.2011.08.021.Secreted.
41. Ishii M, Sun J, Ting M-C, Maxson RE. The development of the calvarial bones and sutures and the pathophysiology of craniosynostosis. Curr Top Dev Biol. 2015;115:131–56. doi:10.1016/bs.ctdb.2015.07.004.
42. Eames BF, Helms JA. Conserved molecular program regulating cranial and appendicular skeletogenesis. Dev Dyn. 2004;231(1):4–13. doi:10.1002/dvdy.20134.
43. Abzhanov A, Rodda SJ, McMahon AP, Tabin CJ. Regulation of skeletogenic differentiation in cranial dermal bone. Development. 2007;134(17):3133–44. doi:10.1242/dev.002709.
44. Bhatt S, Diaz R, Trainor PA, Wu DK, Kelley MW, Tam PL, et al. Signals and switches in mammalian neural crest cell differentiation signals and switches in mammalian neural crest cell differentiation. Cold Spring Harb Perspect Biol. 2013;5:a008326. doi:10.1101/cshperspect.a008326.
45. Thorogood PV, Hinchliffe JR. An analysis of the condensation process during chondrogenesis in the embryonic chick hind limb. J Embryol Exp Morphol. 1975;33(3):581–606.
46. Ducy P, Karsenty G. Genetic control of cell differentiation in the skeleton. Curr Opin Cell Biol. 1998;10(5):614–9. http://www.ncbi.nlm.nih.gov/pubmed/9818172
47. Komori T, Yagi H, Nomura S, Yamaguchi A, Sasaki K, Deguchi K, et al. Targeted disruption of Cbfa1 results in a complete lack of bone formation owing to maturational arrest of osteoblasts. Cell. 1997;89(5):755–64. doi:10.1016/S0092-8674(00)80258-5.
48. Mundlos S, Otto F, Mundlos C, Mulliken JB, Aylsworth AS, Albright S, et al. Mutations involving the transcription factor CBFA1 cause cleidocranial dysplasia. Cell. 1997;89(5):773–9. http://www.ncbi.nlm.nih.gov/pubmed/9182765
49. Otto F, Thornell AP, Crompton T, Denzel A, Gilmour KC, Rosewell IR, et al. Cbfa1, a candidate gene for cleidocranial dysplasia syndrome, is essential for osteoblast differentiation and bone development. Cell. 1997;89(5):765–71. http://www.ncbi.nlm.nih.gov/pubmed/9182764
50. Akiyama H, Chaboissier MC, Martin JF, Schedl A, De Crombrugghe B. The transcription factor Sox9 has essential roles in successive steps of the chondrocyte differentiation pathway and is required for expression of Sox5 and Sox6. Genes Dev. 2002;16(21):2813–28. doi:10.1101/gad.1017802.
51. Bi W, Deng JM, Zhang Z, Behringer RR, de Crombrugghe B. Sox9 is required for cartilage formation. Nat Genet. 1999;22(1):85–9. doi:10.1038/8792.
52. Yan YL, Miller CT, Nissen RM, Singer A, Liu D, Kirn A, et al. A zebrafish sox9 gene required for cartilage morphogenesis. Development. 2002;129(21):5065–79. http://www.ncbi.nlm.nih.gov/pubmed/12397114\n; http://dev.biologists.org/content/129/21/5065.full.pdf
53. Foster JW, Dominguez-Steglich MA, Guioli S, Kwok C, Weller PA, Stevanović M, et al. Campomelic dysplasia and autosomal sex reversal caused by mutations in an SRY-related gene. Nature. 1994;372(6506):525–30. doi:10.1038/372525a0.
54. Kwok C, Weller PA, Guioli S, Foster JW, Mansour S, Zuffardi O, et al. Mutations in SOX9, the gene responsible for campomelic dysplasia and autosomal sex reversal. Am J Hum Genet. 1995;57(5):1028–36.
55. Wagner T, Wirth J, Meyer J, Zabel B, Held M, Zimmer J, et al. Autosomal sex reversal and campomelic dysplasia are caused by mutations in and around the SRY-related gene SOX9. Cell. 1994;79(6):1111–20. http://www.ncbi.nlm.nih.gov/pubmed/8001137
56. Lefebvre V, Huang W, Harley VR, Goodfellow PN, de Crombrugghe B. SOX9 is a potent activator of the chondrocyte-specific enhancer of the pro alpha1(II) collagen gene. Mol Cell Biol. 1997;17(4):2336–46. http://www.pubmedcentral.nih.gov/articlerender.fcgi?artid=232082&tool=pmcentrez&rendertype=abstract

57. Zhang P, Jimenez SA, Stokes DG. Regulation of human COL9A1 gene expression. Activation of the proximal promoter region by SOX9. J Biol Chem. 2003;278(1):117–23. doi:10.1074/jbc.M208049200.
58. Liu Y, Li H, Tanaka K, Tsumaki N, Yamada Y. Identification of an enhancer sequence within the first intron required for cartilage-specific transcription of the α2(XI) collagen gene. J Biol Chem. 2000;275(17):12712–8. doi:10.1074/jbc.275.17.12712.
59. Yang J, Andre P, Ye L, Yang Y-Z. The Hedgehog signalling pathway in bone formation. Int J Oral Sci. 2015;14:73–9. doi:10.1038/ijos.2015.14.
60. Mak KK, Chen M-H, Day TF, Chuang P-T, Yang Y. Wnt/beta-catenin signaling interacts differentially with Ihh signaling in controlling endochondral bone and synovial joint formation. Development. 2006;133(18):3695–707. doi:10.1242/dev.02546.
61. Long F, Chung U, Ohba S, McMahon J, Kronenberg HM, McMahon AP. Ihh signaling is directly required for the osteoblast lineage in the endochondral skeleton. Development. 2004;131(6):1309–18. doi:10.1242/dev.01006.
62. Hojo H, Ohba S, Taniguchi K, Shirai M, Yano F, Saito T, et al. Hedgehog-Gli activators direct osteo-chondrogenic function of bone morphogenetic protein toward osteogenesis in the perichondrium. J Biol Chem. 2013;288(14):9924–32. doi:10.1074/jbc.M112.409342.
63. Yoshida T, Vivatbutsiri P, Morriss-Kay G, Saga Y, Iseki S. Cell lineage in mammalian craniofacial mesenchyme. Mech Dev. 2008;125(9–10):797–808. doi:10.1016/j.mod.2008.06.007.
64. Lenton K, James AW, Manu A, Brugmann SA, Birker D, Nelson ER, et al. Indian hedgehog positively regulates calvarial ossification and modulates bone morphogenetic protein signaling. Genesis. 2011;49(10):784–96. doi:10.1002/dvg.20768.
65. Jenkins D, Seelow D, Jehee F, Perlyn C, Alonso L, Bueno D, et al. RAB23 mutations in Carpenter syndrome imply an unexpected role for hedgehog signaling in cranial-suture development and obesity. Am J Hum Genet. 2007;80(6):1162–70.
66. Rice DPC, Connor EC, Veltmaat JM, Lana-Elola E, Veistinen L, Tanimoto Y, et al. Gli3Xt-J/Xt-J mice exhibit lambdoid suture craniosynostosis which results from altered osteoprogenitor proliferation and differentiation. Hum Mol Genet. 2010;19(17):3457–67. doi:10.1093/hmg/ddq258.
67. Otto F, Kanegane H, Mundlos S. Mutations in the RUNX2 gene in patients with cleidocranial dysplasia. Hum Mutat. 2002;19(3):209–16. doi:10.1002/humu.10043.
68. Sperber G, Sperber SM, Guttmann GD. Craniofacial embryogenetics and development. 2nd ed. Shelton: PMPH; 2010.
69. Dimitriou R, Tsiridis E, Giannoudis PV. Current concepts of molecular aspects of bone healing. Injury. 2005;36(12):1392–404. doi:10.1016/j.injury.2005.07.019.
70. Gerstenfeld LC, Alkhiary YM, Krall EA, Nicholls FH, Stapleton SN, Fitch JL, et al. Three-dimensional reconstruction of fracture callus morphogenesis. J Histochem Cytochem. 2006;54(11):1215–28. doi:10.1369/jhc.6A6959.2006.
71. Ai-Aql ZS, Alagl AS, Graves DT, Gerstenfeld LC, Einhorn TA. Molecular mechanisms controlling bone formation during fracture healing and distraction osteogenesis. J Dent Res. 2008;87(2):107–18. doi:10.1177/154405910808700215.
72. Hankenson K, Zimmermann G, Marcucio RS. Biologic perspectives of delayed fracture healing. Injury. 2014;45(Suppl 2):S8–S15. doi:10.1002/jcp.24872.The.
73. Marsell R, Einhorn TA. The biology of fracture healing. Injury. 2011;42(6):551–5. doi:10.1016/j.injury.2011.03.031.THE.
74. Morgan EF, Mason ZD, Chien KB, Pfeiffer AJ, George L, Einhorn TA, Gerstenfeld LC. Micro-computed tomography assessment of fracture healing: relationships among callus structure, composition, and mechanical function. Bone. 2009;44(2):335–44. doi:10.1016/j.bone.2008.10.039.Micro-Computed.
75. Kon T, Cho TJ, Aizawa T, Yamazaki M, Nooh N, Graves D, et al. Expression of osteoprotegerin, receptor activator of NF-kappaB ligand (osteoprotegerin ligand) and related proinflammatory cytokines during fracture healing. J Bone Miner Res. 2001;16(6):1004–14. doi:10.1359/jbmr.2001.16.6.1004.

76. Sandberg MM, Hannu TA, Vuorio EI. Gene expression during bone repair. Clin Orthop Relat Res. 1993;289:292–312.
77. Bostrom M. Expression of bone morphogenetic proteins in fracture healing. Clin Orthop Relat Res. 1998;(355 Suppl):S116–23. http://www.ncbi.nlm.nih.gov/pubmed/9917632
78. Wang X, Yu YY, Lieu S, Yang F, Lang J, Lu C, et al. MMP9 regulates the cellular response to inflammation after skeletal injury. Bone. 2013;52(1):111–9. doi:10.1016/j.bone.2012.09.018. MMP9.
79. Cho T-J, Gerstenfeld LC, Einhorn T a. Differential temporal expression of members of the transforming growth factor beta superfamily during murine fracture healing. J Bone Miner Res. 2002;17(3):513–20. doi:10.1359/jbmr.2002.17.3.513.
80. Wang Q, Huang C, Xue M, Zhang. Expression of endogenous BMP-2 in periosteal progenitor cells is essential for bone healing. Bone. 2011;48(3):524–32. doi:10.1016/j.bone.2010.10.178.Expression.
81. Colnot C, Thompson Z, Miclau T, Werb Z, Helms JA. Altered fracture repair in the absence of MMP9. Development. 2003;130(17):4123–33. doi:10.1242/dev.00559.
82. Gerstenfeld LC, Cho TJ, Kon T, Aizawa T, Tsay A, Fitch J, et al. Impaired fracture healing in the absence of TNF-alpha signaling: the role of TNF-alpha in endochondral cartilage resorption. J Bone Miner Res. 2003;18(9):1584–92. doi:10.1359/jbmr.2003.18.9.1584.
83. Glass GE, Chan JK, Freidin A, Feldmann M, Horwood NJ, Nanchahal J. TNF-alpha promotes fracture repair by augmenting the recruitment and differentiation of muscle-derived stromal cells. Proc Natl Acad Sci U S A. 2011;108(4):1585–90. doi:10.1073/pnas.1018501108.
84. Cheng H, Jiang W, Phillips FM, Haydon RC, Peng Y, Zhou L, et al. Osteogenic activity of the fourteen types of human bone morphogenetic proteins (BMPs). J Bone Joint Surg Am. 2003;85-A(8):1544–52.
85. Wang X-X, Wang X, Li Z-L. Effects of mandibular distraction osteogenesis on the inferior alveolar nerve: an experimental study in monkeys. Plast Reconstr Surg. 2002;109(7):2373–83. http://www.ncbi.nlm.nih.gov/pubmed/12045565
86. Bodine PVN, Seestaller-Wehr L, Kharode YP, Bex FJ, Komm BS. Bone anabolic effects of parathyroid hormone are blunted by deletion of the Wnt antagonist secreted frizzled-related protein-1. J Cell Physiol. 2007;210(2):352–7. doi:10.1002/jcp.20834.
87. Guo J, Liu M, Yang D, Bouxsein ML, Saito H, Galvin RJS, et al. Suppression of Wnt signaling by Dkk1 attenuates PTH-mediated stromal cell response and new bone formation. Cell Metab. 2010;11(2):161–71. doi:10.1021/ja8019214.Optimization.
88. Jilka RL, Brien CAO, Ali AA, Roberson P, Weinstein RS, Manolagas SC. Formation by actions on post-mitotic. Bone. 2010;44(2):275–86. doi:10.1016/j.bone.2008.10.037. INTERMITTENT.
89. Craft PD, Mani MM, Pazel J, Masters FW. Experimental study of healing in fractures of membranous bone. Plast Reconstr Surg. 1974;55(3):321–5.
90. Paccione MF, Warren SM, Spector JA, Greenwald JA, Bouletreau PJ, Longaker MT. A mouse model of mandibular osteotomy healing. J Craniofac Surg. 2001;12(5):444–50. doi:10.1097/00001665-200109000-00008.
91. Hasegawa T, Miwa M, Sakai Y, Nikura T, Lee SY, Oe K, et al. Mandibular hematoma cells as a potential reservoir for osteoprogenitor cells in fractures. J Oral Maxillofac Surg. 2012;70(3):599–607. doi:10.1016/j.joms.2011.03.043.
92. Oe K, Miwa M, Sakai Y, Lee SY, Kuroda R, Kurosaka M. An in vitro study demonstrating that haematomas found at the site of human fractures contain progenitor cells with multilineage capacity. J Bone Joint Surg Br. 2007;89-B(1):133–8. doi:10.1302/0301-620X.89B1.18286.
93. Spector JA, Luchs JS, Mehrara BJ, Greenwald JA, Smith LP, Longaker MT. Expression of bone morphogenetic proteins during membranous bone healing. Plast Reconstr Surg. 2001;107(1):124–34.
94. Steinbrech DS, Mehrara BJ, Rowe NM, Dudziak ME, Luchs JS, Saadeh PB, et al. Gene expression of TGF-beta, TGF-beta receptor, and extracellular matrix proteins during membranous bone healing in rats. Plast Reconstr Surg. 2000;105(6):2028–38.

95. Aronson J, Good B, Stewart C, Harrison B, Harp J. Preliminary studies of mineralization during distraction osteogenesis. Clin Orthop Relat Res. 1990a;(250):43–9. http://www.ncbi.nlm.nih.gov/pubmed/2293943
96. Aronson J, Good B, Stewart C, Harrison B, Harp J. Preliminary studies of mineralization during distraction osteogenesis. Clin Orthop Relat Res. 1990b;250:43–9.
97. Jazrawi LM, Majeska RJ, Klein ML, Kagel E, Stromberg L, Einhorn TA. Bone and cartilage formation in an experimental model of distraction osteogenesis. J Orthop Trauma. 1998;12(2):111–6.
98. Vauhkonen M, Peltonen J, Karaharju E, Aalto K, Alitalo I. Collagen synthesis and mineralization in the early phase of distraction bone healing. Bone Miner. 1990;10(3):171–81. http://www.ncbi.nlm.nih.gov/pubmed/2224204
99. Sato M, Yasui N, Nakase T, Kawahata H, Sugimoto M, Hirota S, et al. Expression of bone matrix proteins mRNA during distraction osteogenesis. J Bone Miner Res. 1998;13(8):1221–31. doi:10.1359/jbmr.1998.13.8.1221.
100. Yasui N, Sato M, Ochi T, Kimura T, Kawahata H, Kitamura Y, Nomura S. Three modes of ossification during distraction osteogenesis in the rat. J Bone Joint Surg Br. 1997;79(5):824–30. doi:10.1302/0301-620X.79B5.7423.
101. Li G, Virdi AS, Ashhurst DE, Simpson AH, Triffitt JT. Tissues formed during distraction osteogenesis in the rabbit are determined by the distraction rate: localization of the cells that express the mRNAs and the distribution of types I and II collagens. Cell Biol Int. 2000;24(1):25–33. doi:10.1006/cbir.1999.0449.
102. Karaharju EO, Aalto K, Kahri A, Lindberg L-A, Kallio T, Karaharju-Suvanto T, et al. Distraction bone healing. Clin Orthop Relat Res. 1993;297:38–43.
103. Hamanishi C, Yoshii T, Totani Y, Tanaka S. Lengthened callus activated by axial shortening. Clin Orthop Relat Res. 1994;307(307):250–4.
104. Ilizarov GA. Transosseous osteosynthesis. In: Green SA, editor. vol. 1. Berlin: Springer; 1992. doi:10.1017/CBO9781107415324.004
105. Cho T-J, Kim JA, Chung CY, Yoo WJ, Gerstenfeld LC, Einhorn TA, Choi IH. Expression and role of interleukin-6 in distraction osteogenesis. Calcif Tissue Int. 2007;80(3):192–200. doi:10.1007/s00223-006-0240-y.
106. Farhadieh RD, Dickinson R, Yu Y, Gianoutsos MP, Walsh WR. The role of transforming growth factor-beta, insulin-like growth factor I, and basic fibroblast growth factor in distraction osteogenesis of the mandible. J Craniofac Surg. 1999;10(1):80–6.
107. Holbein O, Neidlinger-Wilke C, Suger G, Kinzl L, Claes L. Ilizarov callus distraction produces systemic bone cell mitogens. J Orthop Res. 1995;13(4):629–38. doi:10.1002/jor.1100130420.
108. Lammens J, Liu Z, Aerssens J, Dequeker J, Fabry G. Distraction bone healing versus osteotomy healing: a comparative biochemical analysis. J Bone Miner Res. 1998;13(2):279–86. doi:10.1359/jbmr.1998.13.2.279.
109. Sato M, Ochi T, Nakase T, Hirota S, Kitamura Y, Nomura S, Yasui N. Mechanical tension-stress induces expression of bone morphogenetic protein (BMP)-2 and BMP-4, but not BMP-6, BMP-7, and GDF-5 mRNA, during distraction osteogenesis. J Bone Miner Res. 1999;14(7):1084–95. doi:10.1359/jbmr.1999.14.7.1084.
110. Rauch F, Lauzier D, Croteau S, Travers R, Glorieux FH, Hamdy R. Temporal and spatial expression of bone morphogenetic protein-2, -4, and -7 during distraction osteogenesis in rabbits. Bone. 2000;26(6):611–7.
111. Ashinoff RL, Cetrulo CL, Galiano RD, Dobryansky M, Bhatt KA, Ceradini DJ, et al. Bone morphogenic protein-2 gene therapy for mandibular distraction osteogenesis. Ann Plast Surg. 2004;52(6):585–90; discussion 591. http://www.ncbi.nlm.nih.gov/pubmed/15166991
112. Nuntanaranont T, Suttapreyasri S, Vongvatcharanon S. Quantitative expression of bone-related cytokines induced by mechanical tension-stress during distraction osteogenesis in a rabbit mandible. J Investig Clin Dent. 2014;5(4):255–65. doi:10.1111/jicd.12034.

113. Khanal A, Yoshioka I, Tominaga K, Furuta N, Habu M, Fukuda J. The BMP signaling and its Smads in mandibular distraction osteogenesis. Oral Dis. 2008;14(4):347–55. http://www.ncbi.nlm.nih.gov/pubmed/18449963
114. Mehrara BJ, Longaker MT. New developments in craniofacial surgery research. Cleft Palate Craniofac J. 1999;36(5):377–87. doi:10.1597/1545-1569(1999)036<0377:NDICSR>2.3.CO;2.
115. Pacicca DM, Patel N, Lee C, Salisbury K, Lehmann W, Carvalho R, et al. Expression of angiogenic factors during distraction osteogenesis. Bone. 2003;33(6):889–98. http://www.ncbi.nlm.nih.gov/pubmed/14678848
116. Carvalho RS, Einhorn TA, Lehmann W, Edgar C, Al-Yamani A, Apazidis A, et al. The role of angiogenesis in a murine tibial model of distraction osteogenesis. Bone. 2004;34(5):849–61. doi:10.1016/j.bone.2003.12.027.
117. Choi IH, Chung CY, Cho TJ, Yoo WJ. Angiogenesis and mineralization during distraction osteogenesis. J Korean Med Sci. 2002;17(4):435–47. doi:10.3346/jkms.2002.17.4.435.
118. Pérez-Sayáns M, Somoza-Martín JM, Barros-Angueira F, Rey JMG, García-García A. RANK/RANKL/OPG role in distraction osteogenesis. Oral Surg Oral Med Oral Pathol Oral Radiol Endodontol. 2010;109(5):679–86. doi:10.1016/j.tripleo.2009.10.042.
119. Zhu W-Q, Wang X, Wang X-X, Wang Z-Y. Temporal and spatial expression of osteoprotegerin and receptor activator of nuclear factor -kappaB ligand during mandibular distraction in rats. J Craniomaxillofac Surg. 2007;35(2):103–11. doi:10.1016/j.jcms.2006.12.001.
120. Fang TD, Salim A, Xia W, Nacamuli RP, Guccione S, Song HM, et al. Angiogenesis is required for successful bone induction during distraction osteogenesis. J Bone Miner Res. 2005;20(7):1114–24. doi:10.1359/JBMR.050301.
121. Aronson J. Temporal and spatial increases in blood flow during distraction osteogenesis. Clin Orthop Relat Res. 1994a;(301):124–31. http://www.ncbi.nlm.nih.gov/pubmed/8156663
122. Bragdon B, Lybrand K, Gerstenfeld L. Overview of biological mechanisms and applications of three murine models of bone repair: closed fracture with intramedullary fixation, distraction osteogenesis, and marrow ablation by reaming. Curr Protoc Mouse Biol. 2015;5:21–34. doi:10.1002/9780470942390.mo140166.
123. Matsubara H, Hogan DE, Morgan EF, Mortolock DP, Einhorn TA, Gerstenfeld LC. Vascular tissues are a primary source of BMP2 expression during bone formation induced by distraction osteogenesis. Bone. 2012;51(1):168–80. doi:10.1016/j.drugalcdep.2008.02.002.A.
124. Morgan EF, Hussein AI, Al-Awadhi BA, Hogan DE, Matsubara H, Al-Aql ZS, et al. Vascular development during distraction osteogenesis proceeds by sequential intramuscular arteriogenesis followed by intraosteal angiogenesis. Bone. 2012;51(3):535–45. doi:10.1016/j.bone.2012.05.008.Vascular.
125. Jacobsen KA, Al-Aql ZS, Wan C, Fitch JL, Stapleton SN, Mason ZD, et al. Bone formation during distraction osteogenesis is dependent on both VEGFR1 and VEGFR2 signaling. J Bone Miner Res. 2008;23(5):596–609. doi:10.1359/jbmr.080103.
126. Donneys A, Farberg AS, Tchanque-Fossuo CN, Deshpande SS, Buchman SR. Deferoxamine enhances the vascular response of bone regeneration in mandibular distraction osteogenesis. Plast Reconstr Surg. 2012a;129(4):850–6. doi:10.1097/PRS.0b013e31824422f2.
127. Farberg AS, Sarhaddi D, Donneys A, Deshpande SS, Buchman SR. Deferoxamine enhances bone regeneration in mandibular distraction osteogenesis. Plast Reconstr Surg. 2014;133(3):666–71. doi:10.1097/01.prs.0000438050.36881.a9.
128. Colnot C. Skeletal cell fate decisions within periosteum and bone marrow during bone regeneration. J Bone Miner Res. 2009;24(2):274–82. doi:10.1359/jbmr.081003.
129. Shibazaki R, Maki K, Tachikawa T, Shibasaki Y, Hinton RJ, Carlson DS, Opperman LA. Changes in parathyroid hormone-related protein and 3-dimensional trabecular bone structure of the mandibular condyle following mandibular distraction osteogenesis in growing rats. J Oral Maxillofac Surg. 2005;63(4):505–12. doi:10.1016/j.joms.2004.12.005.

130. Kasaai B, Moffatt P, Al-Salmi L, Lauzier D, Lessard L, Hamdy RC. Spatial and temporal localization of WNT signaling proteins in a mouse model of distraction osteogenesis. J Histochem Cytochem. 2012;60(3):219–28. doi:10.1369/0022155411432010.
131. Nott RL, Stelnicki EJ, Mack JA, Ben Y, Mitchell R, Mooney MP. Changes in the protein expression of hedgehog and patched-1 in perisutural tissues induced by cranial distraction. Plast Reconstr Surg. 2002;110(2):523–32. http://www.ncbi.nlm.nih.gov/pubmed/12142671
132. Lauterburg MT, Exner GU, Jacob HAC. Forces involved in lower limb lengthening: an in vivo biomechanical study. J Orthop Res. 2006;24(9):1815–22. doi:10.1002/jor.20217.
133. Aarnes GT, Steen H, Ludvigsen P, Waanders NA, Huiskes R, Goldstein SA. In vivo assessment of regenerate axial stiffness in distraction osteogenesis. J Orthop Res. 2005;23(2):494–8. doi:10.1016/j.orthres.2004.08.024.
134. Carter DR, Beaupre GS, Giori NJ, Helms JA. Mechanobiology of skeletal regeneration. Clin Orthop Relat Res. 1998;355S:S41–55.
135. Loboa EG, Fang TD, Parker DW, Warren SM, Fong KD, Longaker MT, Carter DR. Mechanobiology of mandibular distraction osteogenesis: finite element analyses with a rat model. J Orthop Res. 2005;23(3):663–70. doi:10.1016/j.orthres.2004.09.010.
136. Loboa EG, Fang TD, Warren SM, Lindsey DP, Fong KD, Longaker MT, Carter DR. Mechanobiology of mandibular distraction osteogenesis: experimental analyses with a rat model. Bone. 2004;34:336–43. doi:10.1016/j.bone.2003.10.012.
137. Shu Z, Xin-sheng C, Bing W. Mechanotransduction in osteoblast and osteocyte regulation***☆○◆. J Clin Rehabil Tissue Eng Res. 2011;15(24):4530–6.
138. Natu SS, Ali I, Alam S, Giri KY, Agarwal A, Kulkarni VA. The biology of distraction osteogenesis for correction of mandibular and craniomaxillofacial defects: a review. Dent Res J. 2014;11(1):16–26. http://www.pubmedcentral.nih.gov/articlerender.fcgi?artid=3955310&tool=pmcentrez&rendertype=abstract
139. Goodman CA, Hornberger TA, Robling AG. Bone and skeletal muscle: key players in mechanotransduction and potential overlapping mechanisms. Bone. 2015;80:24–36. doi:10.1016/j.bone.2015.04.014.
140. Klein-Nulend J, Bakker AD, Bacabac RG, Vatsa A, Weinbaum S. Mechanosensation and transduction in osteocytes. Bone. 2013;54(2):182–90. doi:10.1016/j.bone.2012.10.013.
141. Lanyon LE. Osteocytes, strain detection, bone modeling and remodeling. Calcif Tissue Int. 1993;53 Suppl 1:S102–6; discussion S106–7. http://www.ncbi.nlm.nih.gov/pubmed/8275362
142. Bonivtch AR, Bonewald LF, Nicolella DP. Tissue strain amplification at the osteocyte lacuna: a microstructural finite element analysis. Mater Eng. 2007;40(10):2199–206.
143. Han Y, Cowin SC, Schaffler MB, Weinbaum S. Mechanotransduction and strain amplification in osteocyte cell processes. Proc Natl Acad Sci U S A. 2004;101(47):16689–94. doi:10.1073/pnas.0407429101.
144. Davidson EH, Sultan SM, Butala P, Knobel D, Warren SM. Lacunocanalicular fluid flow transduces mechanical tension stress during distraction osteogenesis. J Craniofac Surg. 2013;24(5):1558–64. doi:10.1097/SCS.0b013e31828f2060.
145. Malone AMD, Anderson CT, Tummala P, Kwon RY, Johnston TR, Stearns T, Jacobs CR. Primary cilia mediate mechanosensing in bone cells by a calcium-independent mechanism. Proc Natl Acad Sci U S A. 2007;104(33):13325–30. doi:10.1073/pnas.0700636104.
146. Li J, Burr DB, Turner CH. Suppression of prostaglandin synthesis with NS-398 has different effects on endocortical and periosteal bone formation induced by mechanical loading. Calcif Tissue Int. 2002;70(4):320–9. doi:10.1007/s00223-001-1025-y.
147. Sawakami K, Robling AG, Ai M, Pitner ND, Liu D, Warden SJ, et al. The Wnt co-receptor LRP5 is essential for skeletal mechanotransduction but not for the anabolic bone response to parathyroid hormone treatment. J Biol Chem. 2006;281(33):23698–711. doi:10.1074/jbc.M601000200.
148. Kesavan C, Wergedal JE, Lau K-HW, Mohan S. Conditional disruption of IGF-I gene in type 1α collagen-expressing cells shows an essential role of IGF-I in skeletal anabolic response to loading. Am J Physiol Endocrinol Metab. 2011;301(6):E1191–7. doi:10.1152/ajpendo.00440.2011.

149. Lau K-HW, Baylink DJ, Zhou X-D, Rodriguez D, Bonewald LF, Li Z, et al. Osteocyte-derived insulin-like growth factor I is essential for determining bone mechanosensitivity. Am J Physiol Endocrinol Metab. 2013;305(2):E271–81. doi:10.1152/ajpendo.00092.2013.
150. Watanuki M, Sakai A, Sakata T, Tsurukami H, Miwa M, Uchida Y, et al. Role of inducible nitric oxide synthase in skeletal adaptation to acute increases in mechanical loading. J Bone Miner Res. 2002;17(6):1015–25. doi:10.1359/jbmr.2002.17.6.1015.
151. Hong P, Boyd D, Beyea SD, Bezuhly M. Enhancement of bone consolidation in mandibular distraction osteogenesis: a contemporary review of experimental studies involving adjuvant therapies. J Plast Reconstr Aesthet Surg. 2013;66(7):883–95. doi:10.1016/j.bjps.2013.03.030.
152. Buchman SR, Ignelzi MA, Radu C, Wilensky J, Rosenthal AH, Tong L, et al. Unique rodent model of distraction osteogenesis of the mandible. Ann Plast Surg. 2002;49(5):511–9. doi:10.1097/01.SAP.0000015490.10557.33.
153. Felice PA, Ahsan S, Perosky JE, Deshpande SS, Nelson NS, Donneys A, et al. Prophylactic amifostine preserves the biomechanical properties of irradiated bone in the murine mandible. Plast Reconstr Surg. 2014;133:314e–21e. doi:10.1097/01.prs.0000438454.29980.f8.
154. Deshpande SS, Gallagher KK, Donneys A, Nelson NS, Guys NP, Felice PA, et al. Stem cells rejuvenate radiation-impaired vasculogenesis in murine distraction osteogenesis. Plast Reconstr Surg. 2015;135(3):799–806. doi:10.1097/PRS.0000000000001024.
155. Fregene A, Jing XL, Monson LA, Buchman SR. Alteration in volumetric bone mineralization density gradation patterns in mandibular distraction osteogenesis following radiation therapy. Plast Reconstr Surg. 2009;124(4):1237–44. doi:10.1097/PRS.0b013e3181b5a42f.
156. Schwarz DA, Jamali AM, Kakwan MS, Fregene A, Arman KG, Buchman SR. Biomechanical assessment of regenerate integrity in irradiated mandibular distraction osteogenesis. Plast Reconstr Surg. 2009;123(2 Suppl 1):114S–22S. doi:10.1097/PRS.0b013e318191c5d2.
157. Tchanque-Fossuo CN, Monson LA, Farberg AS, Donneys A, Zehtabzadeh AJ, Razdolsky ER, Buchman SR. Dose-response effect of human equivalent radiation in the murine mandible: part I. A histomorphometric assessment. Plast Reconstr Surg. 2011;128(1):114–21. doi:10.1097/PRS.0b013e31821741d4.
158. Deshpande SS, Gallagher KK, Donneys A, Tchanque-Fossuo CN, Sarhaddi D, Nelson NS, et al. Parathyroid hormone therapy mollifies radiation-induced biomechanical degradation in murine distraction osteogenesis. Plast Reconstr Surg. 2013a;132(1):91–100. doi:10.1097/PRS.0b013e3182910ae7.
159. Deshpande S, James AW, Blough J, Donneys A, Wang SC, Cederna PS, et al. Reconciling the effects of inflammatory cytokines on mesenchymal cell osteogenic differentiation. J Surg Res. 2013b;185(1):278–85. doi:10.1016/j.jss.2013.06.063.
160. Tchanque-Fossuo CN, Donneys A, Razdolsky ER, Monson LA, Farberg AS, Deshpande SS, et al. Quantitative histologic evidence of amifostine-induced cytoprotection in an irradiated murine model of mandibular distraction osteogenesis. Plast Reconstr Surg. 2012;130(6):1199–207. doi:10.1097/PRS.0b013e31826d2201.

Distraction of the Mandible

3

Joseph G. McCarthy and Roberto L. Flores

The original experimental studies and clinical experiences in craniofacial distraction were focused on the mandible. Ilizarov [1] had popularized the modern concept of bone lengthening or distraction osteogenesis of the appendicular skeleton but had ignored the craniofacial skeleton. While there had been experimental reports of attempts at mandibular lengthening [2, 3], it was the detailed canine studies from New York University [4, 5] that first raised the clinical feasibility of mandibular distraction, later confirmed by the original 1989 cases reported in 1992 [6]. The Mexico City group, led by Molina and Ortiz-Monasterio, reported a larger series of mandibular distraction cases in 1995 [7].

The development of mandibular distraction represented a significant paradigm shift in the evolution of craniofacial surgery. It permitted surgery on infants and young patients without the need for maxillomandibular fixation (MMF) or the harvest of bone grafts. Moreover, morbidity rates were lowered, and operating times and hospital stays were shortened. It is a gradual treatment process, not a dramatic acute intraoperative skeletal/soft tissue movement. Consequently, there was less skeletal relapse, and there was also remodeling or enlarging of the associated soft tissues (distraction histogenesis). On the other hand, the surgeon must stay actively involved with the patient for a minimum of 2 months, and a second surgery may be required for device removal. In mandibular distraction, the relationship with the team orthodontist is critical and continues during the entire treatment period. Team organization is important, especially in airway management, and the otolaryngologist, pulmonologist, and anesthesiologist must work in a collaborative fashion with the craniofacial surgeon. Other key members of the clinical team are the geneticist, nurse clinician/practitioner, pediatrician/internist, psychologist, social worker, and speech therapist.

J.G. McCarthy, M.D. (✉) • R.L. Flores, M.D.
Wyss Department of Plastic Surgery, NYU Langone Medical Center, New York, NY, USA
e-mail: Joseph.mccarthy@nyumc.org

J.G. McCarthy (ed.), *Craniofacial Distraction*,
DOI 10.1007/978-3-319-52564-8_3

In the early days of mandibular distraction, the concept won wide acceptance for patients with bilateral mandibular deficiency, especially those with Pierre Robin sequence (PRS), because of the possibility of correction of the airway problems and avoidance of tracheotomy.

In the chapter organization, the first section will deal with bilateral mandibular distraction, i.e., patients with Pierre Robin sequence (PRS), bilateral craniofacial microsomia (BCFM), and Treacher Collins syndrome (TCS). A later section will be devoted to unilateral mandibular distraction, usually employed in the patient with unilateral craniofacial microsomia (UCFM) as well as some patients with unilateral temporomandibular ankylosis. This section will also discuss combined maxillo-mandibular distraction.

3.1 Bilateral Mandibular Distraction

3.1.1 Pathology

It should be emphasized that there are both skeletal and soft tissue deficiencies in congenital mandibular deficiencies. This recognition is especially important when one considers the functional matrix theory of Moss [8] which states that craniofacial skeletal development is dependent on the function of the associated soft tissues and spaces. The corollary is that mandibular distraction should not be regard solely as "bone carpentry." There is also a true soft tissue deficiency, and one advantage of distraction osteogenesis is that there is enlargement of the associated soft tissues such as the muscles of mastication (distraction histogenesis) [9]. The patients may also benefit from soft tissue augmentation with autogenous fat injections or microvascular flap transfers.

The mandibular skeletal deficiency is traditionally rated according to the Kaban modification of the Pruzansky classification [10, 11] (Fig. 3.1). In this classification, type 1 represents a mandible in which all of the components are present but are diminished in size. In type 2a, there is significant deficiency of the body and ramus, but the vertical plane of the ramus and condyle aligns with the glenoid fossa. In type 2b, the vertical axis is displaced laterally. In type 3, there is absence of the ramus or only a ramal remnant; there is no condyle.

There are three main diagnoses of patients undergoing bilateral mandibular distraction, and each condition has a different surgical plan and outcome:

3.1.1.1 Pierre Robin Sequence (PRS)

Pierre Robin Sequence is defined by micrognathia causing glossoptosis and subsequence airway obstruction. The body of the mandible is usually reduced, and the ramus and condyle can be of normal size. Cleft palate is commonly present, but does not define the presence of this disorder. The maxilla is not affected, but there is usually soft tissue deficiency in the chin and submental area. Many patients can have "catch-up" growth of the mandible with resolution of the micrognathia and

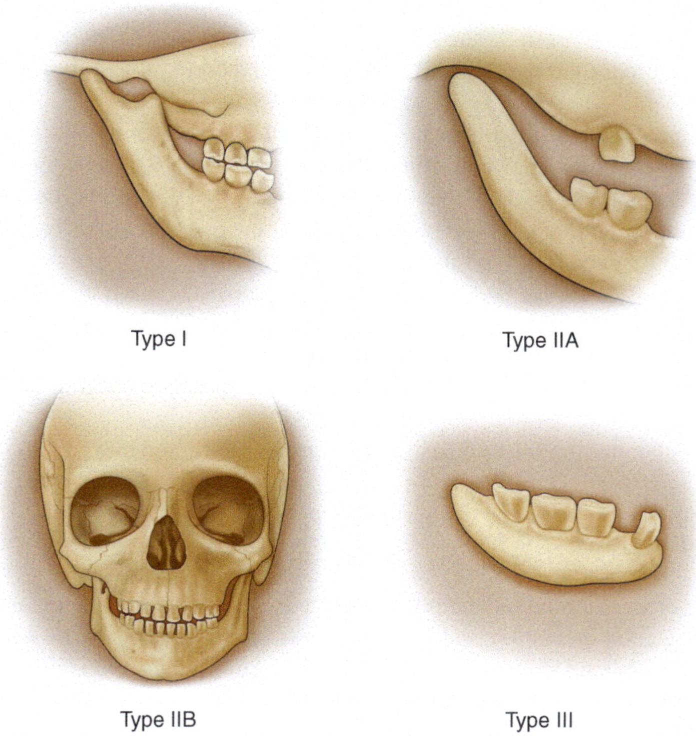

Fig. 3.1 The Pruzansky-Kaban classification. See text for details (Reprinted from Craniofacial Distraction, McCarthy, J. G., Springer, 1999)

respiratory problems; others require surgical intervention to relieve life-threatening airway obstruction.

3.1.1.2 Bilateral Craniofacial Microsomia (BCFM)

In this condition, the pathology is highly variable. The deficiency is predominantly in the ramus but also in the body of the mandible. There can also be a type 3 deformity. The mandibular deformity is usually symmetric and respiratory obstruction can occur. There is little, if any, catch-up growth.

The soft tissue deficiencies are more significant, especially in the cheeks where there can even be a number 7 Tessier cleft. There is soft tissue deficiency in the chin and submental areas. There are external ear anomalies as well as deficits in branches of the facial nerve. The most commonly used classification, the OMENS system, rates five facial areas by severity on a 0–3 scale. Each area represents one letter of the acronym: orbital asymmetry, mandibular hypoplasia, ear deformity, nerve dysfunction, and soft tissue deficiency [12].

3.1.1.3 Treacher Collins Syndrome (TCS)

This condition has the most severe skeletal and soft tissue deficiency and can pose the greatest challenge in mandibular reconstruction and correction of the respiratory obstruction.

The skeletal deficiency involves the ramus which is significantly shortened, and occasionally there is a type 3 deformity. There is a characteristic antegonial notch with a steep mandibular plane angle. The chin is retruded but has vertical excess. The maxilla has a unique posterior vertical deficiency, and there is a characteristic associated orbitozygomatic hypoplasia with orbital clefting. The zygomatic arch is often absent.

The soft tissue deficiencies are pronounced and are especially noticeable in the cheeks, orbitozygomatic, and eyelid regions where there can be eyelid colobomata. The chin and submental area are likewise deficient. There are varying degrees of microtia.

The dentoalveolar findings in these conditions are discussed in Chap. 4.

3.1.2 Indications

The main or most common indication is correction of the airway obstruction. There can be associated alimentation problems, but these can be corrected with resolution of the airway problem [15]. Another indication is dysmorphism, especially because of the associated psychosocial problems. One could also argue that mandibular distraction in the growing patient results in augmentation of the bony volume of the lower jaw in preparation for later orthodontic therapy and definitive orthognathic surgery. The postoperative change is noted not only in mandibular skeletal volume but also in position. As noted earlier, there is also in augmentation of soft tissue volume [9].

3.1.2.1 Absolute Indications

1. Growing Patient
   (a) Obstructive sleep apnea (OSA): Airway obstruction must be endoscopically or radiographically documented, and sleep studies are important diagnostic aids. The AHI must be greater than 10. The patient usually shows evidence of weight loss, somnolence, and, in extreme examples, cardiac problems. The surgical decision is best arrived at as a team recommendation by the craniofacial surgeon, otolaryngologist, pulmonologist, and anesthesiologist.
   (b) Severe dysmorphism: This is a more challenging indication to establish, and there is a lack of hard data or metrics to be used as supportive evidence. The argument is that it provides improved psychosocial functioning in the critical development years before definitive surgery can be done at the time of skeletal maturity. This benefit must be weighed against the risks of reconstruction and the patient investment into the treatment plan.
   (c) Severe micrognathia with overjet: Usually, patients with this condition have findings of obstructive sleep apnea. Lengthening and augmentation of the

bony volume also facilitate dental and orthodontic rehabilitation that are critical for definitive orthognathic surgery.

2. Adult or Craniofacially Mature Patient
   (a) Overjet greater than 12 mm, especially with evidence of obstructive sleep apnea. Moreover, the relapse rate is especially high when the mandible is corrected by acute advancement osteotomy such as the bilateral sagittal split osteotomy.
   (b) Micrognathia with restrictive and deficient soft tissues in the chin and submental area, findings that predispose to relapse, as discussed above. This is usually associated with severe micrognathia.
   (c) Patients with previous unsuccessful mandibular advancement surgery.

This topic is discussed in more detail in Chap. 5.

3.1.2.2 Controversial Indications

1. Growing Patient
   (a) Mild/moderate dysmorphism without evidence of obstructive sleep apnea. It is known that these patients will require definitive surgery at skeletal maturity. If mandibular distraction is performed during the period of growth and development, the child may require two surgical interventions. This is more likely in patients with bilateral craniofacial macrosomia, Treacher Collins syndrome, and Pierre Robin sequence. The counterargument is that the psychosocial functioning of the patient should be improved during the critical development years before 18 years of age. This is discussed in more detail in Section 3.5.2.
2. Patient in the 12–15 Year Age Group
   (a) In general, distraction is deferred in these patients until skeletal maturity is reached; the remaining interval is only a few years in length. It should also be emphasized that at skeletal maturity, the mandatory endpoint of distraction is that a class 1 occlusion must be achieved.
3. Adult or Craniofacially Mature Patient
   This subject is discussed in Chap. 5.

3.1.3 Preoperative Assessment

A functioning and well-organized clinical team is essential. It should include the craniofacial surgeon, orthodontist, otolaryngologist, pulmonologist, anesthesiologist, nurse clinician, psychologist, and social worker. In the preoperative assessment, there are multiple variables that must be carefully considered.

3.1.3.1 Age of Patient/Patient and Family Cooperation

The difficult years are ages 1–3 because of the challenge of patient cooperation. The roles of the pediatric nurse, psychologist, and social worker are invaluable in determining when the young patient is ready for distraction of the mandible.

Family cooperation is likewise essential as they are usually responsible for device activation and care. As mentioned earlier, distraction is usually deferred in the patient aged 14–17, unless there is evidence of obstructive sleep apnea. Of course, patients with skeletal maturity rarely pose a problem in decision making as to cooperation.

3.1.3.2 Health of Patient

The patient must demonstrate stable health without critical cardiac or other systemic problems. If the airway is unstable, consideration should be given to tracheostomy. Nutritional status and weight of the patient must be considered. Medical clearance by a pediatrician or primary care physician is required.

3.1.3.3 Respiratory Status/OSA

The relevant team members evaluate and make decisions regarding the respiratory status of the patient after endoscopic, radiographic, and sleep studies [13]. The respiratory obstruction is usually retroglossal in location, but one must remember that there are other potential sites of airway obstruction, as in the nose or other areas of the respiratory tract, tonsils/adenoids, hypopharynx, and trachea (tracheomalacia). It is notable that secondary airway anomalies (in addition to tongue-based airway obstruction) are common in Pierre Robin sequence and Treacher Collins syndrome [14]. The AHI values tend to be the determinant metric for or against the use of distraction, provided that there is no central sleep apnea or a critical secondary airway anomaly precluding success of mandibular distraction.

The patient can present with different respiratory scenarios, such as an indwelling tracheotomy or a non-life-threatening obstructive sleep apnea. In these situations, the surgical decision is elective in nature. The most challenging patient is the one with a dangerously obstructed airway and impending tracheotomy. In these situations, it may be safer to perform a temporary tracheotomy and provide control of the airway throughout the distraction process. In the newborn with a challenging airway obstruction, the tendency has been to intubate the child and proceed with rapid (2 mm/day) mandibular distraction while the patient remains intubated.

3.1.3.4 Alimentation

Many patients who present with obstructive sleep apnea are thin and malnourished and often have an indwelling gastrostomy tube. The nutritional problem usually improves with correction of the airway obstruction (see [15]) in children with isolated airway anomalies; however, the outcome in syndromic patients is less clear.

3.1.3.5 Bone Volume and Blood Supply

The Pruzansky-Kaban classification is usually used to define the mandibular skeletal pathology. Patients with a type 3 cannot undergo distraction but must first have restoration of the ramus and condyle with some type of bone transfer, nonvascular or vascularized [16–20].

Patients can present with history of a previous mandibular distraction or a previous osteotomy. Patients can also have a history of a bone graft restoration of the ramus and condyles or a vascularized composite flap. Distraction can be recommended for these patients, provided there is adequate bone volume with sufficient blood supply/attached soft tissue. If there is evidence of rib graft reconstruction of the ramus, and the grafts are small in caliber, distraction is contraindicated because of the likelihood of fibrous union (Fig. 3.2) (see [17]; see [19, 20]). In these scenarios, distraction of the native bone away from the rib graft is recommended [21, 22]. The indications for distraction of the radiated bone are not codified. Although mandibular distraction in the radiated field can be successful, the complication rate is increased, likely due to the decreased blood supply at the surgical site.

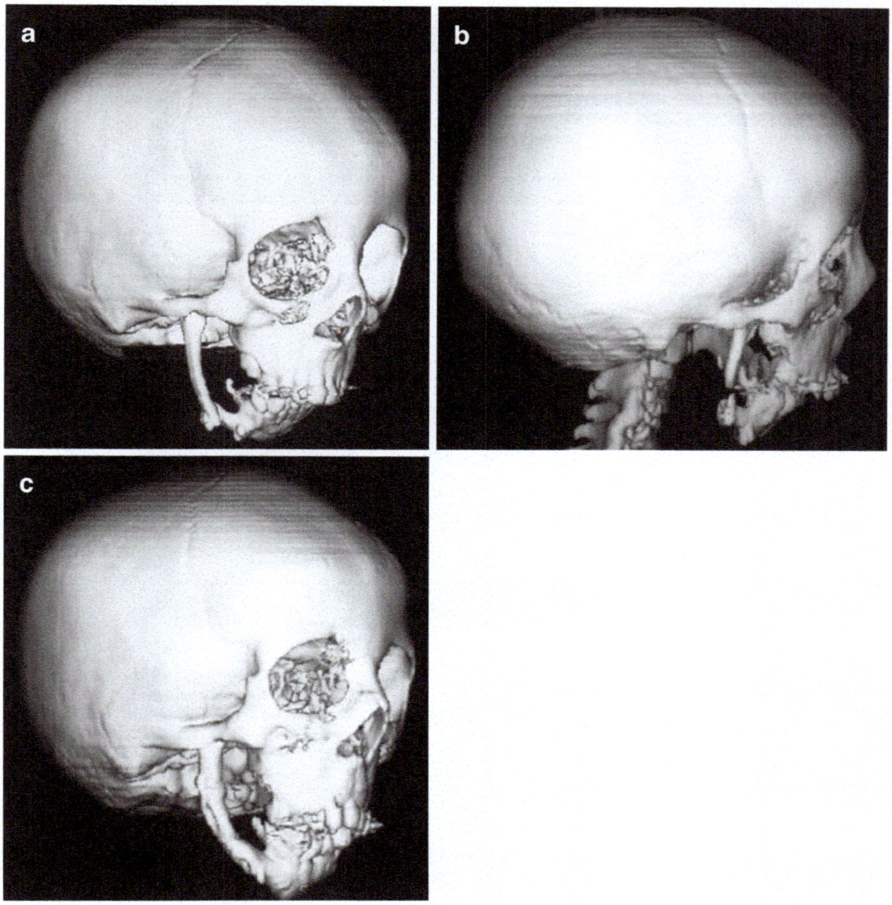

Fig. 3.2 Serial CT scans. (**a**) Following reconstruction of the ramus/body of the mandible with an autogenous rib graft. (**b**) Following distraction (osteotomy in the rib graft) with development of fibrous union. (**c**) Following successful secondary distraction of a larger iliac bone graft reconstruction of the mandibular defect

3.1.3.6 Dentition

There can be teeth or tooth follicles at the site of the planned osteotomy. If this problem is not addressed and distraction is performed, it will be unsuccessful, and there will also be injury of the involved teeth. It is preferable to remove the teeth or tooth follicles and wait at least 4 months before performing the osteotomy at the appropriate edentulous site [23] (Figs. 3.3, 3.4, and 3.5).

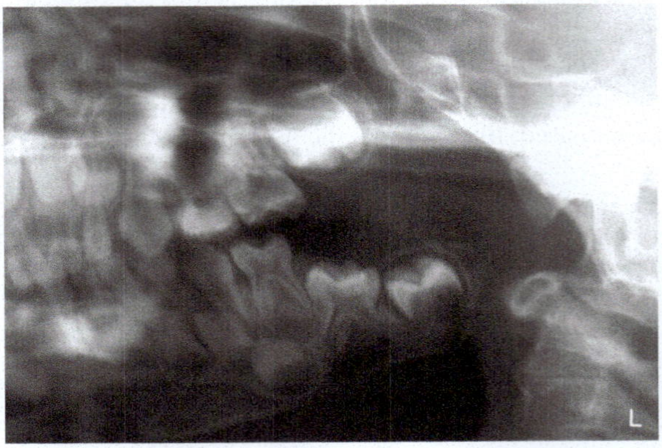

Fig. 3.3 Removal of a tooth follicle prior to mandibular distraction. Panorex showing a deficient mandible with a terminal tooth follicle

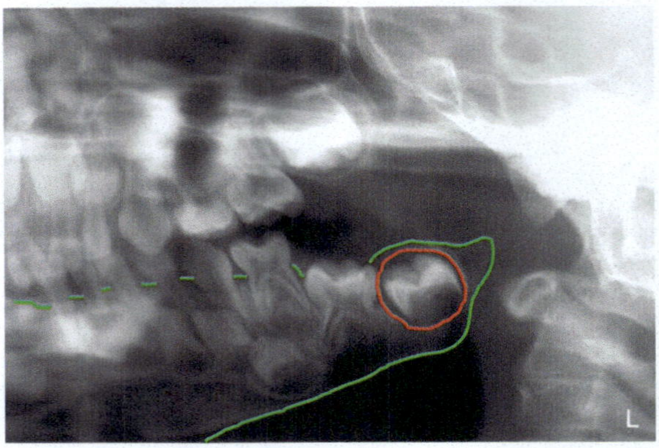

Fig. 3.4 Outline of the mandible (*green*) and the tooth follicle (*red*)

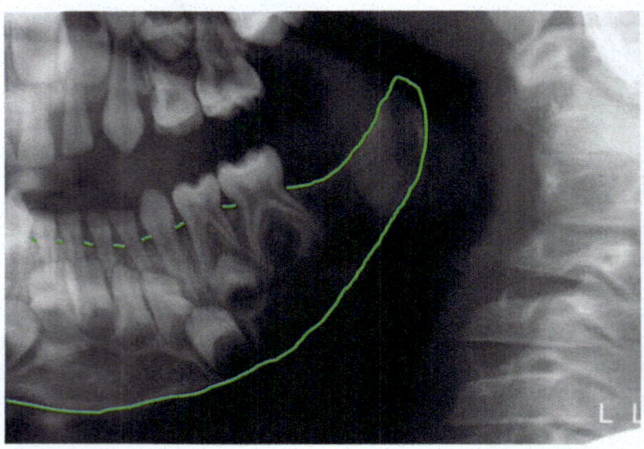

Fig. 3.5 Successful distraction 6 months after removal of the tooth follicle with elongation of the ramus

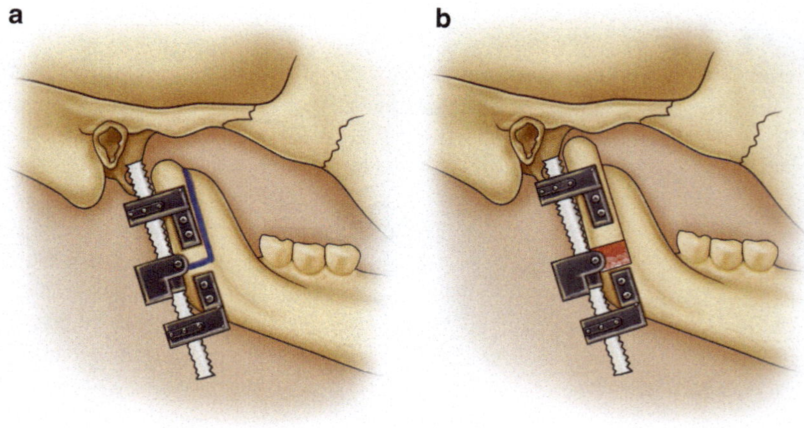

Fig. 3.6 Reconstruction of the TMJ with transport distraction. (**a**) Line of osteotomy and application of device. Note the defect from the gap arthroplasty. (**b**) With activation, the transport segment was moved toward the glenoid fossa with the leading edge covered by a fibrocartilaginous cap. Note the generated bone behind the transport segment (Reprinted from Stucki-McCormick, S. V. et al. Semin. Oxford War 1999: 5(1): 59–63)

3.1.3.7 Concomitant Temporomandibular Joint Disorder (TMJD) or TMJ Ankylosis

In the patient with a history of temporomandibular joint disorder or pain and arthritis, the TMJ can be protected with an orthodontic device that permits condylar unloading [24]. The unresolved question is in what order to treat the patient who presents with a true indication for mandibular distraction in the presence of TMJ ankyloses [25, 26]. It is the authors' preference to perform the distraction first and then wait 6 months after device removal to consider several treatment possibilities, such as the following: gap arthroplasty, Matthews device [27], costochondral grafts (see [17]; see [19, 20]), fibular transfer with cartilage cap, and transport distraction [28–32] (Figs. 3.6 and 3.7). TMJ ankylosis combined with retrognathia poses one of the more formidable reconstructive dilemmas. Although it is certainly possible to elongate the mandible, sustainable release of the fused TMJ remains elusive. Procedures designed to release bony ankylosis have a significant recurrence risk and may result in mandibular setback resulting in recurrent airway obstruction.

3.1.3.8 Associated Maxillary Deficiency

This is more of a problem in the patient with unilateral craniofacial macrosomia, but in the patient with Treacher Collins syndrome, there is a pathognomonic posterior maxillary deficiency that requires special attention when considering mandibular advancement [33].

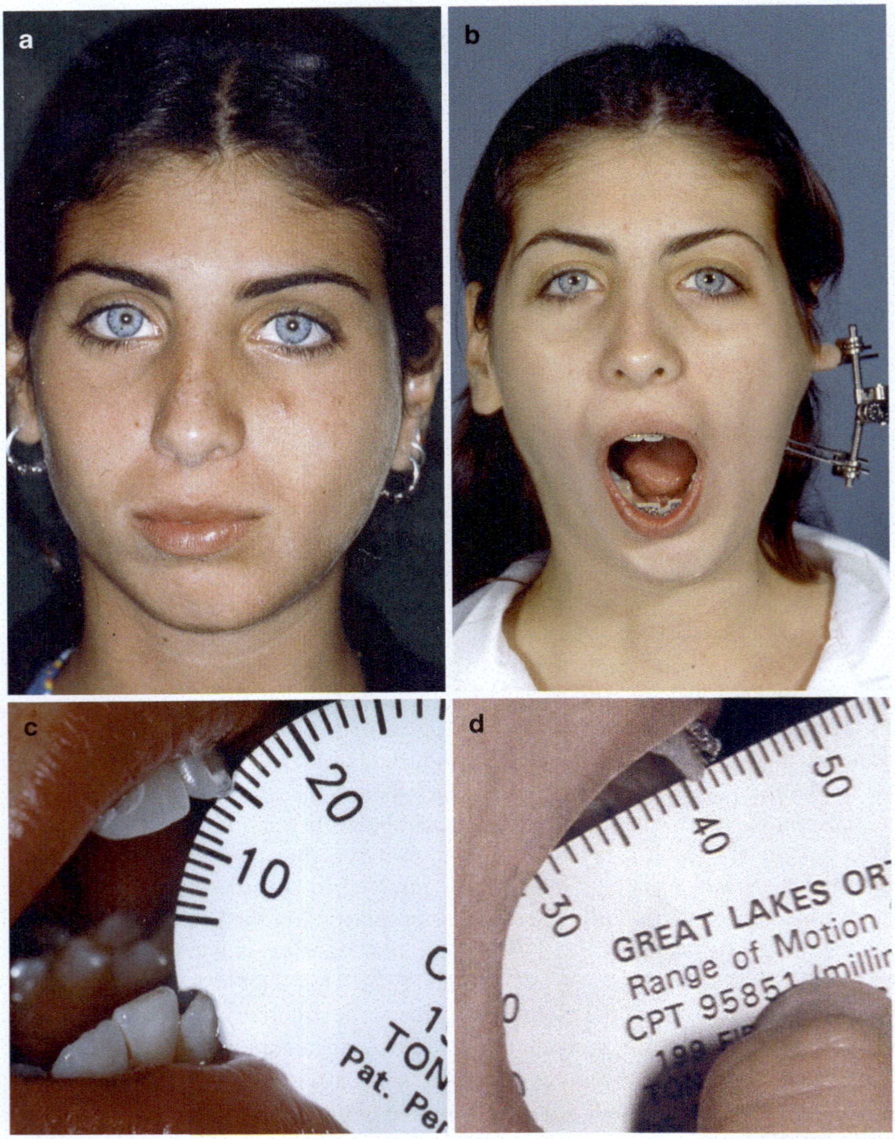

Fig. 3.7 A 17-year-old female following a mandibular fracture and left-sided TMJ ankylosis. (**a**) Preoperative appearance with only 10 mm of interincisal opening. (**b**) Interincisal opening following gap arthroplasty and transport distraction with an external device. (**c**) Preoperative interincisal measurement (goniometer in a dental space). (**d**) Postoperative measurement

3.2 Orthodontic Assessment

This is discussed in detail in Chap. 4.

3.2.1 Preoperative Planning

A clinical examination is the first step. This should be done carefully with the head in a neutral position, and the examiner should observe the patient in all dimensions, paying special attention to the soft tissues, occlusion, and temporomandibular function or interincisal opening with all findings recorded.

The respiratory status is evaluated by the otolaryngologist, pulmonologist, and anesthesiologist, in conjunction with the craniofacial surgeon. As previously stated, multisited airway pathology is common, and patients with suspected airway stenosis should undergo laryngoscopy/bronchoscopy in addition to polysomnography.

Photographs are obtained, and the views include frontal, oblique, profile, submental, bird's eye, and occlusal.

Cephalograms (posteroanterior, lateral and basilar views) and panoramic radiographs are especially indicated preoperatively and can also be used postoperatively to document the progress of the distraction and stability/growth over the long term. In general, children under 3 years of age are not cooperative in terms of obtaining a satisfactory cephalograms.

CT scans are obtained on all patients, and the introduction of the ICAT has simplified the process. Bony stock, tooth location, and condition of the condyle/TMJ are preoperatively assessed.

Vector and device selection/placement are considered together [34–36].

The vectors (Fig. 3.8) are defined by the relationship of the long arms of the distraction device to the maxillary occlusal plane as follows: vertical vector has an angle of approximately 90°–60° and tends to be indicated in the patient with a predominant ramal deficiency; the oblique vector has an angle of 60°–45° and is used for lengthening of the ramus and body, whereas the horizontal vector has an angle less than 45° and is especially indicated in the patient with severe deficiency of the body of the mandible (Fig. 3.9). In general, a single vector, if properly planned with device placement, can correct a multidimensional mandibular deficiency.

The osteotomy is preferably planned at right angles to the device activation rod, and care must be taken to avoid injury to the teeth or follicles. An inverted L osteotomy can be useful in preserving the developing and permanent teeth. The osteotomy should be performed at the site of adequate bone volume. In other words, the divided edges of the bone at the osteotomy site should be as broad and thick as possible to promote bone formation in the distraction zone.

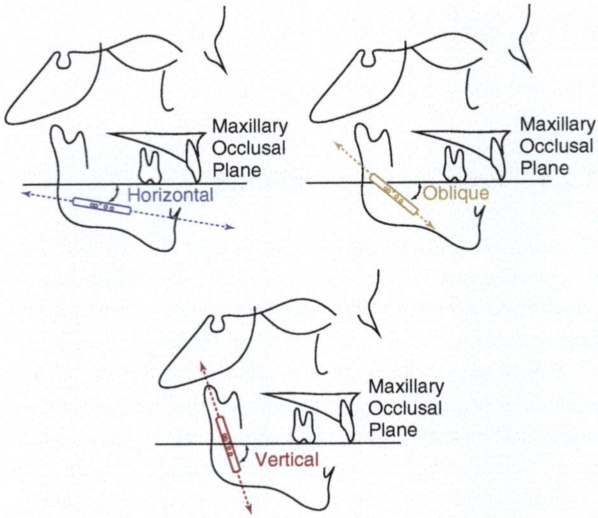

Fig. 3.8 The vectors of distraction are related to the maxillary occlusal plane: horizontal, oblique, and vertical

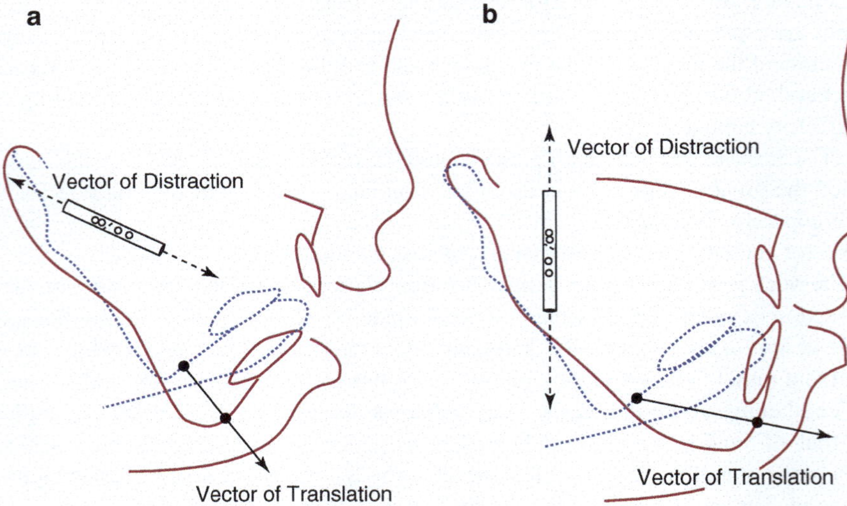

Fig. 3.9 Vectors of distraction. (**a**) With an oblique vector in mandibular distraction, the chin point is translated in an inferior direction without closing of the anterior open bite. (**b**) With a vertical vector, there is counterclockwise rotation of the mandible. Note the projection of the chin and closure of the anterior open bite. (*Blue*), pre-distraction; (*Red*), post-distraction

Device placement and selection are dictated by bone volume and tooth position, especially in the pediatric patient. Depending on the hypoplasty and deficiency of the mandible, there may be little room for variation in device orientation. Device placement must be absolutely rigid with secure screw/pin fixation. Screws must be bicortical and should not injure teeth or tooth follicles.

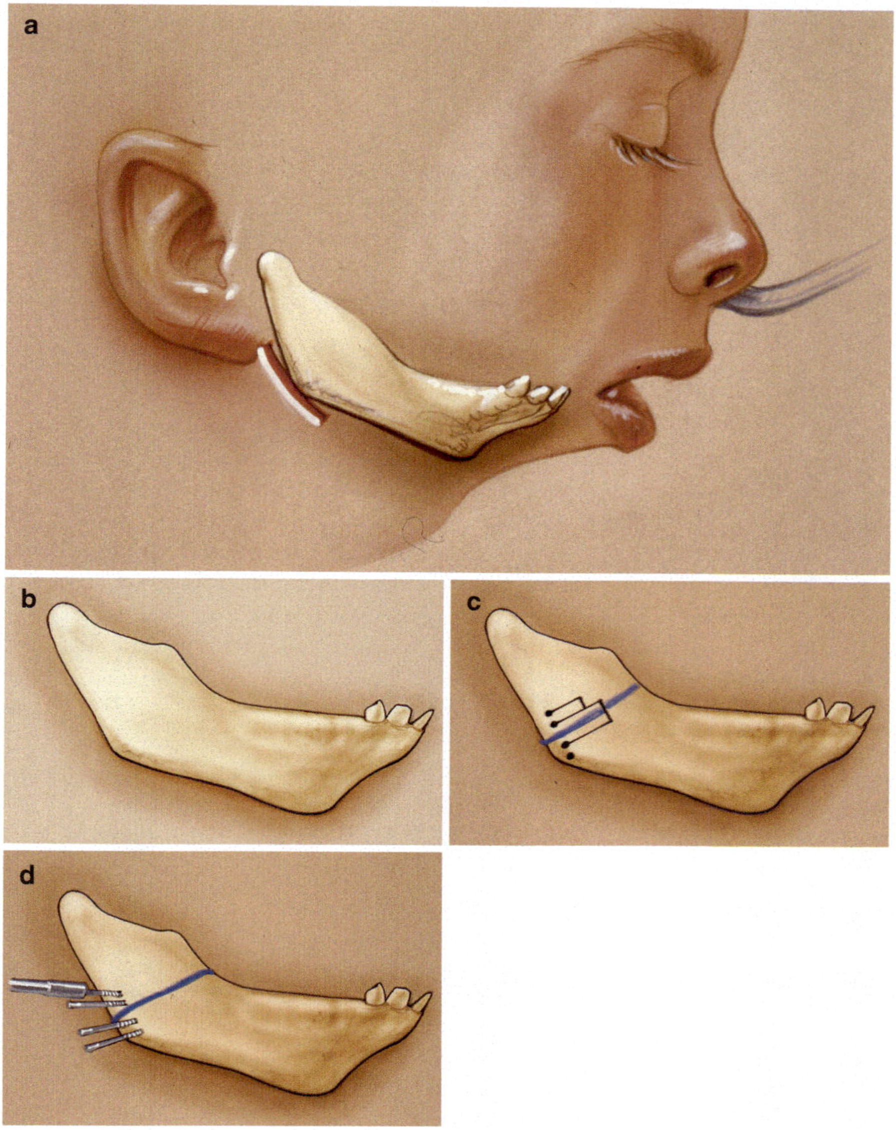

Fig. 3.10 External mandibular distraction device technique. (**a**) Submandibular incision. The incision should be placed lower than illustrated. (**b**) Outline of the hypoplastic mandible. (**c**) Proposed line of osteotomy (*blue*) and pin sites. (**d**) Insertion of pins (Figures 3.10 and 3.11 reprinted from Thorne, C.H. Grabb & Smith, Plastic Surgery, J.B Lippincott, Philadelphia, 2007)

The original mandibular distraction devices were *external* with the pins introduced percutaneously (Figs. 3.10 and 3.11) [6]. There have been subsequent reports of *internal* devices introduced intraorally, either linear [37] (Fig. 3.12) or curvilinear [38–40]. The *semi-buried* is the authors' preference since it allows the application of a vertical vector [41] and easy access for device activation (Figs. 3.13 and 3.14).

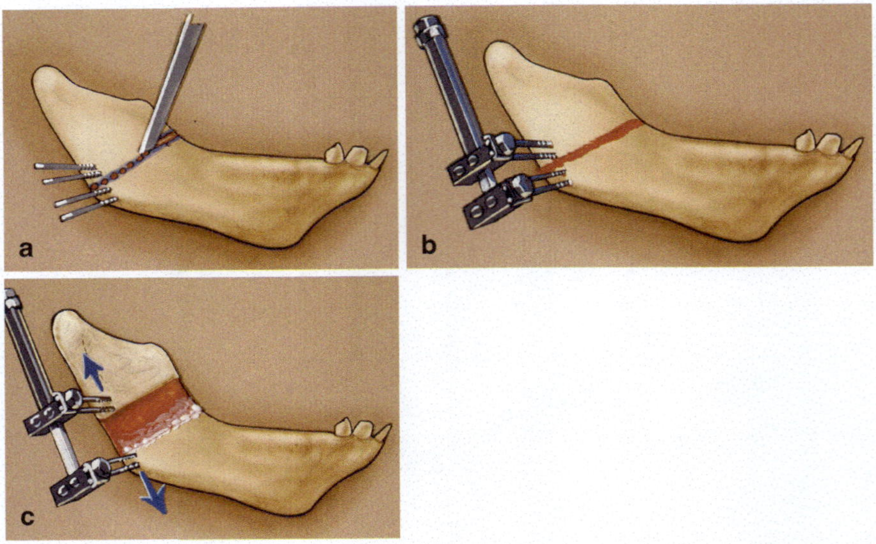

Fig. 3.11 (**a**) Completion of osteotomy. (**b**) Application of device. (**c**) Activation of device and generation of bone (*red*)

Fig. 3.12 Internal mandibular distraction device (Drawing adapted from Diner PA, Kollar EM, Martinez H, Vazquez MP. Intraoral distraction for mandibular lengthening: a technical innovation. J Craniomaxillofac Surg. 1996 Apr;24(2):92–5)

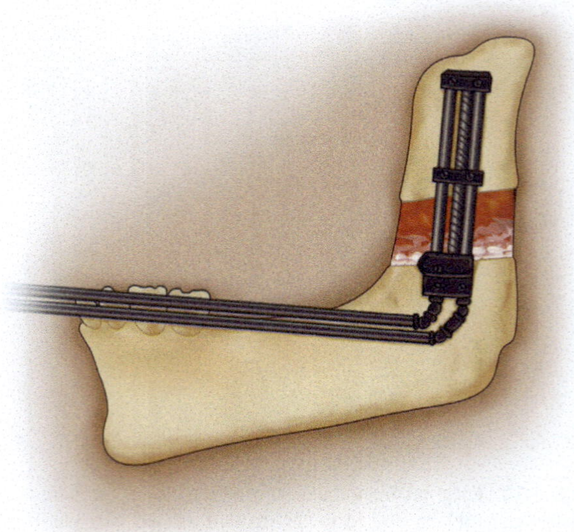

The *external* devices in which the pins are inserted percutaneously require less bone stock and have the advantage that, if there is device failure, the device can be replaced in the outpatient setting. In addition, they allow molding of the regenerate. However, the external devices are associated with the least satisfactory scar because it often is not located in the natural skin lines.

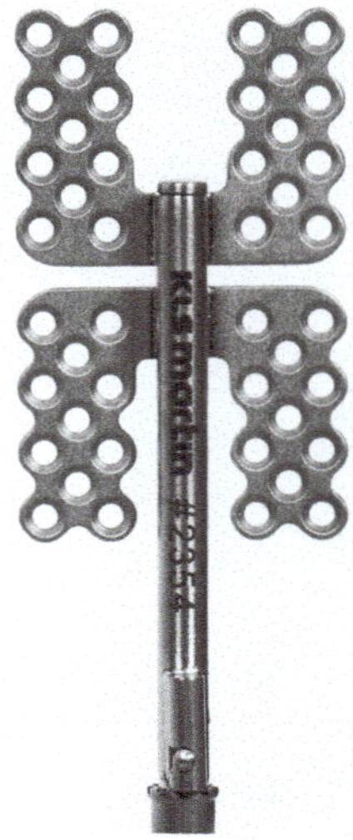

Fig. 3.13 Semi-buried device. The foot plates can be modified and reduced. The activation arm is passed through a separate skin incision (KLS Martin®)

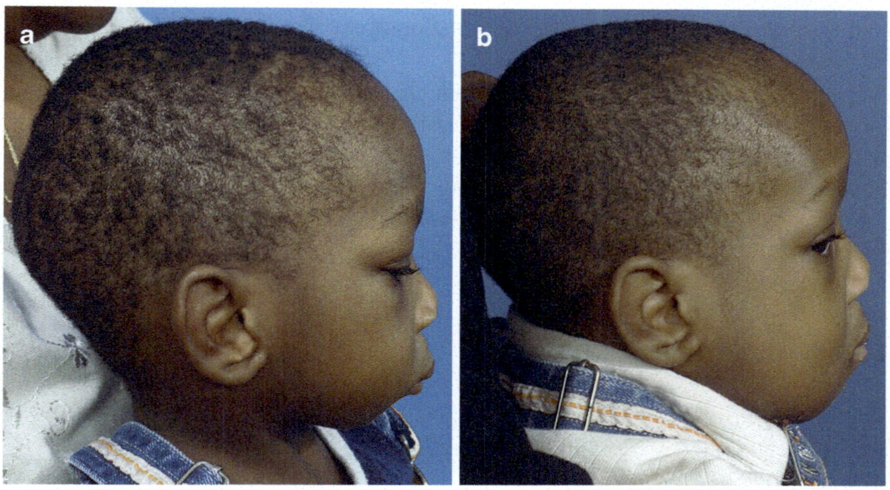

Fig. 3.14 Example of the semi-buried mandibular distraction device. (**a**) An 8-year-old boy with micrognathia and obstructive sleep apnea. (**b**) Following mandibular distraction. (**c**) Lateral cephalogram following osteotomy and device application but before activation. (**d**) At the completion of activation. Note the expansion of the airway and counterclockwise rotation of the devices. There has been overcorrection with a deliberate class III dental relationship

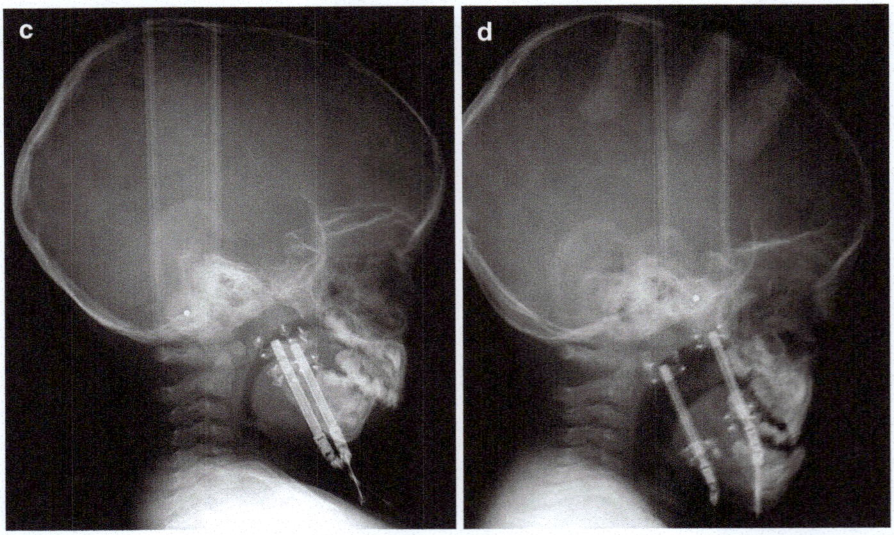

Fig. 3.14 (continued)

The *intraoral* devices leave no scar but suffer the disadvantage that they require a large amount of bone volume for application of the plates, and vector selection is limited (see Chap. 5 for more details).

The *semi-buried* devices, the preference of the authors, are especially indicated for the vertical vector. One may argue that the scar is unsatisfactory. However this problem can be obviated as they can be inserted through a low submandibular incision (Risdon) that allows the plates to be applied intimately and securely to the bone.

Virtual surgical planning has been reported but at this time has a limited role in planning a distraction procedure.

3.2.2 Operative Technique

There are multiple types of incisions or surgical approaches, but all are dependent on tooth/follicle position, bone volume, desired vector, and size and shape of the distraction device.

As mentioned earlier, with *external* devices, the pins are inserted percutaneously, and this type of approach is indicated in the patient with a relatively hypoplastic mandible. The buccal aspect of the mandible is exposed in the subperiosteal plane after an incision is made either below the mandible border (Risdon) or along the oblique line of the ramus (Fig. 3.15). Illuminated retractors allow precise placement of the percutaneous pins (self-drilling). The surgeon's finger placed extramucosally on the lingual side ensures bicortical placement without soft tissue penetration. After one pin on either side of the osteotomy is passed through the device and

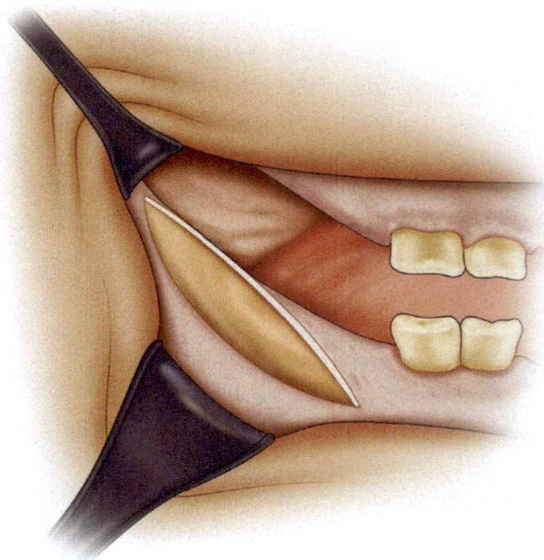

Fig. 3.15 Intraoral incision along the oblique line of the mandible

secured to the bone (bicortical), the maneuver is repeated with the remaining pins (see Fig. 3.10). The osteotomy is made with a saw/osteotome ideally at a right angle to the distraction vector (device). The device must be stable with four pins and should be seated only a few millimeters above the skin. The wound is irrigated and closed with sutures.

In the intraoral approach or incision, the incision is made along the oblique line, and the buccal aspect of the ramus is exposed with lighted retractors (see Fig. 3.15). The subject is discussed in more detail in Chap. 5.

The semi-buried devices are inserted through a low Risdon incision, care taken to avoid injury to the marginal mandibular nerve (see Fig. 3.13). Subperiosteal exposure is obtained, only large enough to perform the osteotomy and place and secure the distraction device.

The osteotomy has to be complete. There had been discussion in the early days of mandibular distraction whether it should be a corticotomy (as proposed by Ilizarov) or complete osteotomy. However, with the passage of time, all workers agree the osteotomy should be complete. The preference is to make the osteotomy perpendicular to the activation rod. Some authors have recommended a sagittal split, but this is a more complicated osteotomy, especially in a hypoplastic ramus (see Chap. 5).

One must take every step to avoid injury to the inferior alveolar nerve. The osteotomies are initiated with a saw along the buccal cortex, saline copiously irrigated at the osteotomy site. The saw cut is extended along the anterior and posterior borders and lingual aspect. Rotation of a broad osteotome inserted into the buccal cortex completes the osteotomy. Again, an inverted L osteotomy may prove useful in preserving sensibility to the lower lip.

Device placement determines vector orientation. The device must be rigidly applied to the mandible. Lack of rigidity probably represents the number one cause of distraction failure. It must be emphasized that there should be multiple screws inserted on each side of the activation rod. In either pin or screw insertion, they must have bicortical attachment. The osteotomy must be verified. This is done by activating and lengthening the distraction device, confirming completion of the osteotomy by direct visualization and palpation, and then closing it to place the bony edges in apposition. With the semi-buried device, a separate small incision is made for exit of the activation rod.

3.2.3 Postoperative Management

Latency is the period after osteotomy but prior to device activation. In the original papers of Ilizarov, latency was defined as 5 days to allow the ingress of inflammatory cells and development of a micro-vasculature at the osteotomy site. In general, a latency of 5 days is recommended for mandibular distraction. However, this can be reduced or even avoided in neonates or infants with respiratory distress who are intubated.

Activation is that period when the device is being turned ("activated") to lengthen the mandible on a daily basis. The usual *rate* is 1 mm a day but can be increased to 2 mm a day in infants and neonates. The *rhythm* is the number of times per day the device is turned. The rhythm is once or twice a day, but this is not a critical variable.

The *end point* of activation is age dependent, but in the growing patient undergoing bilateral mandibular distraction, the end point is a class 3 malocclusion, provided the orthodontist feels there is still a functioning bite (see Fig. 3.14). The role of lateral cephalograms is helpful in deciding when to discontinue activation.

Consolidation is that period following activation and usually lasts 8 weeks. Cephalograms at that point usually show radiographic evidence of mineralization in the distraction zone.

Orthodontic therapy and molding of the generate during the periods of activation and consolidation [42] are discussed in Chap. 4 (see Fig. 3.20).

3.3 Case Examples (Figs. 3.16, 3.17, 3.18, 3.19, 3.20, 3.21, and 3.22)

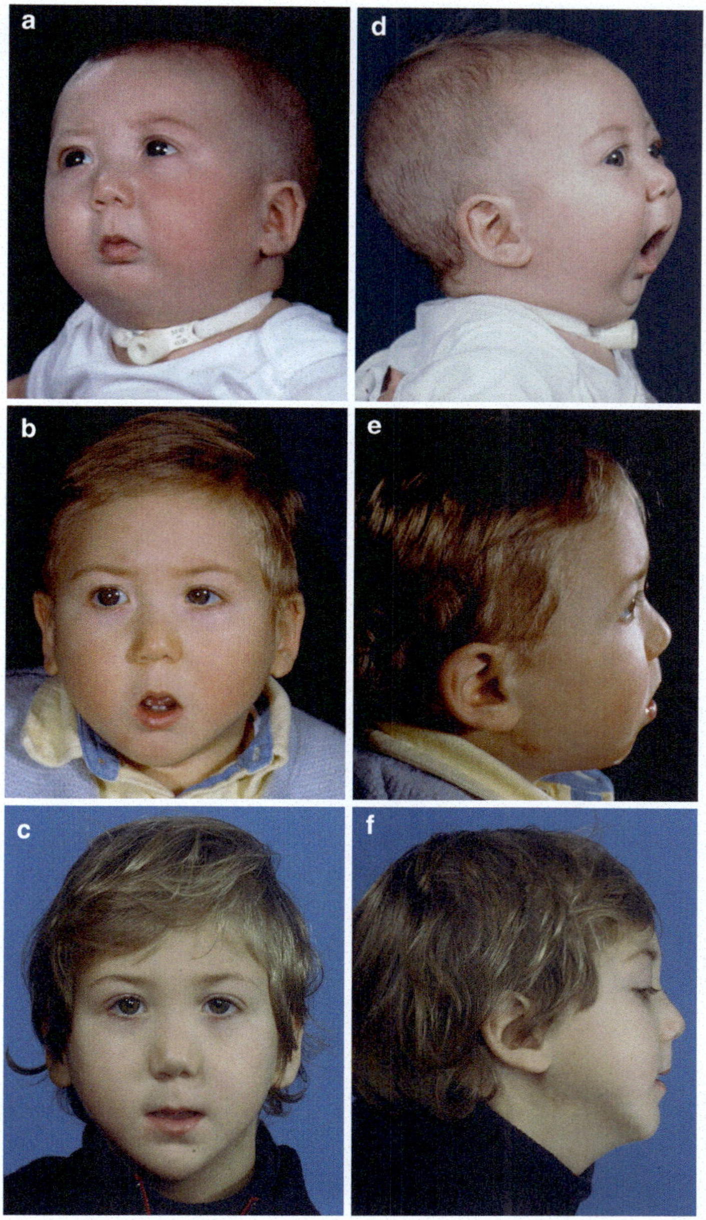

Fig. 3.16 An infant with Stickler syndrome and life-threatening obstructive sleep apnea requiring a neonatal tracheotomy. (**a**) Preoperative appearance. Note the tracheotomy and micrognathia. (**b**) One year after bilateral mandibular distraction. The tracheotomy has been decannulated. (**c**) Four years postoperative. (**d**) Preoperative profile. (**e**) Profile 1 year postoperative. (**f**) Profile 4 years postoperative with maintenance of airway function and mandibular projection.

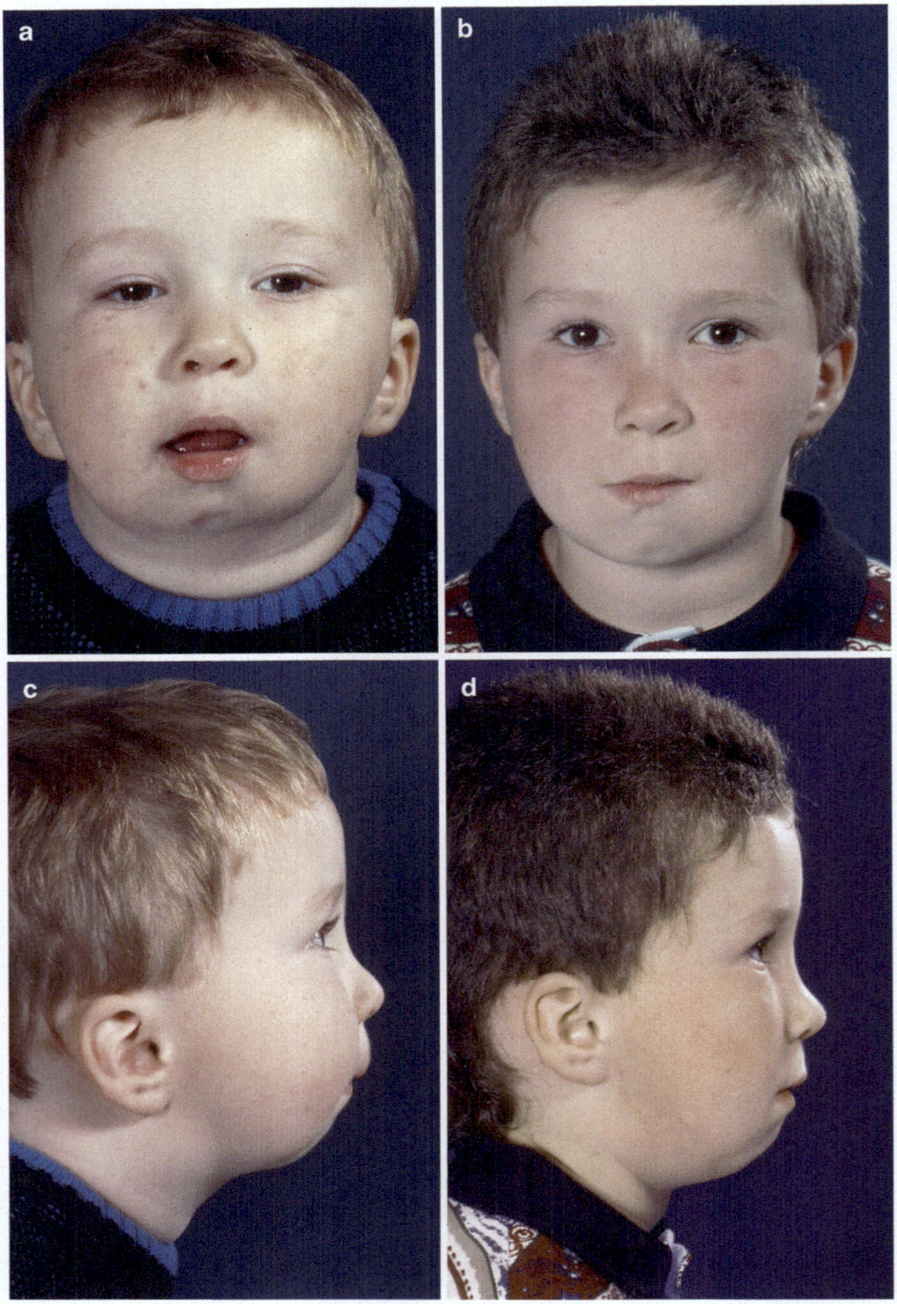

Fig. 3.17 A 4-year-old boy with micrognathia and obstructive sleep apnea. (**a**) Preoperative frontal view. (**b**) Postoperative frontal view 3 years after bilateral mandibular distraction (external devices). (**c**) Preoperative profile. (**d**) Postoperative profile

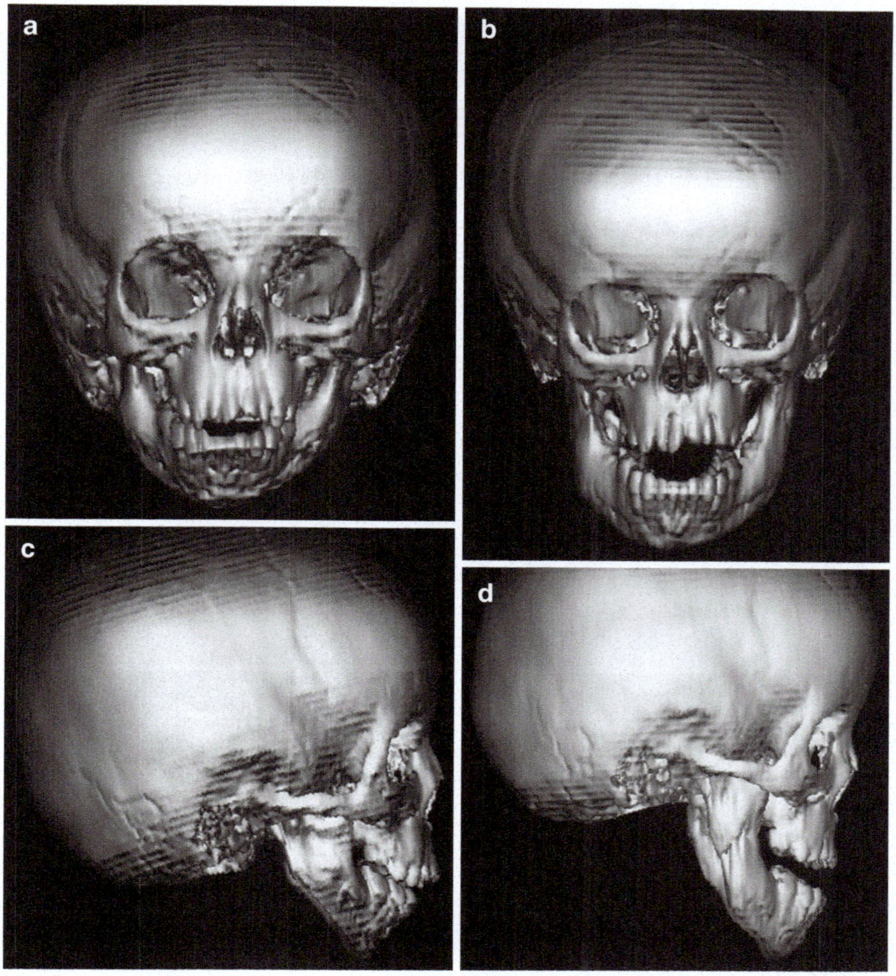

Fig. 3.18 CT scans of patient illustrated in Fig. 3.17. (**a**) Frontal view before bilateral mandibular distraction. (**b**) Postoperative frontal view. (**c**) Preoperative lateral view. (**d**) Postoperative lateral view. Note the volume of bone generated in the mandibular ramus and body with an increase in chin projection

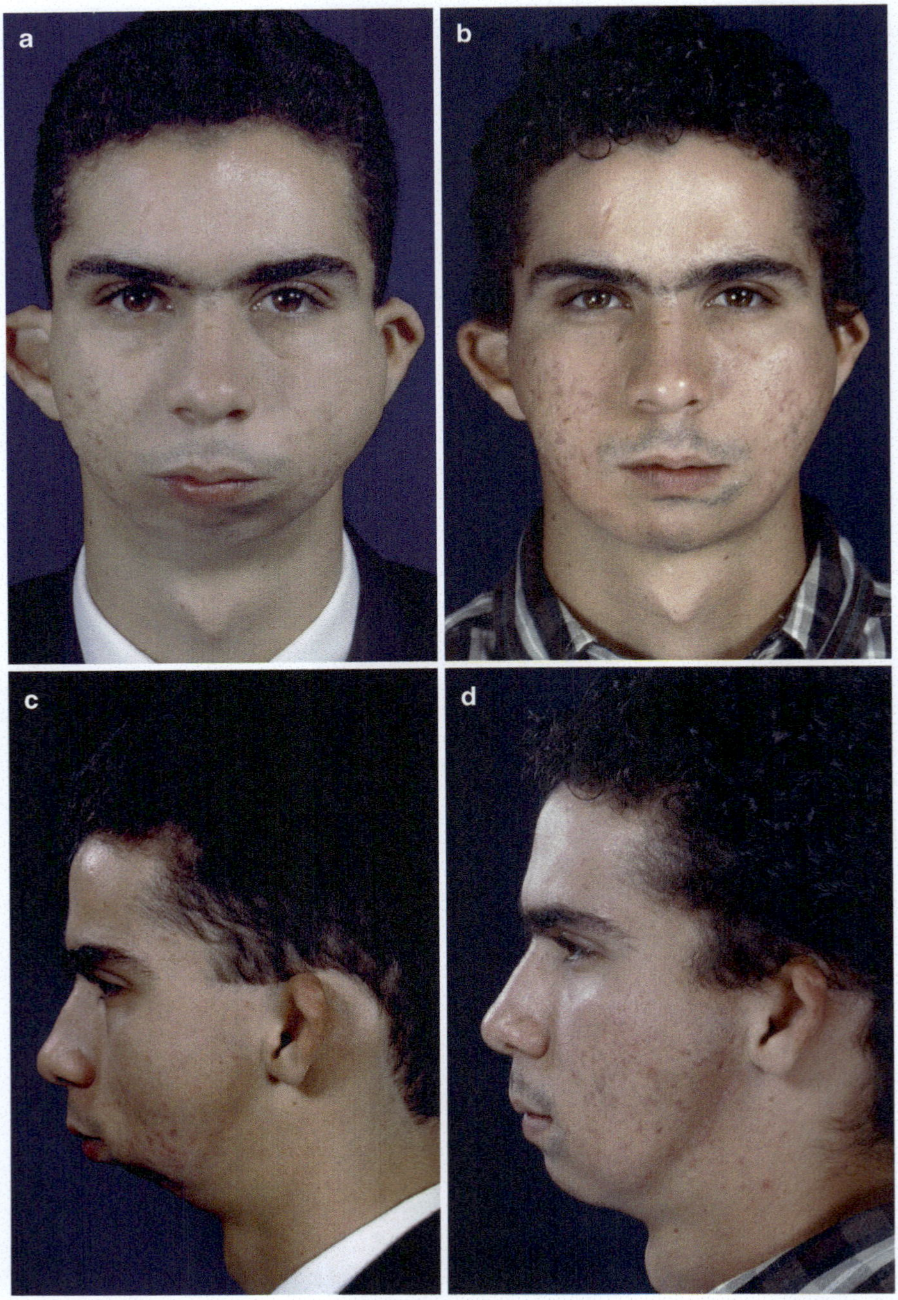

Fig. 3.19 An adult male with severe micrognathia and obstructive sleep apnea who underwent bilateral mandibular distraction. (**a**) Preoperative frontal view. (**b**) Postoperative frontal view. (**c**) Preoperative profile. (**d**) Postoperative profile. He also had an osseous genioplasty as a second stage procedure. Note the satisfactory submandibular scar with an external distraction device

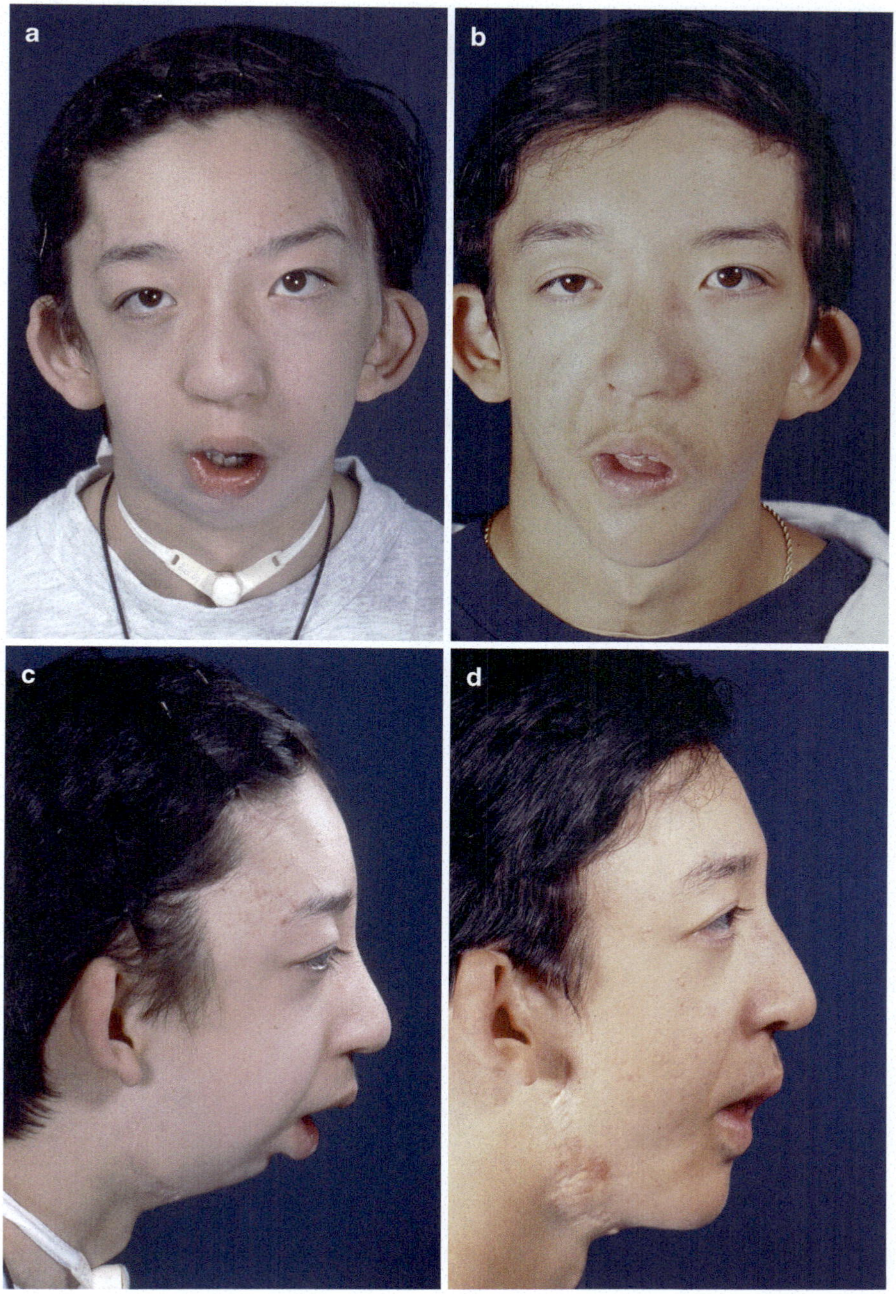

Fig. 3.20 A 14-year-old boy with micrognathia, indwelling tracheotomy, and history of failed efforts at mandibular reconstruction at another institution. (**a**) Preoperative frontal view. (**b**) Postoperative view after bilateral mandibular distraction and molding of the generate. The tracheotomy has been removed. (**c**) Preoperative profile. (**d**) Postoperative profile

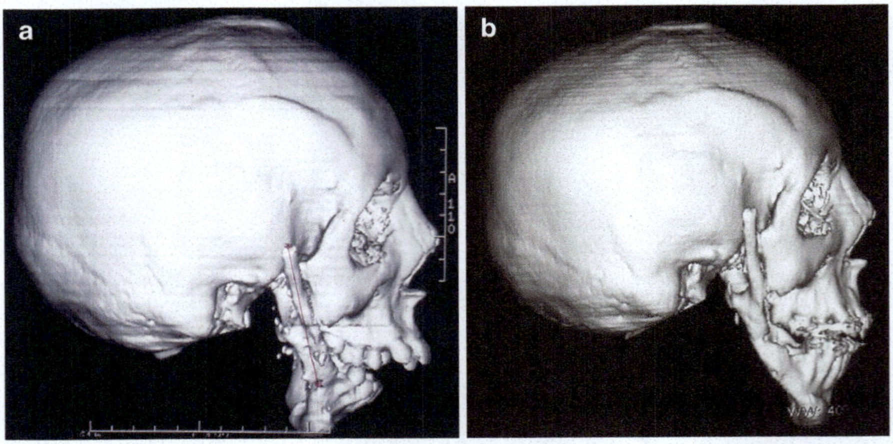

Fig. 3.21 CT scans of patient illustrated in Fig. 3.20. (**a**) Preoperative CT scan. Note the severe micrognathia, anterior open bite, class II malocclusion, and residual rib graft (failed reconstruction at another institution). (**b**) Postoperative CT scan after bilateral mandibular distraction and molding of the generate. Note the elongation and counterclockwise rotation of the mandible and closure of the anterior bite

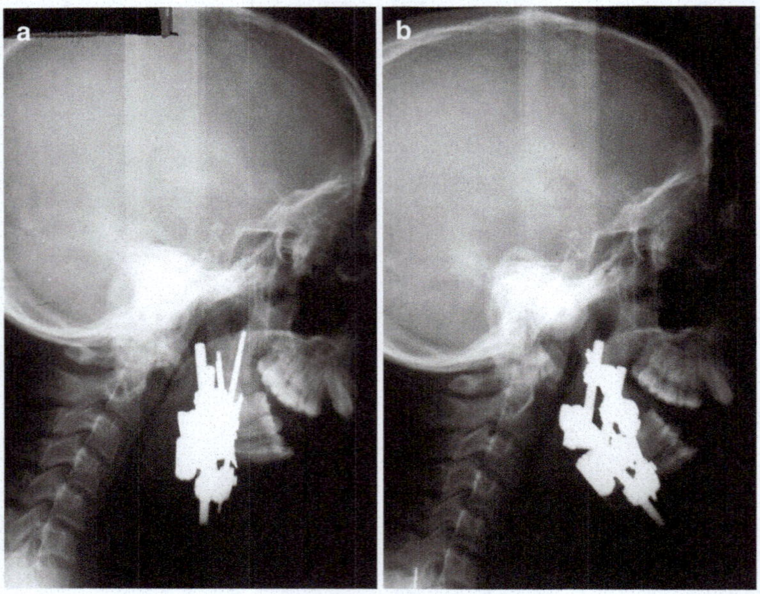

Fig. 3.22 Serial lateral cephalograms. (**a**) Following osteotomies and application of external distraction devices and before activation. (**b**) With activation and angulation of the external devices, there has been elongation and counterclockwise rotation of the mandible. (**c**) Larger distraction devices were applied and activation continued. (**d**) At the completion of activation and device angulation, the bite has been closed (also with the aid of wires between the maxillary and mandibular dentition). Note the expansion of airway space

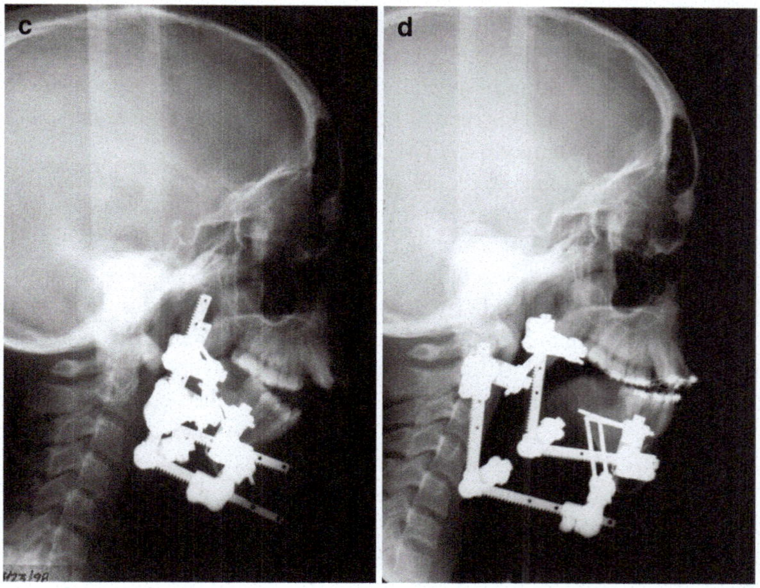

Fig. 3.22 (continued)

3.3.1 Complications

As in any surgical procedure, complications must be considered. In evaluating clinical outcomes, one must consider the following variables: diagnosis or syndrome, type of distraction device, age of patient, volume of mandibular bone, radiation to the operative field, and previous mandibular surgery. One must also distinguish among the treatments required to resolve the complication (medical vs. surgical intervention) and, finally, a complication that resolved with therapy and one that did not resolve and impacted negatively on outcome [43]. The literature is confusing, as some papers are based only on a survey of multiple centers, often with limited clinical experience, and, in addition, the above distinctions are not made.

There are several possible complications following mandibular distraction. Device failure has been reported. It is critical that the device is tested before application in the patient and also after fixation at completion of the osteotomy. The external device has the advantage that, if there is a failure, the device can be exchanged in the outpatient setting. Infection has been reported, usually at the incision or device site. Most usually resolve with oral or intravenous antibiotics and do not impact negatively on the outcome. However, removal of all hardware would be indicated if conservative therapy fails.

Hypertrophic or unsightly scars are more likely with the external device or after a wound infection. Nerve injury has been reported, usually of the inferior alveolar and the marginal mandibular and buccal branches of the facial nerve. They are usually temporary and resolve satisfactorily.

Tooth injury usually occurs at the time of the osteotomy/pin or screw insertion and can be avoided with prior extraction of the teeth or follicles.

Fractures are most common especially when the mandibular osteotomy is made close to the sigmoid notch. This type of fracture isolates the condyle and can lead to temporomandibular joint ankylosis (TMJ).

Temporomandibular joint problems include pain during the activation process, especially when a vertical vector is employed. This can be avoided or lessened with an orthodontic device to unload the condyle (see [24]). Trismus or TMJ ankylosis usually is secondary to an inadvertent osteotomy and isolation of the condylar fragment.

Relapse must first be defined. The term is often misused to describe a condition where one side of the mandible grows less than the contralateral side. Relapse is a term that should be reserved to define translation of the advanced skeletal unit backward from its most forward postoperative position. It is often confused with craniofacial asymmetry or differential growth between both sides of the mandible or between the maxilla and the distracted mandible. Causes of relapse include fibrous union because of insufficient bone at the distraction site (see [17, 19, 20]) (see Fig. 3.2) or overly rapid distraction.

In a stratification of complications after mandibular distraction of 226 sided procedures in 141 patients (unilateral in 56 patients and bilateral in 85 patients), the sample was divided into distraction performed on grafted bone and native bone and distraction performed with external vs. internal devices (see [43]). The major incident rate (treatment outcome compromised) was 5.31%. Literature reviews have also been reported for complications after mandibular distraction. In one review of 565 patients, 11% had complications that resolved spontaneously, 10.8% had conservatively managed complications without hospitalization, and permanent complications were observed in 9.6% of patients [44]. In another study, albeit a literature review, the following incidence of complications was reported: tooth injury 22.5%, hypertrophic scarring 15.6%, nerve injury 11.4%, infection 9.5%, device failure 7.9%, and TMJ injury 0.7% [45]. Literature surveys regrettably incorporate papers reflecting surgical inexperience and limited number of patients.

3.3.2 Outcomes/Longitudinal Studies

In evaluating outcomes, one must document whether there was the need for additional surgery such as tonsillectomy, tongue suspension, secondary distraction, definitive orthognathic surgery at the time of skeletal maturity, or microvascular free flap for soft tissue augmentation [46].

One must distinguish among the various syndromes (PRS, BCFM, and TCS) because the treatments or outcomes can vary among them [20, 47]. The goals, as mentioned earlier, include improving the respiratory status of the patient and any associated alimentary problems, correcting severe malocclusions, and reducing craniofacial dysmorphism. Most workers in the field would agree there are distinct differences in outcomes among the three syndromes (PRS, BCFM, TCS) [20, 47].

In PRS, the outcomes after mandibular distraction have been dramatic in neonatal patients whose respiratory problems were resistant to conservative measures [48]. One study noted that the most important predictor of failure in outcome (tracheostomy) was the GERD- need for Nissen fundoplication and the absence of a cleft palate. Syndromic diagnoses, as well as cardiac and respiratory anomalies, were not associated with failure [49] as defined by tracheostomy or incomplete amelioration of AHI (never reduced below 20). Moreover, a study from the same center showed that PRS patients weighing under 4 kg with severe airway obstruction were no more at risk for complications and treatment efficacy than a similar cohort weighing more than 4 kg [21, 22]. In a three-dimensional airway reconstruction before and after mandibular distraction for respiratory distress in patients with micrognathia, volume and surface area of the airway increased by an average of 279.2% and 89.4%, respectively. Of 12 patients, tracheostomy was avoided in one patient, and it was removed in 10 of 11 patients who had tracheostomy in the preoperative period [50].

While both PRS and TCS have retrognathia and glossoptosis causing airway obstruction, each has a distinct or unique pathologic anatomy and pathophysiology that result in a lower rate of success and a higher rate of complications in the TCS cohort (see [47]). The greater challenges to success in TCS are likely related to the increased complexity of the mandibular pathology which can include a deficient ramus, absent condyle, clockwise rotation of the mandibular body, foreshortened strap muscles, and decreased posterior maxillary height.

BCFM patients probably lie between the PRS and TCS patients in terms of successful outcomes and complication rate. Both BCFM and TCS patients tend to have greater mandibular skeletal deficiencies. However, the anatomic basis of the TCS airway is unique with a posteriorly reduced maxilla and an oblique mandibular plane angle and a more cephalically positioned retrognathia.

Pearls and Pitfalls

- Importance of a functioning clinical team.
- A low positioned Risdon incision is better for exposure and can result in a satisfactory scar.
- With a hypoplastic mandible and dental crowding, consider tooth follicle removal.
- In a patient with a Pruzansky-Kaban III mandible, the first stage must be a nonvascularized or vascularized bony transfer.
- Modify or reduce the size of the foot plates in a buried device, but be sure there is device rigidity (screws on either side of the activation rod) and plates on either side of the osteotomy.
- In general, a vertical vector is the workhorse, and the uniplanar device can result in multidimensional movement of the mandible.
- Consider accelerated activation (2 mm per day) and avoidance of latency period in neonates and infants.

3.4 Unilateral Mandibular Distraction

Many of the principles and protocols discussed in bilateral mandibular distraction are applicable to the patient undergoing unilateral distraction. However, there are unique differences:

- The most common diagnosis is unilateral craniofacial microsomia (UCFM).
- The deformity is asymmetric.
- Treatment is commonly directed at one side of the craniofacial skeleton, and the challenge is to restore symmetry.
- Unilateral mandibular distraction as therapy also affects the position of the non-distracted side of the mandible and dentoalveolus (see Chap. 4 for the orthodontic measures required).
- Usually, an associated maxillary vertical deficiency also has to be addressed in the treatment plan.
- The post-distraction posterior open bite must be orthodontically managed (see Chap. 4).
- Respiratory problems are less common in UCFM.

3.4.1 Pathology

The most common diagnosis for the patient undergoing unilateral mandibular distraction is UCFM (Fig. 3.23). There are some patients who have sustained mandibular fracture and have post-traumatic TMJ ankylosis.

The mandibular skeletal deficiency is best defined by the Pruzansky-Kaban classification as described earlier in this chapter (see Fig. 3.1).

The affected ramus/condyle is vertically deficient, and the chin point is deviated to the affected side (Fig. 3.23). The inferior border of the ipsilateral mandible is elevated or displaced in the cephalic direction. The dentoalveolar deformity usually includes dental crowding in the body and ramus of the affected mandible. In the upper jaw, the ipsilateral dentoalveolus is likewise hypoplastic with dental crowding, and there is a marked occlusal cant upward on the affected side. There can be an ipsilateral orbital dystopia with frontal bone flattening; the mastoid can be hypoplastic.

The soft tissue deformities are also significant. The chin pad is hypoplastic and deviated to the affected side. The submental soft tissue is deficient and constrictive. The affected cheek soft tissue is especially hypoplastic, and there can be a cleft extending from the affected oral commissure to the auricular remnant (Tessier #7).

The underlying muscles of mastication are affected and, as emphasized in the functional matrix theory of Moss [8], these findings impact on the vitality and function of the mandible. The facial nerve may be affected, especially the marginal mandibular and buccal branches. The external ear is variably affected in the form of minor preauricular skin remnants, ipsilateral auricular hypoplasia, and microtia/anotia.

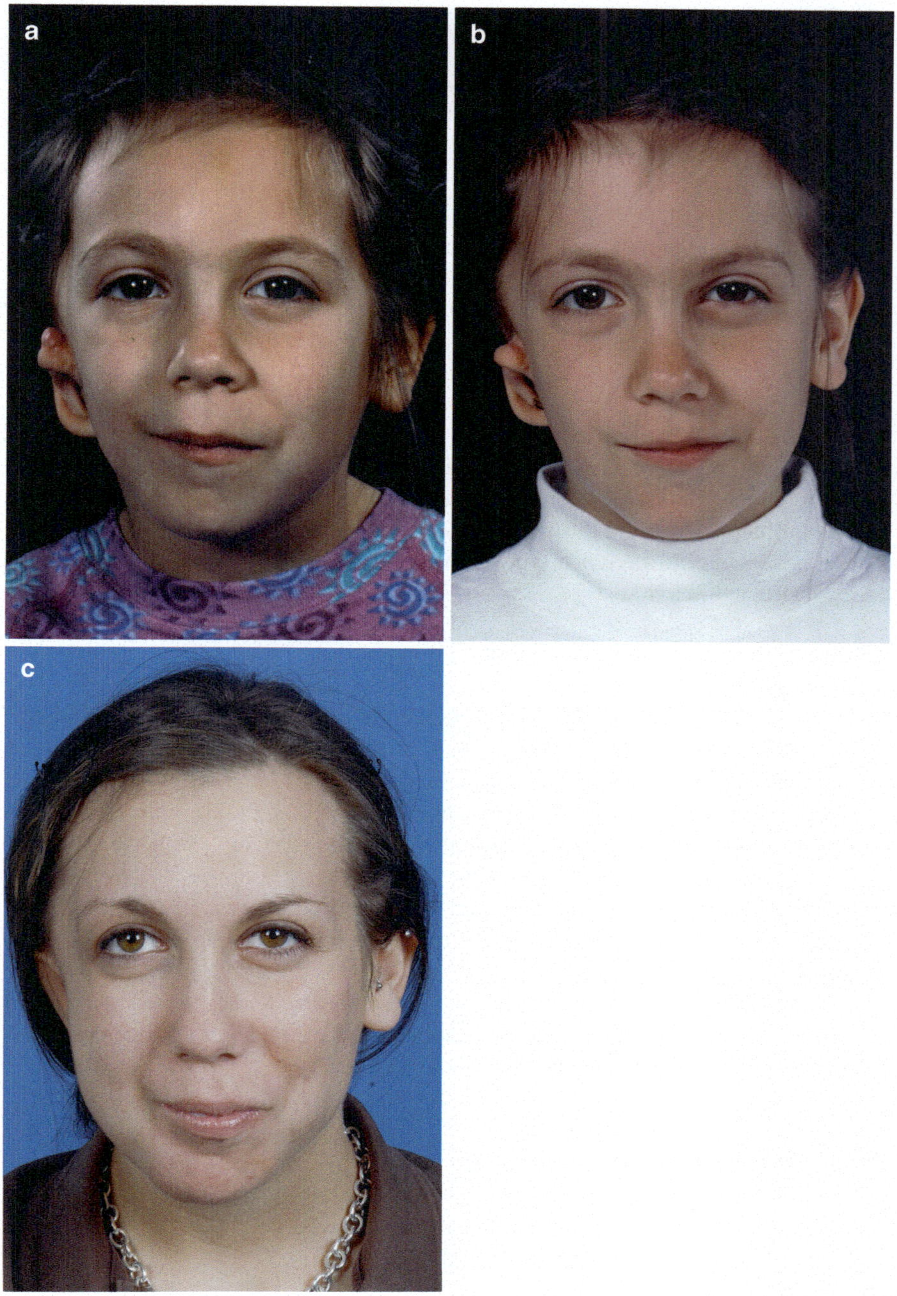

Fig. 3.23 Longitudinal follow-up after unilateral mandibular distraction. (**a**) A 7-year-old girl with right-sided craniofacial microsomia. (**b**) Appearance 16 months following unilateral mandibular distraction. Note the lowering of the oral commissure and inferior border of the mandible on the affected side. The chin is midline and there is more cheek fullness. (**c**) Appearance 13 years postoperative without additional jaw surgery

3.4.2 Indications

1. Airway/Associated Alimentary Problems
   Unilateral craniofacial microsomia patients can present with airway obstruction. Tongue-based airway stenosis is more commonly associated with a Pruzansky type IIB and III mandible. [51].
2. Dysmorphism
   The goal is to attempt to reduce the craniofacial asymmetry.
3. Augmentation of Mandibular Bony Volume
   One could consider unilateral mandibular distraction in such a patient for bony augmentation in preparation for eventual orthodontic therapy and orthognathic surgery at the time of skeletal maturity.

3.4.2.1 Absolute Indications

1. Growing and Craniofacially Mature Patients
   In growing and mature patients with unilateral craniofacial microsomia and airway problems, or severe dysmorphism, the indication for mandibular reconstruction is absolute. If there is a type III deformity, the ramus and condyle must be reconstructed in a first stage.

3.4.2.2 Controversial Indications

1. Growing Patients
   In the growing patient with mild to moderate dysmorphism, without findings of obstructive sleep apnea, there is lack of agreement as to the indications for mandibular distraction. This stands in contrast to patients with obstructive sleep apnea. The argument favoring distraction is that a preliminary mandibular distraction in the growing patient would improve or lessen the dysmorphism and provide the child with an interval of improved psychosocial functioning. Moreover, the increased bony volume allows orthodontic/dental intervention in anticipation of definitive orthognathic surgery at skeletal maturity.

   In the patient of approximately 13–17 years of age without signs of obstructive sleep apnea, it would be controversial not to wait a few years for definitive orthognathic surgery at the time of skeletal maturity.

3.4.3 Preoperative Assessment

The reader is referred to the discussion earlier in the chapter.

3.4.4 Orthodontic Assessment

The reader is referred to Chap. 4.

3.4.5 Preoperative Planning

The reader is referred to the previous section in bilateral mandibular distraction. However, it should be noted that the semi-buried technique is preferred in unilateral mandibular distraction as it is particularly suited when the vertical-oblique vectors are indicated.

Unlike patients undergoing bilateral mandibular distraction, maxillary pathology is a prominent part of the planning in the patient scheduled for unilateral mandibular distraction. Management of the maxilla is age dependent:

0–4 years: The maxilla descends spontaneously as the affected mandible is lengthened in the vertical dimension during the activation period. Orthodontic treatment is usually not required.

4–9 years: It is in this age group that intensive orthodontic therapy with cross tongue elastics and bite block therapy is indicated (see Chap. 4).

9–14 years: One could consider maxillomandibular distraction. The technique was popularized by the Mexico City group [52] and reported by others [53–57]. It entails the previously described procedure for mandibular distraction combined with maxillary (Le Fort I) distraction to increase the vertical height of the maxillary dentoalveolus and correct the occlusal cant. There are, however, several caveats. The Le Fort I osteotomy must be carefully performed in order to avoid damage to unerupted maxillary teeth. Maxillomandibular fixation (MMF) is required, and this can be challenging for the younger patient. The technique of combined maxillomandibular distraction is also more painful than that of mandibular distraction alone.

3.4.6 Operative Technique

The reader is referred to the technical details in the section on bilateral mandibular distraction. In general, it is preferable that a low Risdon (submandibular) is made and access gained to the ramal-body remnant in a subperiosteal plane. In general, a vertical vector is preferred in the placement of the distraction device on the ramal remnant (Fig. 3.24).

3.4.7 Postoperative Management

The reader is referred to the previous section in bilateral mandibular distraction. In the *activation* phase, the following clinical endpoints must be achieved in the growing child. The chin point must cross the midline to the contralateral side, and the occlusal plane must be lower on the distracted side (Fig. 3.25). The inferior border of the mandible and the affected oral commissure on the distracted side must be lower than their contralateral counterparts. In other words, activation should not be discontinued until there is evidence of "overcorrection" (see Fig. 3.14). Failure to do so will require secondary distraction (Fig. 3.26).

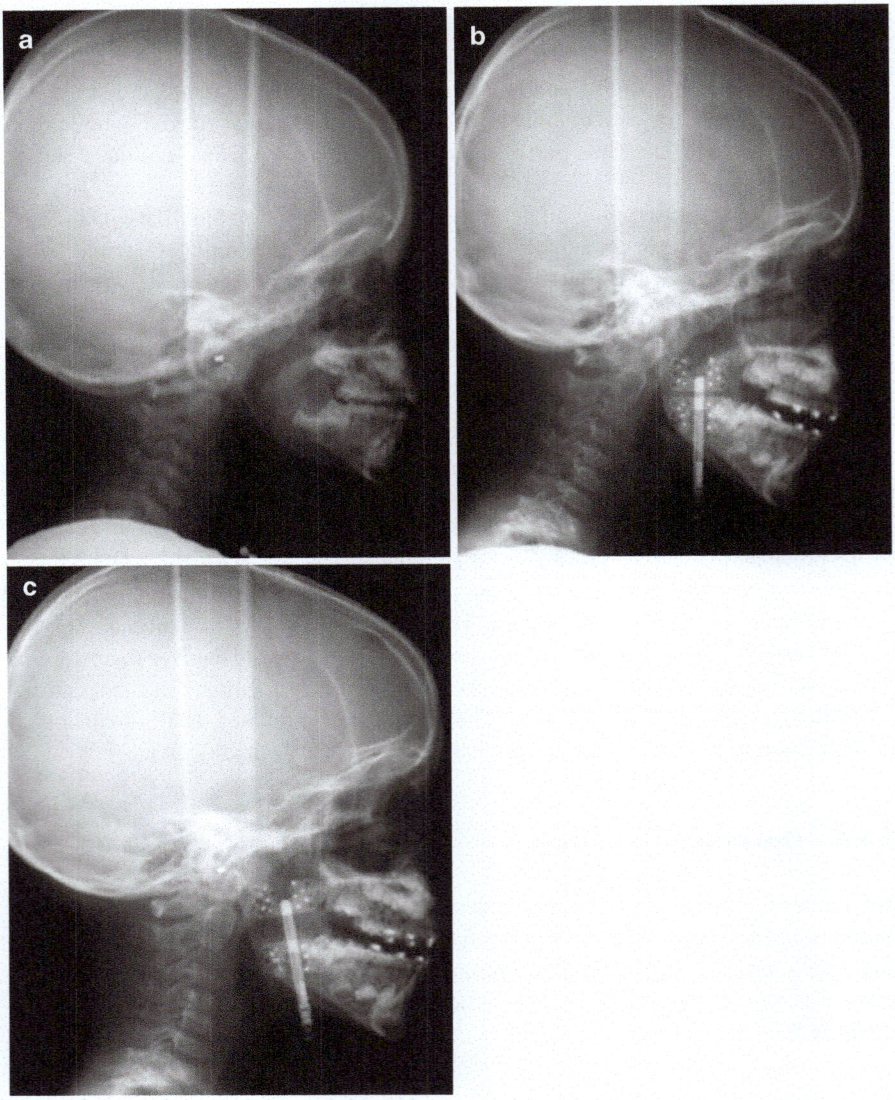

Fig. 3.24 Serial lateral cephalograms. (**a**) Preoperative view. (**b**) After osteotomy and device application but before activation. The vector is vertical. (**c**) During activation. Note the counter-clockwise rotation of the mandible and distraction device (semi-buried) and increased projection of the chin. There is also a marked expansion of the retroglossal airway. The bony generate is apparent between the device foot plates

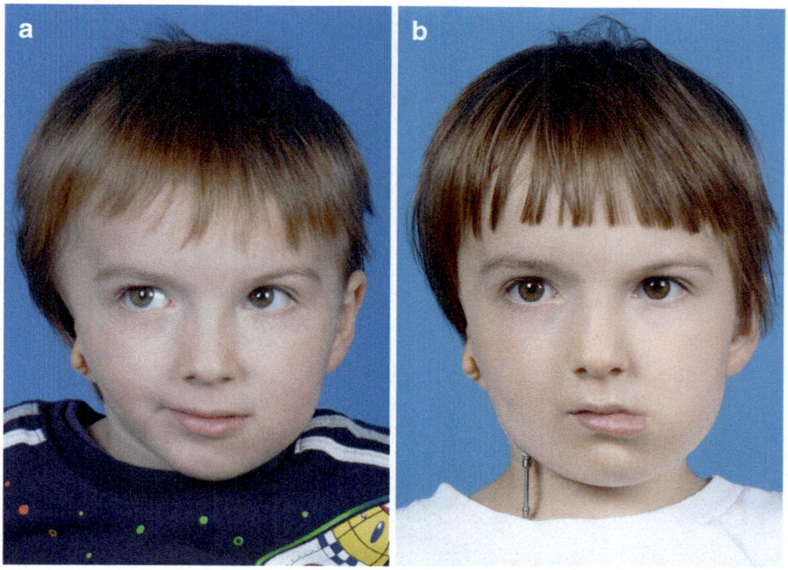

Fig. 3.25 The end points of unilateral mandibular distraction. (**a**) A young boy with right-sided craniofacial microsomia. (**b**) Following unilateral mandibular activation with a semi-buried device (note the activation toggle). The affected oral commissure, occlusal plane, and inferior border of the mandible have been lowered and the chin point driven to the contralateral side. Note the increased fullness of the affected cheek

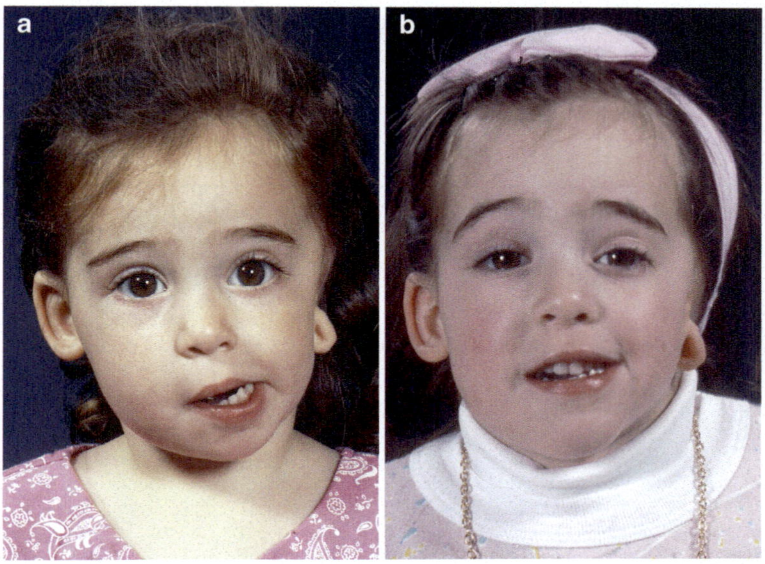

Fig. 3.26 (**a**) A 3-year-old girl with left-sided craniofacial microsomia and severe occlusal cant. (**b**) Following inadequate left-sided mandibular distraction. While improved, the chin point remains on the affected side and the commissure is still elevated. There is a residual occlusal cant, and the affected inferior border of the mandible is elevated. (**c**) At the conclusion of activation with secondary mandibular distraction, the occlusal cant has been corrected (see tongue blade), and the chin point is across the midline. The inferior mandible border on the affected side is lower

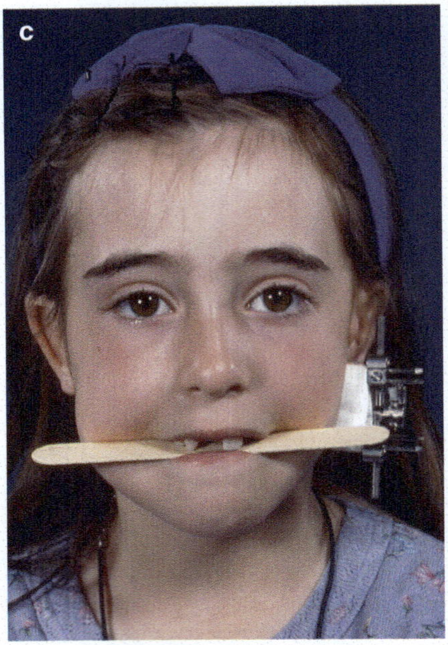

Fig. 3.26 (continued)

The *consolidation* phase lasts for 8 weeks, following which the distraction device is removed.

The role of the orthodontist, as discussed in Chap. 4, is critically important in mandibular distraction, especially because of the management of the associated maxillary deformity. Bite block therapy after device removal is critical to prevent relapse of the lengthened ramus. In bilateral mandibular distraction, the latter can be a problem only in the Treacher Collins syndrome (bilateral posterior maxillary deficiency).

3.5 Case Examples (Figs. 3.27, 3.28, 3.29, and 3.30)

3.5.1 Complications

This subject is discussed earlier in the chapter.

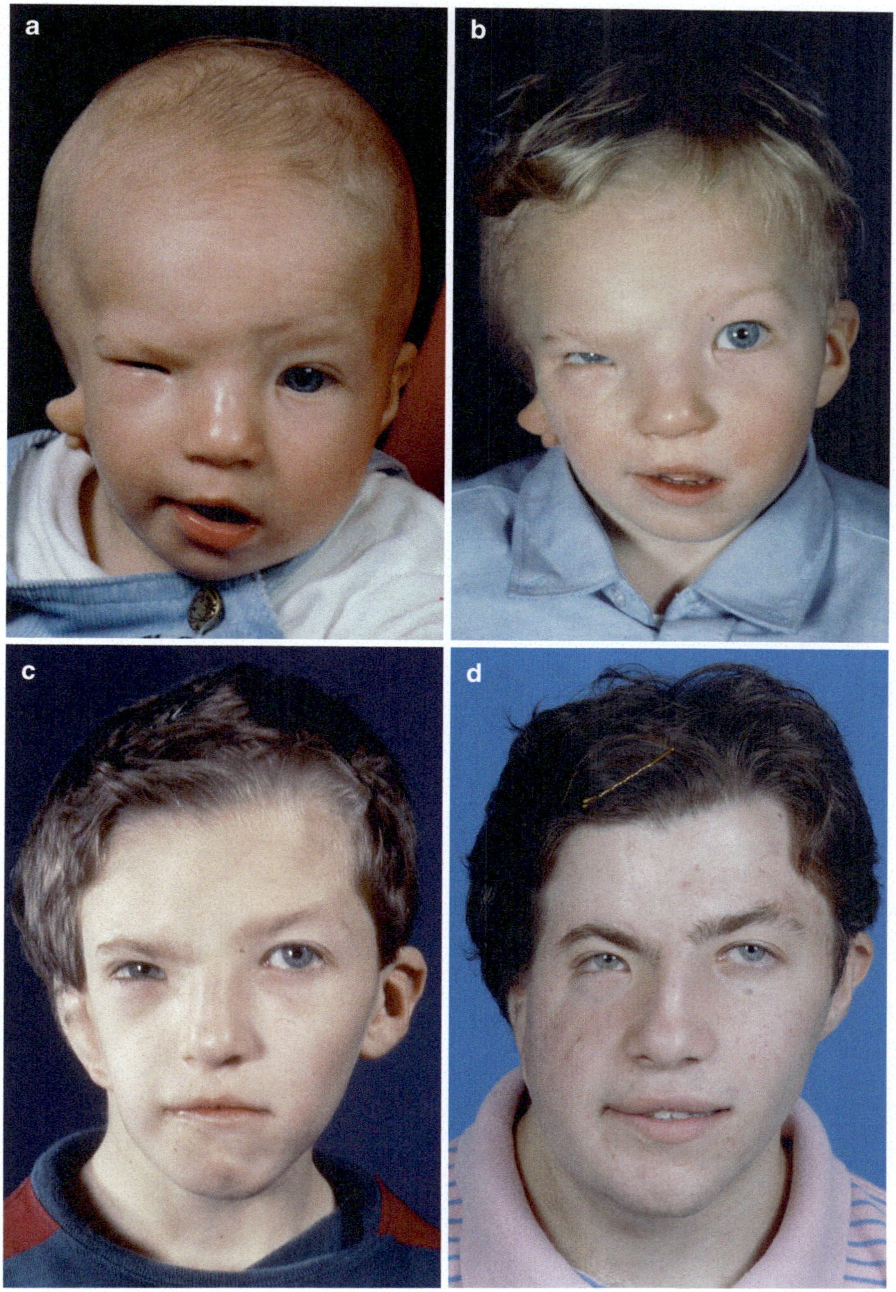

Fig. 3.27 An 18-month-old boy with right-sided craniofacial microsomia who underwent the first mandibular distraction (unilateral) in 1989. (**a**) Preoperative appearance. (**b**) Postoperative appearance at age 2 years. Note the improvement in chin position and cheek fullness. (**c**) Appearance at 6 years postoperative. (**d**) Appearance at 20 years of age. He had undergone microsurgical reconstruction of the affected cheek soft tissue, Le Fort I osteotomy, bilateral ramal osteotomies, and osseous genioplasty

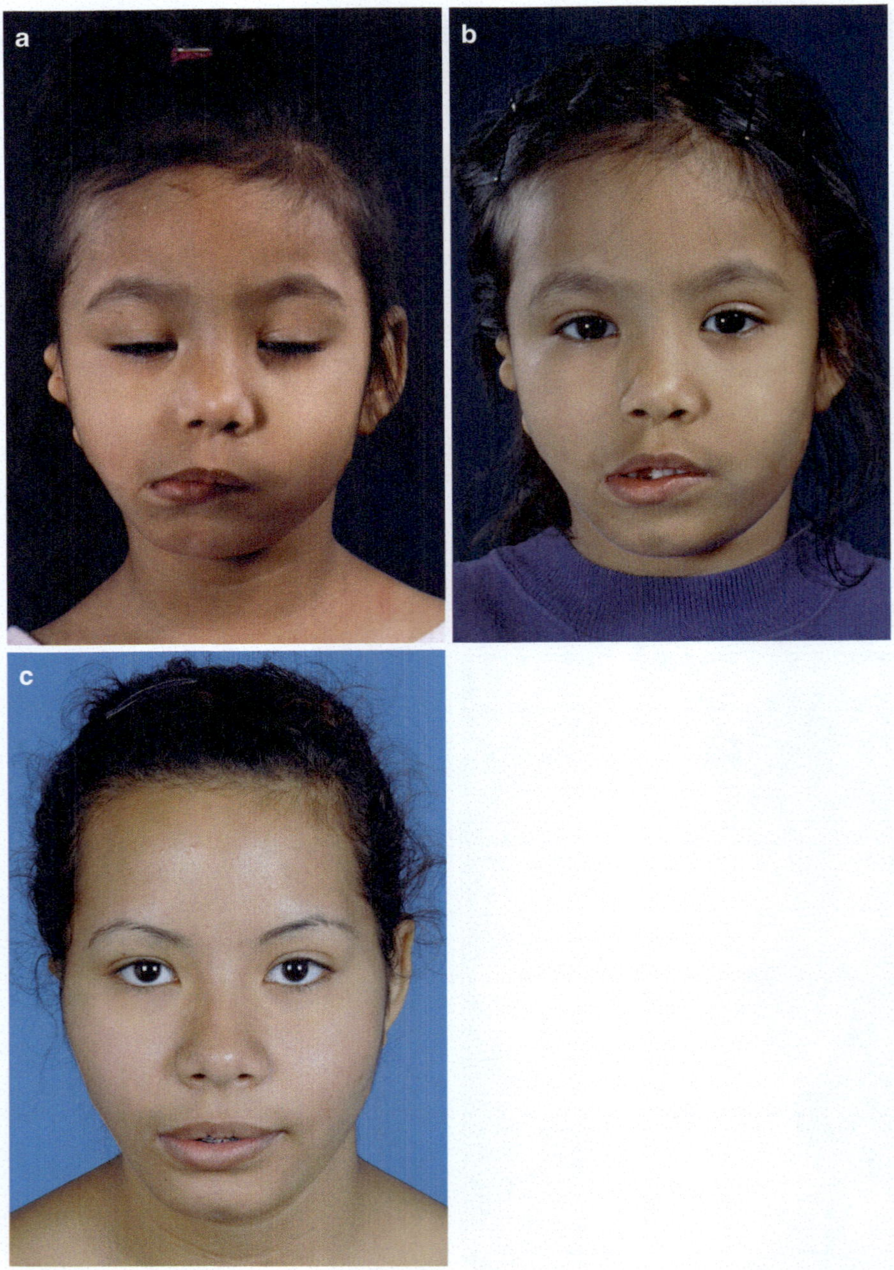

Fig. 3.28 A 4-year-old girl with unilateral craniofacial microsomia who underwent right-sided mandibular distraction. (**a**) Preoperative appearance. (**b**) One year following mandibular distraction. Note the lowering of the oral commissure and inferior border of the mandible and projection and movement of the chin to the unaffected side. (**c**) Appearance 15 years postoperative without additional jaw surgery

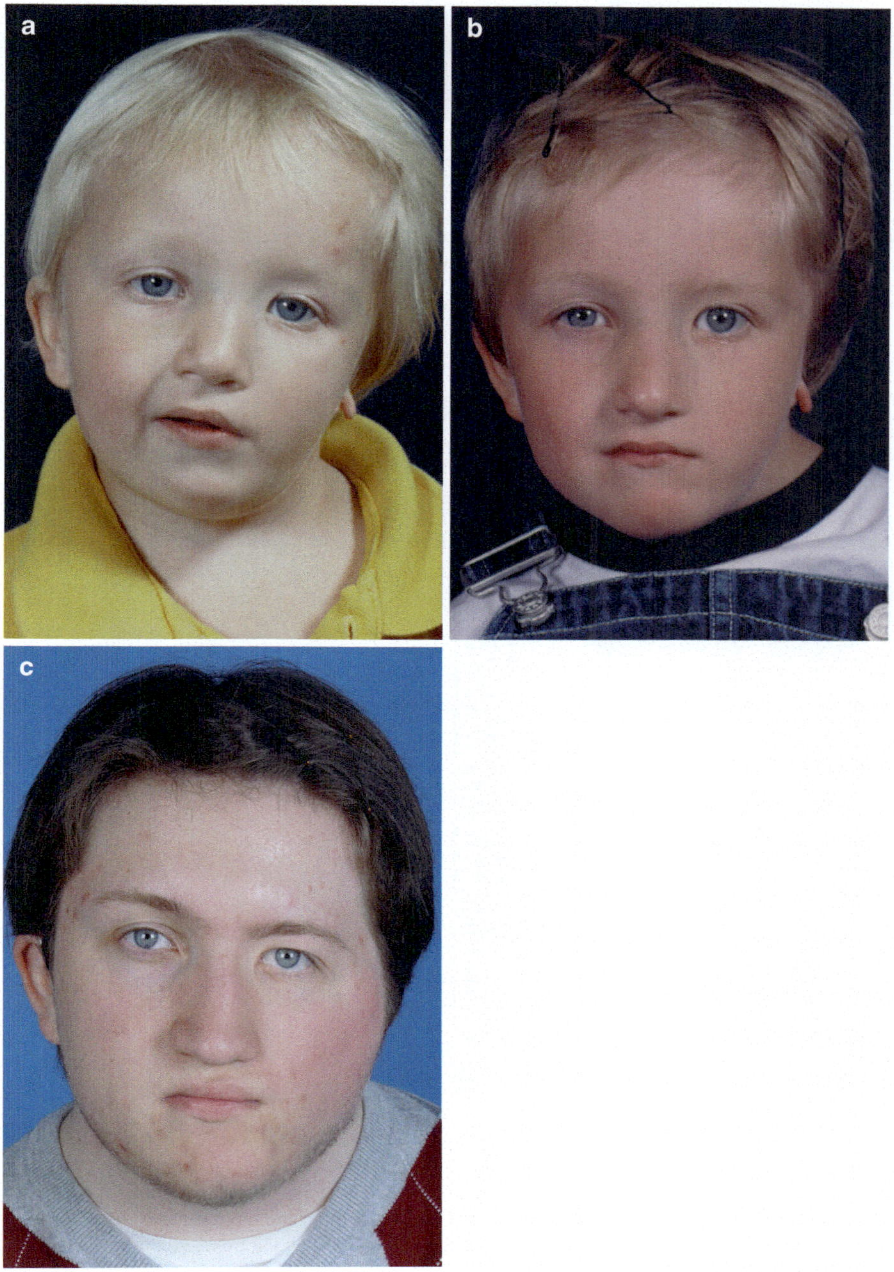

Fig. 3.29 A 3-year-old boy with left-sided craniofacial microsomia who underwent unilateral mandibular distraction. (**a**) Preoperative appearance. The head tilt is secondary to a cervical vertebral anomaly. (**b**) One year following unilateral mandibular distraction. Note the chin is midline, and there is increased cheek fullness. (**c**) Appearance 15 years postoperative without additional jaw surgery

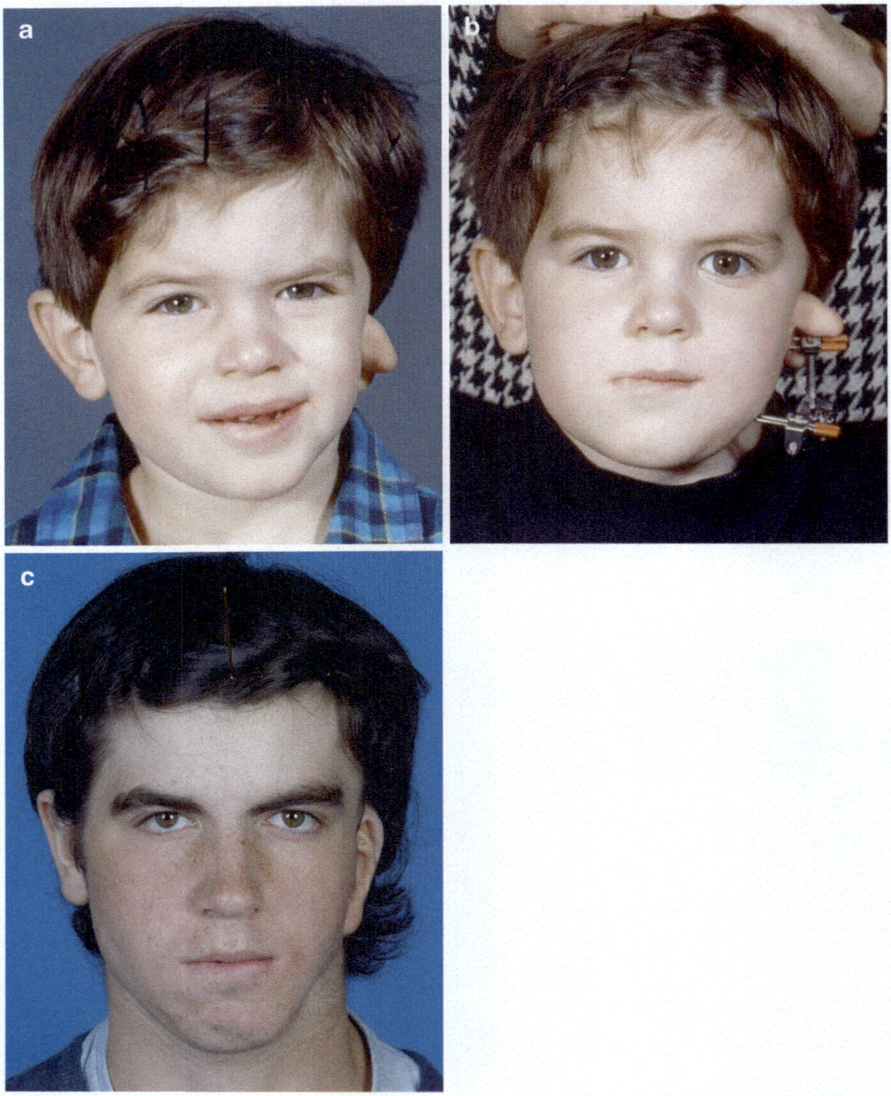

Fig. 3.30 Longitudinal follow-up after unilateral mandibular distraction. A 4-year-old boy with left-sided craniofacial microsomia. (**a**) Preoperative appearance. (**b**) At the completion of activation with an external device. Note the lowering of the affected oral commissure and inferior border of the mandible. The chin point is on the affected side of midline, and there is more cheek fullness on the affected side. (**c**) Appearance 12 years postoperative without additional jaw surgery. The ear has been reconstructed

3.5.2 Outcomes/Longitudinal Studies

There are several goals in unilateral mandibular distraction.

1. Aesthetic
   The aesthetic goals are the amelioration of craniofacial asymmetry characterized by ipsilateral cheek deficiency, elevated oral commissure, elevated body of the mandible, and deviation of the chin point to the affected side. The chin lacks adequate projection.
2. Occlusal/Dental
   The goals are correction of the occlusal cant and promotion of maxillary and mandibular teeth eruption. Despite active partnership with a craniofacial orthodontist, final correction of the occlusal cant commonly occurs at the time of definitive orthognathic surgery.
3. Skeletal
   The goal of distraction is to increase the vertical height of the ramus and augment the body as well as move the chin point to the opposite side. The goal of maxillary treatment is to lower the dentoalveolus on the affected side and to reestablish a level occlusal plane.
4. Respiratory
   In the unusual patient with respiratory insufficiency, the goal is to bring the AHI into a normal range.

It should be noted that, especially in the growing patient, there can be need for additional surgery. Secondary distraction may be indicated, and it is usually due to undercorrection and lack of orthodontic involvement at the time of the primary distraction (see Fig. 3.26). Definitive orthognathic surgery is usually required at the time of skeletal maturity. Soft tissue augmentation can be achieved with serial autogenous fat grafts in the patient with mild to moderate soft tissue deficiency, but a microvascular free flap (see [46]) may be indicated in the patient with severe deficiency.

Commissuroplasty may be indicated when there is a macrostomia or a true #7 Tessier cleft. In older patients without prior treatment, the lowering of the affected oral commissure is less successful than when mandibular distraction is performed in the younger patient.

The literature dealing with mandibular distraction in the treatment of unilateral craniofacial microsomia is less than robust. Regrettably, case reports are lacking adequate sample size and longitudinal follow-up.

Relapse during the early postoperative year is a loosely defined term often inaccurately used to describe a tendency for diminished post-distraction growth of the mandible on the affected side [58]. Others argue that distraction osteogenesis is not effective over the long term. Despite initial improvement in skeletal morphology, patients tend to "relapse" with growth and development. One study showed 90% recurrence with a mean postsurgical time of 44 months; however, the study lacked objective data such as cephalometric studies, and follow-up was limited to only clinical examination [59]. Another study of 26 patients with follow-up of 11 years reported that after distraction, mandibular horizontal and vertical changes had an eventual return to baseline [60]; however, the authors failed to document a clinical commitment to obtain overcorrection before discontinuing activation. Oral commissure symmetry (not overcorrection) was the accepted endpoint, and there was no mention of the position of the chin point or the use of post-distraction orthodontic treatment to manage the posterior open bite following unilateral mandibular distraction. In a systematic review, another group reported that the surgical treatment of craniofacial microsomia is patient and not treatment dependent; however, this study suffers the same study deficiencies noted above [61]. Another report showed no statistical evidence to support early distraction osteogenesis in unilateral craniofacial microsomia and therefore questioned the rationale for treatment [62], but this paper also was limited by a variable length of follow-up, lack of strict definition of indications, and failure to employ the Pruzansky-Kaban classification or the use of orthodontic therapy.

In a recent long-term report of 19 growing patients with mild to moderate deformity undergoing unilateral mandibular distraction from the NYU Craniofacial Group [63], 12 patients reached skeletal maturity with *satisfactory* skeletal and soft tissue position and without any additional therapy (see Figs. 3.28, 3.29, and 3.30). The study documented the critical treatment factors contributing to successful distraction in this unique patient population: overcorrection and rigorous orthodontic therapy to deal with the posterior open bite and maxillary dentoalveolar deficiency. Moreover, while some patients may show "relapse," they still maintain satisfactory results provided there is significant overcorrection at the time of the primary distraction. While many patients may require secondary surgery when they reach skeletal maturity, the impact of improved appearance in the growing child during the critical years of psychosocial development cannot be overemphasized (Fig. 3.31). Moreover, early distraction does not impact negatively on the volume of bone stock available for secondary or definitive orthognathic surgery. Previous studies have demonstrated that mandibular bone volume is increased after distraction, and there is an associated, albeit variable, improvement in soft tissue anatomy [64, 65]. It remains for craniofacial centers to conduct prospective, well-documented studies on patients undergoing unilateral mandibular distraction and to maintain a strict treatment protocol with specific guidelines for overcorrection and rigorous orthodontic post-distraction management.

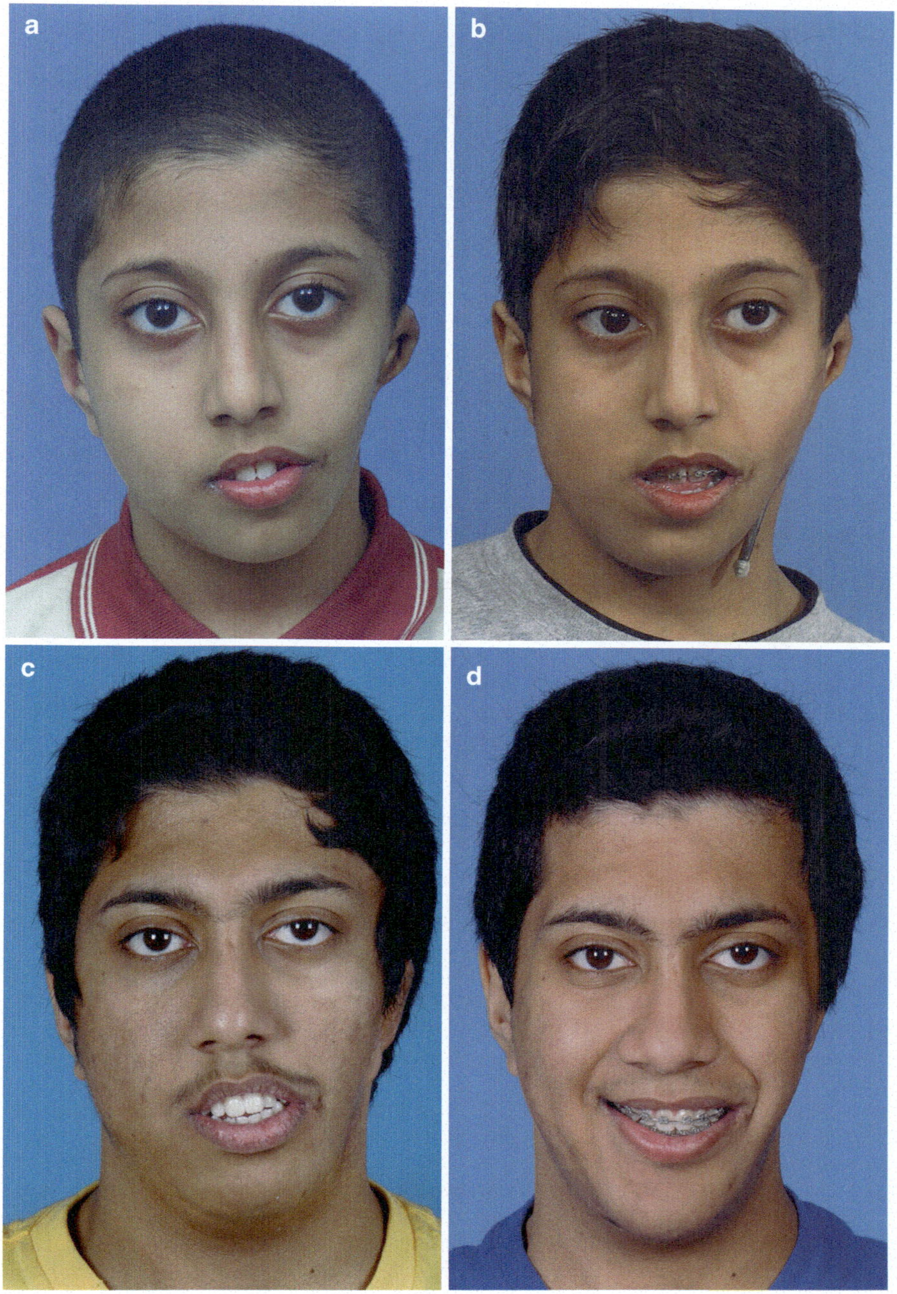

Fig. 3.31 Longitudinal follow-up after unilateral mandibular distraction. (**a**) A 7-year-old male with left-sided craniofacial microsomia. (**b**) At the completion of activation (semi-buried device). (**c**) Appearance 4 years postoperative. (**d**) Appearance after Le Fort I osteotomy and bilateral ramal osteotomies (bone graft insertion on *left side*). An osseous genioplasty was also performed

References

1. Ilizarov GA. The tension-stress effect on the genesis and growth of tissues: I. The influence of stability of fixation and soft-tissue preservation. Clin Orthop. 1989;239:264.
2. Snyder CC, Levine GA, Swanson HM, Browne Jr EZ. Mandibular lengthening by gradual distraction. Preliminary report. Plast Reconstr Surg. 1973;51(5):506–8.
3. Michieli S, Miotti B. Lengthening of mandibular body by gradual surgical-orthodontic distraction. J Oral Surg. 1977;35(3):187–92.
4. Karp NS, Thorne CHM, McCarthy JG, Sissons HA. Bone lengthening in the craniofacial skeleton. Ann Plast Surg. 1990;24:231.
5. Karp NS, McCarthy JG, Schreiber JS, Sissons HA, Thorne CHM. Membranous bone lengthening: a serial histologic study. Ann Plast Surg. 1992;29:2.
6. McCarthv JG, Schreiber J, Karp N, Thorne CH, Gravson BH. Lengthening the human mandible by gradual distraction. Plast Reconstr Surg. 1992;89(l):1–8; discussion 9–10.
7. Molina F, Ortiz Monasterio F. Mandibular elongation and remodeling by distraction: a farewell to major osteotomies. Plast Reconstr Surg. 1995;96(4):825–40.
8. Moss ML. The functional matrix. In: Kraus B, Riedel R, editors. Vistas in orthodontics. Philadelphia: Lea & Febiger; 1962. p. 85–98.
9. Mackool RJ, Hopper RA, Grayson BH, Hollidav R, McCarthy JG. Volumetric change of the medial pterygoid following distraction osteogenesis of the mandible: an example of the associated soft-tissue changes. Plast Reconstr Surg. 2003;111(6):1804–7.
10. Pruzansky S. Not all dwarfed mandibles are alike. Birth Defects. 1969;5:120.
11. Kaban LB, Moses MH, Mulliken JB. Surgical correction of hemifacial microsomia in the growing child. Plast Reconstr Surg. 1988;82:9.
12. Vento AR, LaBrie RA, Mulliken JB. The O.M.E.N.S. classification of hemifacial microsomia. Cleft Palate Craniofac J. 1991;28:68.
13. Ma X, Forte AJ, Persing JA, Alonso N, Berlin NL, Steinbacher DM. Reduced three-dimensional airway volume is a function of skeletal dysmorphology in Treacher Collins syndrome. Plast Reconstr Surg. 2015;135(2):382e–92e.
14. Murage KP, Tholpady SS, Friel M, Havlik RJ, Flores RL. Outcomes analysis of mandibular distraction osteogenesis for the treatment of Pierre Robin sequence. Plast Reconstr Surg. 2013;132(2):419–21.
15. Monasterio FO, Molina F, Berlanga F, et al. Swallowing disorders in Pierre Robin sequence: its correction by distraction. J Craniofac Surg. 2004;15(6):934–41.
16. Eski M, Turegun LY, Deveci M, Gokce HS, Sengezer M. Vertical distraction osteogenesis of fibular bone flap in reconstructed mandible. Ann Plast Surg. 2006;57(6):631–6.
17. Corcoran J, Hubli EH, Salyer KE. Distraction osteogenesis of costochondral neomandibles: a clinical experience. Plast Reconstr Surg. 1997;100(2):311–5; discussion 316–7.
18. Stelnicki EJ, Bovd JB, Nott RL, Barnavon Y, Uecker C, Henson T. Early treatment of severe mandibular hypoplasia with distraction mesenchymogenesis and bilateral free fibula flaps. J Craniofac Surg. 2001;12(4):337–48.
19. Stelnicki EJ, Hollier L, Lee C, Lin WY, Gravson B, McCarthv JG. Distraction osteogenesis of costochondral bone grafts in the mandible. Plast Reconstr Surg. 2002a;109(3):925–33; discussion 934–5.
20. Stelnicki EJ, Lin WY, Lee C, Gravson BH, McCarthv JG. Long-term outcome study of bilateral mandibular distraction: a comparison of Treacher Collins and Nager syndromes to other types of micrognathia. Plast Reconstr Surg. 2002b;109(6):1819–25. discussion 1826–7
21. Tahiri Y, Chang CS, Tuin J, Paliga JT, Lowe KM, Taylor JA, Bartlett SP. Costochondral grafting in craniofacial microsomia. Plast Reconstr Surg. 2015a;135(2):530–41.
22. Tahiri Y, Greathouse ST, Tholpady SS, Havlik R, Sood R, Flores RL. Mandibular distraction osteogenesis in low-weight neonates with Robin sequence: is it safe? Plast Reconstr Surg. 2015b;136(5):1037–44.
23. Regev E, Jensen JN, McCarthv JG, Gravson BH, Eski M. Removal of mandibular tooth follicles before distraction osteogenesis. Plast Reconstr Surg. 2004;113(7):1910–5.

24. Fan K, Andrews BT, Liao E, Allam K, Raposo Amaral CA, Bradlev JP. Protection of the temporomandibular joint during syndromic neonatal mandibular distraction using condylar unloading. Plast Reconstr Surg. 2012;129(5):1151–61.
25. Yadav R, Bhutia O, Shukla G, Rovchoudhurv A. Distraction osteogenesis for management of obstructive sleep apnoea in temporomandibular joint ankylosis patients before the release of joint. J Craniomaxillofac Surg. 2014;42(5):588–94.
26. Anantanarayanan P. Mandibular distraction as a first stage procedure prior to gap arthroplasty for the management of obstructive sleep apnoea secondary to TMJ ankylosis—not a new protocol. Int J Oral Maxillofac Surg. 2014;43(11):1411.
27. Gabbay JS, Heller JB, Song YY, Wasson KL, Harrington H, Bradlev JP. Temporomandibular joint bony ankylosis: comparison of treatment with transport distraction osteogenesis or the Matthews device arthroplasty. J Craniofac Surg. 2006;17(3):516–22.
28. Stucki-McCormick SU, Fox RM, Mizrahi RD. Reconstruction of a neocondyle using transport distraction osteogenesis. Semin Orthod. 1999;5(1):59–63.
29. Rao K, Kumar S, Kumar V, Singh AK, Bhatnagar SK. The role of simultaneous gap arthroplasty and distraction osteogenesis in the management of temporo-mandibular joint ankylosis with mandibular deformity in children. J Craniomaxillofac Surg. 2004;32(1):38–42.
30. Cheung LK. The long-term effect of transport distraction in the management of temporomandibular joint ankylosis. Plast Reconstr Surg. 2007;119(3):1003–9.
31. Eski M, Deveci M, Zor F, Sengezer M. Treatment of temporomandibular joint ankylosis and facial asymmetry with bidirectional transport distraction osteogenesis technique. J Craniofac Surg. 2008;19(3):732–9.
32. Yu H, Shen G, Zhang S, Wang X. Gap arthroplasty combined with distraction osteogenesis in the treatment of unilateral ankylosis of the temporomandibular joint and micrognathia. Br J Oral Maxillofac Surg. 2009;47(3):200–4.
33. Hopper RA. Personal communication. 2016.
34. Gravson BH, McCormick S, Santiago PE, McCarthy JG. Vector of device placement and trajectory of mandibular distraction. J Craniofac Surg. 1997;8(6):473–80; discussion 461–2.
35. Vendittelli BL, Dec W, Warren SM, Garfinkle JS, Gravson BH, McCarthv JG. The importance of vector selection in preoperative planning of bilateral mandibular distraction. Plast Reconstr Surg. 2008;122(4):1144–53.
36. Dec W, Peltomaki T, Warren SM, Garfinkle JS, Gravson BH, McCarthv JG. The importance of vector selection in preoperative planning of unilateral mandibular distraction. Plast Reconstr Surg. 2008;121(6):2084–92; discussion 2093–4.
37. Diner PA, Kollar EM, Martinez H, Vazquez MP. Intraoral distraction for mandibular lengthening: a technical innovation. J Craniomaxillofac Surg. 1996;24(2):92–5.
38. Schendel SA, Linck III DW. Mandibular distraction osteogenesis by sagittal split osteotomy and intraoral curvilinear distraction. J Craniofac Surg. 2004;15(4):631–5.
39. Kaban LB, Seldin EB, Kikinis R, Yeshwant K, Padwa BL, Troulis MJ. Clinical application of curvilinear distraction osteogenesis for correction of mandibular deformities. J Oral Maxillofac Surg. 2009;67(5):996–1008.
40. Aizenbud D, Hazan-Molina H, Thimmappa B, Hopkins EM, Schendel SA. Curvilinear mandibular distraction results and long-term stability effects in a group of 40 patients. Plast Reconstr Surg. 2010;125(6):1771–80.
41. Davidson EH, Brown D, Shetye PR, Greig AV, Grayson BH, Warren SM, McCarthv JG. The evolution of mandibular distraction: device selection. Plast Reconst Surg. 2010;126(6):2061–70.
42. McCarthv JG, Hopper RA, Hollier Jr LH, Peltomaki T, Katzen T, Grayson BH. Molding of the regenerate in mandibular distraction: clinical experience. Plast Reconstr Surg. 2003;112(5):1239–46.
43. Shetye PR, Warren SM, Brown D, Garfinkle JS, Gravson BH, McCarthv JG. Documentation of the incidents associated with mandibular distraction: introduction of a new stratification system. Plast Reconstr Surg. 2009;123(2):1627–34.
44. Verlinden CR, van de Vijfeijken SE, Tuinzing DB, Jansma EP, Becking AG, Swennen GR. Complications of mandibular distraction osteogenesis for developmental deformities: a systematic review of the literature. Int J Oral Maxillofac Surg. 2015;44(1):44–9.

45. Master DL, Hanson PR, Gosain AK. Complications of mandibular distraction osteogenesis. J Cranio Surg. 2010;21(5):1565–70.
46. Spector JA, Warren SM, Singh SP, McCarthv JG, Siebert JW. Marriage of hard and soft tissues of the face revisited: when distraction meets microsurgery. Ann Plast Surg. 2007;59(l):1–5. discussion 5
47. Nardini G, Staffenberg D, Seo L, et al. Treacher Collins syndrome and tracheostomy: decannulation utilizing mandibular distraction osteogenesis. Plast and Reconstr Surg. 2015;136(4 Suppl):47.
48. Flores RL. Neonatal mandibular distraction osteogenesis. Semin Plast Surg. 2014;28(4):199–206.
49. Flores RL, Greathouse ST, Costa M, Tahiri Y, Soleimani T, Tholpadv SS. Defining failure and its predictors in mandibular distraction for Robin sequence. J Craniomaxillofac Surg. 2015;43(8):1614–9.
50. Spinelli G, Agostini T, Arcuri F, Conti M, Raffaini M. Three-dimensional airways reconstruction in syndromic pediatric patients following mandibular distraction osteogenesis. J Craniofac Surg. 2015;26(3):650–4.
51. Szpalski C, Vandegrift M, Patel PA, Appelboom G, Fisher M, Marcus J, McCarthy JG, Shetye PR, Warren SM. Unilateral craniofacial microsomia: unrecognized cause of pediatric obstructive sleep apnea. J Craniofac Surg. 2015;26(4):1277–82.
52. Molina F. Combined maxillary and mandibular distraction osteogenesis. Semin Orthod. 1999;5(1):41–5.
53. Shehata EA, Medra AM. Modified bimaxillary distraction osteogenesis: a technique to correct facial asymmetry. Br J Oral Maxillofac Surg. 2007;45(6):471–7.
54. Satoh K, Suzuki H, Uemura T, Hosaka Y. Maxillo-mandibular distraction osteogenesis for hemifacial microsomia in children. Ann Plast Surg. 2002;49(6):572–8. discussion 578–9
55. Vu HL, Panchal J, Levine N. Combined simultaneous distraction osteogenesis of the maxilla and mandible using a single distraction device in hemifacial microsomia. J Craniofac Surg. 2001;12(3):253–8.
56. Schendel SA, Hazan-Molina H, Aizenbud D. Combined orthognathic distraction procedure: Le Fort I maxillary technique for craniofacial management. Plast Reconstr Surg. 2014;133(4):874–7.
57. Santa Anna EF, Lau GW, Marquezan M, de Souza Araujo MT, Pollev JW, Figueroa AA. Combined maxillary and mandibular distraction osteogenesis in patients with hemifacial microsomia. Am J Orthod Dentofac Orthop. 2015;147(5):566–77.
58. Shetve PR, Gravson BH, Mackool RJ, McCarthv JG. Long-term stability and growth following unilateral mandibular distraction in growing children with craniofacial microsomia. Plast Reconstr Surg. 2006;118(4):985–95.
59. Ascenço AS, Balbinot P, Junior IM, D'Oro U, Busato L, da Silva Freitas R. Mandibular distraction in hemifacial microsomia is not a permanent treatment: a long-term evaluation. J Craniofac Surg. 2014;25(2):352–4.
60. Suh J, Choi TH, Baek SH, Kim JC, Kim S. Mandibular distraction in unilateral craniofacial microsomia: longitudinal results until the completion of growth. Plast Reconstr Surg. 2013;132(5):1244–52.
61. Pluijmers BI, Caron CJJM, Dunaway DJ, Wolvius EB, Koudstaal MJ. Mandibular reconstruction in the growing patient with unilateral craniofacial microsomia: a systematic review. Int J Oral Maxillofac Surg. 2014;43:286–95.
62. Nagy K, Kuijpers-Jagtman AM, Monmaerts MY. No evidence for long-term effectiveness of early osteodistraction in hemifacial microsomia. Plast Reconstr Surg. 2009;124(6):2061–71.
63. Weichman K, Jacobs JMS, Patel PA, et al. Early distraction for mild to moderate unilateral craniofacial microsomia (UCFM): long-term follow-up outcomes and recommendations. Plast Reconstr Surg. 2017;139(4):941e–953e.
64. MacKool RJ, Grayson BH, McCarthy JG. Volumetric assessment of the distracted human mandible. A new CT analytic technique. J Craniofac Surg. 2004;15:745.
65. Altug-Atac AT, Gravson BH, McCarthv JG. Comparison of skeletal and soft-tissue changes following unilateral mandibular distraction osteogenesis. Plast Reconstr Surg. 2008;121(5):1751–9.

Mandibular Distraction, Orthodontic Considerations

4

Pradip R. Shetye and Barry H. Grayson

4.1 Introduction

Mandibular distraction has been successfully used to correct mandibular hypoplasia in all three dimensions since its introduction in 1989 by McCarthy and NYU colleagues [1]. Patients with craniofacial microsomia, Nager syndrome, Treacher Collins syndrome, Robin sequence, temporomandibular joint ankylosis, posttraumatic growth disturbances, and a variety of other mandibular developmental disturbances have significantly benefited from this technique. As with traditional orthognathic surgery, pre- and post-distraction orthodontic therapy is an integral part of the successful outcome of distraction. The goals of pre- and post-distraction orthodontics therapy include the following: preoperative evaluation of the craniofacial skeletal and dental relationships, preparation of the dentition prior to the placement of a distraction device, collaboration with the surgeon on the placement of the distraction device for the optimal vector of distraction, monitoring of the skeletal changes during the activation phase, molding of the generate during the activation and consolidation phase, the management of post-distraction occlusion for long-term stability, and continued longitudinal follow-up.

4.2 Preoperative Evaluation

Patients planning to undergo mandibular distraction must first have a comprehensive craniofacial dental and skeletal evaluation. The soft and hard tissues should be examined, including the upper and lower lip relationship, occlusal cant, interocclusal relationships, mandibular range of motion, inter-incisal opening, and path of

P.R. Shetye, D.D.S., B.D.S., M.D.S. (✉) • B.H. Grayson, D.D.S.
Wyss Department of Plastic Surgery, NYU Langone Medical Center, New York, NY 10016, USA
e-mail: pradip.shetye@nyumc.org

J.G. McCarthy (ed.), *Craniofacial Distraction*,
DOI 10.1007/978-3-319-52564-8_4

mandibular opening and closing. The function of the temporomandibular joint, along with motor and sensory nerve function, should also be examined. The patient must be seen by a dentist to rule out dental decay and reinforce satisfactory oral hygiene during and after distraction process.

4.2.1 Diagnostic Records

The craniofacial skeletal relationship should be documented with medical-grade CT or cone beam CT (CBCT). three-dimensional (3D) and 2D photographs, and dental study models. With current orthodontic imaging software, such as Dolphin, a traditional lateral cephalogram, panorex, and posterioanterior cephalogram can be generated from a 3D CT or CBCT scan. These records become important tools in evaluating a patient's craniofacial morphology as well as in planning the placement of a distraction device with an optimal vector.

4.3 Selection of Distraction Device

Two types of distraction devices are available: external and semiburied distraction devices. The external distraction device is advantageous in a severely hypoplastic mandible and in a patient who has had his or her mandible reconstructed using a bone graft. The main disadvantages of the external distraction device are scar formation, obvious visibility and vulnerability to traumatic dislodgement. The use of the semiburied distraction technique reduces the scarring burden. Moreover, there is also a mechanical advantage: the distraction force is directly transferred to the underlying bone due to the close proximity of the distraction device to the bone. It is also ideally suited for optimal device placement for a vertical vector. The most common disadvantage of the semiburied distraction device is that the device cannot be used if the mandible remnant is extremely hypoplastic [2].

4.4 Pre-distraction Orthodontic Therapy

Following a clinical examination and the evaluation of the diagnostic records, patients are prepared orthodontically for the placement of distraction devices. Prior to device placement, a patient may require decompensation of his or her malocclusion. This may include maxillary and mandibular arch coordination, dental arch alignment, and the uprighting of the maxillary and mandibular anterior teeth. A patient with a mandibular deficiency often has narrow transverse maxillary width. If a maxillary transverse deficiency is noted, it is important to correct the transverse deficiency with maxillary expansion prior to mandibular distraction. Prior correction of the transverse maxillary deficiency allows for more optimal and stable maxillo-mandibular occlusal relationship following completion of the distraction process (Fig. 4.1).

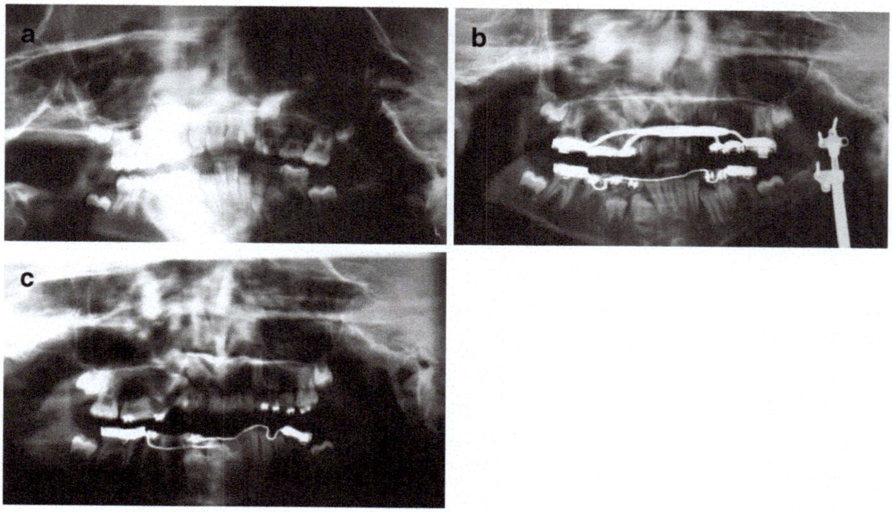

Fig. 4.1 (**a**–**c**) Panoramic radiograph series before (**a**), during (**b**), and after (**c**) the left-side unilateral mandibular distraction. Note that the patient has a maxillary expansion appliance, and a tooth bud was enucleated 6 months prior to making the osteotomy and device placement. Following device removal, there is a resulting posterior open bite on the operated side

One of the challenges in the placement of a distraction device in a growing child is the location of the developing mandibular second and third molar tooth buds. As the location of the tooth buds may not allow sufficient bone to perform the osteotomy and to secure the distraction device, the tooth follicles may be enucleated at least 6 months prior to distraction device placement. This allows adequate time for the formation of new bone in the site of the enucleation (Fig. 4.1).

4.5 Selection of Vectors of Distraction

For an optimal result, it is important that the distraction devices are placed with proper vectors in order to create favorable bony morphology during activation. A successful distraction is dependent on careful preoperative planning and accurate prediction of outcomes [3–5]. The device orientation is described in relation to the stable and unmoving maxillary occlusal plane.

4.5.1 Horizontal Vector Device Placement

The distraction device is placed parallel to the maxillary occlusal plane (Fig. 4.2). The horizontal vector of distraction produces a marked mandibular midline shift but minimal elongation of the affected ramus. It is especially indicated in the patient with Robin sequence.

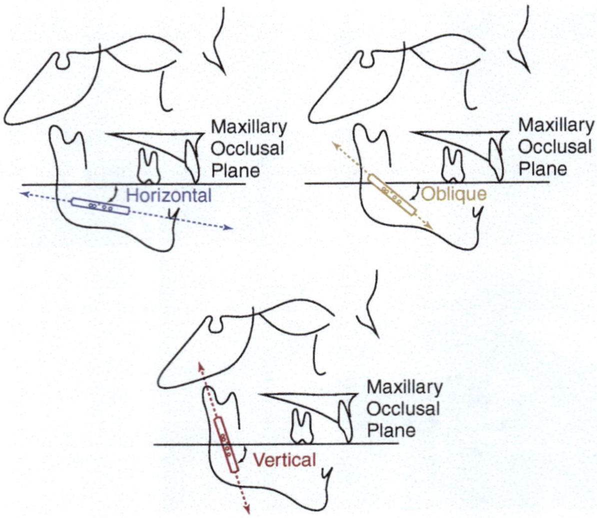

Fig. 4.2 Vectors of distraction as defined by device placement in relation to the maxillary occlusal plane

4.5.2 Vertical Vector Device Placement

Vertical device placement promotes increase in the vertical ramus height, and therefore, this type of placement is ideal for patients with vertical ramus deficiency, as in craniofacial microsomia and Treacher Collins syndrome (Fig. 4.2). A vertical vector of distraction results in a minimal mandibular midline shift but marked ramus elongation [5]. There is a counterclockwise rotation of the mandible with consequent projection of the pogonion. After the completion of unilateral distraction, the patient will develop a lateral open bite on the side of the distraction, and in bilateral patients, there will be a tendency to develop a bilateral open bite. This opening has to be managed orthodontically by using bite-block therapy following distraction.

4.5.3 Oblique Vector Device Placement

Oblique device placement results in an increase in both the vertical and horizontal dimensions of the ramus and the body (Fig. 4.2). An oblique vector of distraction produces an intermediate amount of ramus lengthening and a marked amount of a mandibular midline shift [5].

4.6 3D Planning of Distraction

With current digital technology and the use of a 3D CT scan, it is now possible to virtually simulate the placement of a distraction device as well as the distraction vector. The 3D CT provides a visualization of the inferior alveolar nerve, the tooth buds, and the roots of developing teeth. The planning software has a library of virtual distraction devices of different shapes and sizes, and the surgeon can select the appropriate distraction device based on the anatomy of the mandible and the specific requirements of the patients. Cutting guides and distraction placement guides can be constructed from a pretreatment CT scan for a more accurate placement of a distraction device. However, the simulation of the distraction and the actual result may vary, as soft tissue resistance and muscle pull cannot be accurately predicted.

4.7 Orthodontic Therapy During the Activation Phase

Following surgical osteotomy and fixation of the device, a latency period of 5–6 days is observed prior to the start of the activation phase. During the activation phase, the device is activated at a rate of 1 mm per day (rhythm of 0.5 mm twice a day). Activation is continued until the clinical goals are achieved for each individual patient. A unilateral mandibular distraction involves the lowering of the affected oral commissure, the movement of the chin point to the midline or beyond (especially in a young patient), and the leveling or lowering of the ipsilateral occlusal plane (Fig. 4.3). Overcorrection is recommended to account for future relapse and lack of mandibular growth. In bilateral mandibular distraction, care should be taken

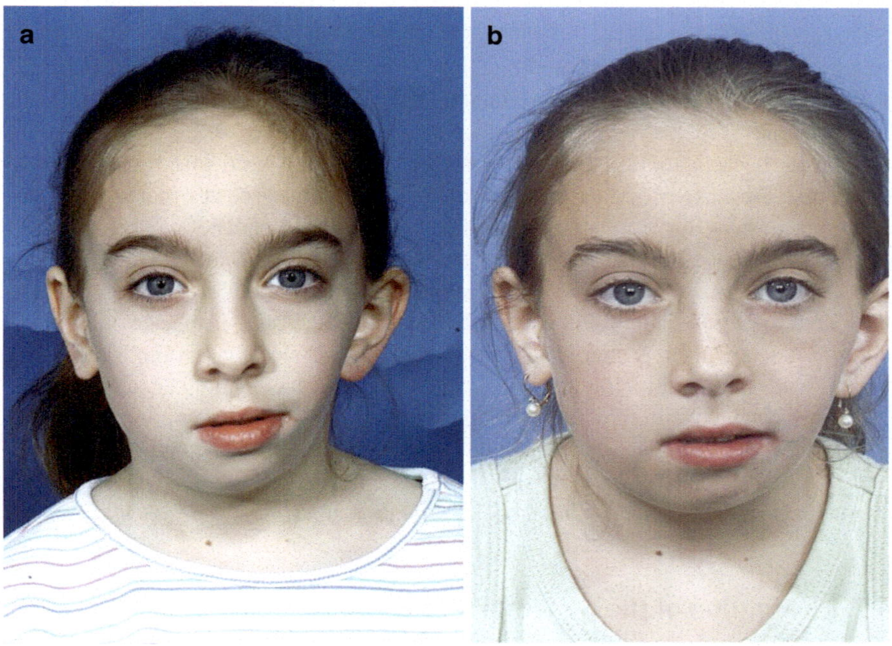

Fig. 4.3 (**a**, **b**) Frontal view of a patient before (**a**) and following (**b**) left-sided unilateral mandibular distraction. Note the overcorrection accomplished by moving the chin to the contralateral side and lowering of the affected oral commissure and inferior mandibular border

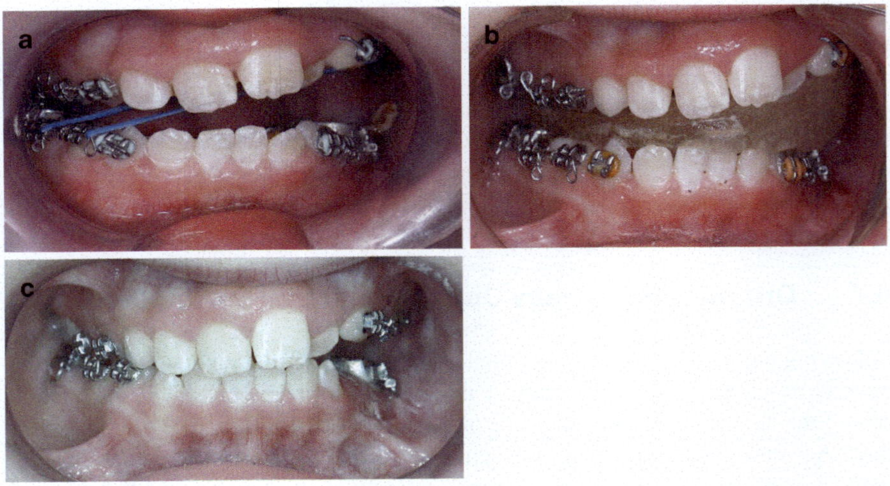

Fig. 4.4 (**a**) Intraoral view of a patient undergoing left-sided unilateral mandibular distraction. Cross tongue elastics are used to redirect the vectors of distraction noting the resulting posterior open bite. (**b**) Intraoral view demonstrating placement of a orthodontic acrylic bite block to stabilize the lateral open bite formed secondary to device activation (unilateral). (**c**) Over the following year, the bite block is gradually reduced to allow for supra-eruption of the maxillary teeth to fill the void

so that both devices are activated equally. After the completion of activation, the mean consolidation period is approximately 8 weeks before the devices are removed in the operating room.

During the activation phase, the vectors of distraction need to be progressively monitored. Because of unfavorable muscle pull and soft tissue resistance, the bony segments may not displace in the anticipated direction. This tendency can be overcome by adding orthodontic elastics to redirect the vectors of distraction in a favorable direction. To enable the placement of elastics, one can use orthodontic brackets, bonded orthodontic splits with hooks, or temporary anchorage devices. The placement of orthodontic attachments in primary and permanent dentition is easily accomplished. For a patient with multiple missing teeth or short clinical crowns, bonding an acrylic splint with hooks may be preferred. An alternative technique is the use of temporary anchorage devices (TADS). Elastics can then be placed directly on the TADS. Intermaxillary elastics can efficiently modify the vector of distraction to achieve the desired skeletal movements and a reasonable dental occlusal relationship (Fig. 4.4).

4.7.1 Molding of the Generate

Animal studies and clinical investigations have suggested that the bony generate can be successfully "molded" during the activation and consolidation phase of mandibular distraction [6, 7]. The generate can be molded with the use of intermaxillary/

interdental elastics. When using elastic traction to close an anterior open bite, care must be taken to minimize the extrusion of individual teeth by distributing the force over the entire dental arch, especially the basilar portions of the jaws. To prevent unwanted dentoalveolar changes from occurring during elastic traction, skeletal rather than dental fixation of the elastics is recommended. Intrusive mechanics may be incorporated into the orthodontic appliances to balance the extrusive force by the molding elastics. TAD screws inserted in the basilar portion of the mandible and maxilla for retention of rubber bands are effective in molding the generate. The molding of the regenerate can be successfully accomplished not only during device activation but also early in the consolidation period [8].

4.8 Orthodontic Therapy During the Consolidation Phase

During the consolidation phase of a distraction, it is important to maintain the stability of the newly distracted bone. The consolidation phase is approximately 8 weeks in length. During this phase, if a patient following unilateral mandibular distraction has developed a posterior open bite, a stabilizing bite block appliance must be fabricated. A bite registration will be needed to mount the study models to the new post-distraction occlusion. The mounted models will be used to construct the appliance that will fit passively to the upper and lower dentition. The bite-bock appliance, made of acrylic, provides occlusal contact in the areas where the maxillary and mandibular teeth are not touching (Fig. 4.4). Thus, it serves to provide balanced posterior occlusion while at the same time relieving compressive force on the newly created generate. The occlusal bite block can be removable and attached with clasps or bonded to the teeth with orthodontic cement. A removal appliance has the advantage of being able to be removed for oral hygiene and laboratory adjustment.

4.9 Orthodontic Therapy Post-Consolidation Phase

When undergoing a unilateral mandibular distraction, the patient often develops a lateral open bite secondary to a vertical ramus elongation. The open bite should be corrected after the consolidation period of distraction by allowing supra-eruption of the maxillary teeth (Fig. 4.5) while preventing supra-eruption of the mandibular teeth. Passive eruption is accomplished by progressively reducing the acrylic on the bite block under the occlusal surface of the maxillary dentition, allowing the latter to supra-erupt downward towards the mandibular occlusal plane. Active eruption is accomplished by placing fixed braces on the primary and adult teeth. Vertical elastics can be used to extrude the teeth to close the open bite. However, caution must be used to selectively achieve eruption of the maxillary dentition downward towards the mandibular occlusal plane. The process of closing the open bite may take 6 months to 1 year. After the closure of the open bite, the orthodontic appliance can be removed, and the patient can be followed up for future growth.

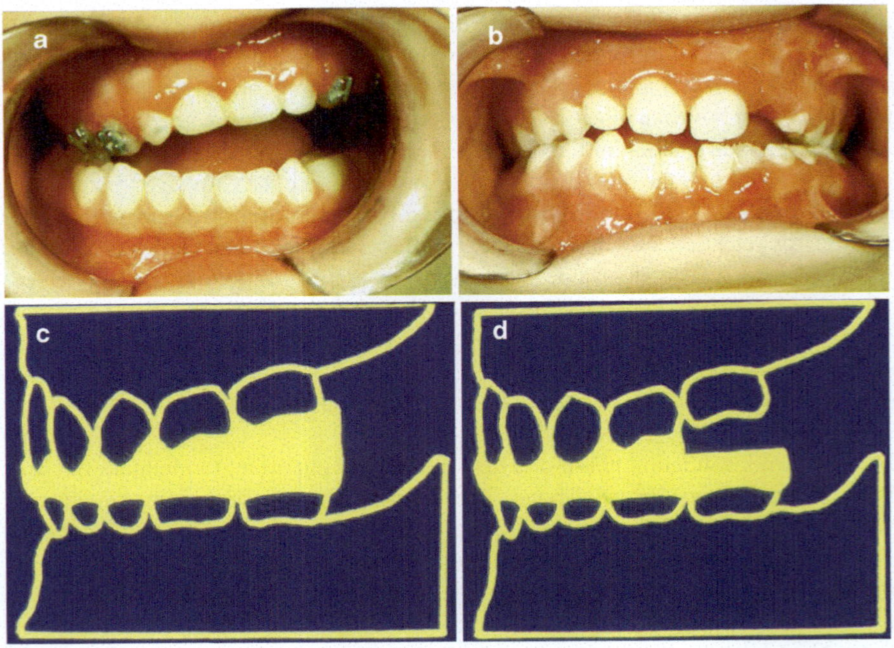

Fig. 4.5 (**a**) Left lateral open bite secondary to the vertical ramus lengthening after left unilateral mandibular distraction. (**b**) The open bite corrected after the consolidation period by allowing supra-eruption of the maxillary teeth while preventing supra-eruption of the mandibular teeth. (**c**) Bite block in position during consolidation period. (**d**) Passive eruption is accomplished by progressively reducing the acrylic on the bite block under the occlusal surface of the maxillary dentition, allowing the latter to supra-erupt downward towards the mandibular occlusal plane to close the open bite

4.10 Long-Term Outcome of Mandibular Distraction

In a retrospective longitudinal study of 12 consecutive growing children (N = 9 males, N = 3 females) with unilateral craniofacial microsomia, who underwent mandibular distraction, long-term skeletal stability and growth were recorded [9]. They had a range of 5–10 years of post-distraction follow-up. Records included clinical photographs, dental study models, lateral and posteroanterior (PA) cephalograms, and panoramic radiographs obtained before distraction, at the time of device removal, and 1, 5, and 10 years post distraction. The mean age of patients at the time of distraction was 48 months. The device was activated an average of 21.7 mm at the rate of 1 mm per day. The mean latency period was 6.1 days, and the consolidation period was 60.6 days. Post distraction, all patients underwent orthodontic treatment with bite-block therapy to close the posterior open bite by bringing the maxillary occlusal plane down to the mandibular occlusal plane. Fifty-two parameters were examined at each of the five time intervals. The result showed on average that the ramal length (Co-Go) increased 13.04 mm in the distracted rami.

At 1 year following distraction, this dimension decreased by 3.46 mm. The study concluded that mandibular distraction in growing children with unilateral craniofacial microsomia, on average, increased the ramal length by 13.04 mm, which was reduced by 3.46 mm during the first year following distraction. This loss of 3.46 mm may be a result of the reduction in the length or volume of the generated bone or the remodeling of the landmarks condylion and gonion, both of which are used to measure the ramus height. Our observations have suggested that these landmarks are remodeled due to the changes in the direction of the soft tissue muscle pull on the mandible. To understand the actual relapse of the distracted bone independently of local surface remodeling, it would be necessary to place bone markers near the distal and proximal areas of the distracted bone and use these as landmarks for measurement. *It must be emphasized that the remodeling of the condyle and gonion (the key cephalometric reference points) gives an exaggerated representation of "relapse"* [9].

At 5 and 10 years following distraction, the average Co-Go dimension increased by 3.83 and 3.10 mm, respectively, with an average growth rate of 0.77 mm per year; during the same period, the unaffected ramus grew 1.3 mm per year. The distraction technique does not eliminate the inherent growth characteristics of the affected mandibular side. The facial asymmetry is significantly improved following distraction, and despite a mild relapse observed during the first year, the surgical correction is stable in the later years of follow-up. However, due to the intrinsic differences in growth rate of the affected and unaffected mandibular rami, the post-distraction symmetry may change over time.

The findings suggest that the primary mandibular distraction should be continued until there is evidence of overcorrection, i.e., chin point driven to the unaffected side. Early distraction definitely reduces the severity of the deformity, promotes psychosocial functioning, and makes secondary correction a less extensive and challenging procedure.

A recent long-term follow-up study demonstrated that mandibular distraction is successful in patients with mild to moderate dysmorphism provided there is a comprehensive clinical program emphasizing adequate mandibular bone stock, proper vector selection, planned overcorrection, and comprehensive orthodontic involvement [10].

Pearls and Pitfalls

- Overcorrection in the growing child.
- Observe the endpoints of activation.
- Management of ipsilateral open bite with bite blocks and cross elastics.
- Molding of generate during activation and consolidation.
- Consider extraction of teeth/tooth buds where the bone is insufficient for optimal device placement.
- Long-term follow-up is essential.
- Distinguish between true relapse and differences in growth rate of the affected and unaffected mandibular sides.

References

1. McCarthy JG, et al. Lengthening the human mandible by gradual distraction. Plast Reconstr Surg. 1992;89(1):1–8; discussion 9–10.
2. Davidson EH, et al. The evolution of mandibular distraction: device selection. Plast Reconstr Surg. 126(6):2061–70.
3. Grayson BH, Santiago PE. Treatment planning and biomechanics of distraction osteogenesis from an orthodontic perspective. Semin Orthod. 1999;5(1):9–24.
4. Dec W, et al. The importance of vector selection in preoperative planning of unilateral mandibular distraction. Plast Reconstr Surg. 2008;121(6):2084–92; discussion 2093–4.
5. Vendittelli BL, et al. The importance of vector selection in preoperative planning of bilateral mandibular distraction. Plast Reconstr Surg. 2008;122(4):1144–53.
6. Vendittelli BL. Moldability of the callus after distraction osteogenesis. J Oral Maxillofac Surg. 2000;58(7):828.
7. McCarthy JG, et al. Molding of the regenerate in mandibular distraction: clinical experience. Plast Reconstr Surg. 2003;112(5):1239–46.
8. Peltomaki T, et al. Moulding of the generate to control open bite during mandibular distraction osteogenesis. Eur J Orthod. 2002;24(6):639–45.
9. Shetye PR, et al. Long-term stability and growth following unilateral mandibular distraction in growing children with craniofacial microsomia. Plast Reconstr Surg. 2006;118(4):985–95.
10. Weichman K, et al. Early distraction for mild to moderate unilateral craniofacial microsomia (UCFM): long-term follow-up outcomes and recommendations. Plast Reconstr Surg. 2017;139(4):941e–53e.

Intraoral Mandibular Distraction

5

Cesar A. Guerrero, William H. Bell, Gisela I. Contasti-Bocco,
Aura M. Rodriguez, and Rafael V. Contasti

The aim of this chapter is to review the indications and biomechanics of intraoral mandibular distraction and focus on the clinical outcomes and innovations utilizing intraoral distraction devices.

The key variables with mandibular distraction remain the following: controlling the vector of distraction, determination of the ideal distraction site, selection of the proper distraction device, optimization of the regenerate, management of postoperative occlusion, and avoidance of possible damage to nerves, muscles, and teeth. Studies on long-term follow-up of these surgical interventions permit the clinicians to develop predictable surgical protocols for patients with severe malformations or deformations.

C.A. Guerrero, D.D.S. (✉)
Assistant Professor, Division of Oral And Maxillofacial Surgery,
University of Texas, Medical Branch, Galveston, Texas, USA
e-mail: drcesarguerrero@gmail.com

W.H. Bell, D.D.S.
Retired Professor, Oral and Maxillofacial Division, Deparment of Surgery,
University of Texas Southwestern Medical School, Parkland Memorial Hospital,
Dallas, Texas, USA

G.I. Contasi-Bocco, D.D.S.
Associated Professor, Department of Orthodontics, Nova Southeastern University,
Fort-Lauderdale, Florida, USA

A.M. Rodriguez, D.D.S.
Private Practice in Orthodontics, Santa Cruz de Tenerife, Canary Islands, Spain

R.V. Contasti, M.D
Plastic and Reconstructive Surgery, Santa Rosa Plastic Surgery Center, Caracas, Venezuela

J.G. McCarthy (ed.), *Craniofacial Distraction*,
DOI 10.1007/978-3-319-52564-8_5

5.1 Mandibular Widening by Distraction

Severe dental crowding is usually a component of a micrognathia, including a deficiency in the three planes of space: anteroposterior, transverse, and vertical. During childhood, the deformity may cause severe airway obstruction, limitations in feeding, and temporomandibular joint disorder (TMJD). Most patients with light or moderate deficiencies are currently treated by orthodontics alone with limited results, teeth moved outside the alveolar bone, gingival recession, premolar extractions, and unsatisfactory facial esthetics and smile [1–5].

Indications [2, 5–7]:

- Narrow V-shaped mandible
- Severe mandibular crowding to avoid dental extractions
- Scissor bite (Brodie syndrome)
- Maxillomandibular transverse deficiency ("tunnel smile," "crocodile bite")
- Impacted anterior teeth
- Treatment after bicuspid extractions
- Congenital absence of the teeth

5.1.1 Preoperative Assessment

5.1.1.1 Dental Model Analysis

The amount of widening required is calculated according to the following variables: available space versus required space, inclination of the incisors (1 MPa = 90°), deep bite, or a marked curve of Spee, intermolar width, and size of the incisors.

5.1.1.2 Soft Tissue Skeletal Analysis

There should be a healthy periodontium around the teeth where the osteotomy will be performed, with at least 1 mm of the bone protecting the roots on either side of the osteotomy, to produce bone generate in the distraction process. The lack of bone at the osteotomy level can lead to delayed healing or periodontal defects. The osteotomy design and site are selected based on bone quantity between the roots and the inclination of the teeth. A Bolton discrepancy analysis is also performed to calculate the amount of widening required and to predict the final maxillomandibular anterior teeth overjet and overbite [6–10].

5.1.2 Surgical Planning

A variety of devices for mandibular widening have been developed. The tooth-borne lingual appliance or the uni-arm devices are the best options. The recently developed uni-arm device can be applied on the buccal or the lingual side [2–10]. The bone-borne device to widen the mandible has limited use because of associated costs and the need for a secondary stage for device removal; equal surgical outcomes can be obtained with dental-borne, bone-borne, or hybrid devices [5–10].

To avoid complications with the dental-borne appliance during or after surgery, several steps are fundamental to prevent device dislodgment. First, dental bands are selected one size larger than indicated, because in the welding process, the metal bands contract. Second, the orthodontist must place the device under the equator of the teeth, closer to the gingival margin. Third, the device must be fixed to the teeth-utilizing glass ionomer cement. Fourth, attention must be given to the passiveness of the dental-borne appliance as well as to the parallelism to the occlusal plane [10, 11].

Presurgical orthodontic therapy includes complete maxillary arch alignment and leveling. After the maxillary teeth are ideally positioned, a final diagnosis and reevaluation are made to plan the deconstructed mandibular arch as wide as the new maxillary alignment. Until that time, no braces are placed on the mandible unless there is a need to open an interdental space for the osteotomy to avoid damaging the dental roots. The orthodontist selects the optimal appliance according to the requirements already mentioned and, more importantly, calculates the amount of widening required, as based on the occlusogram. Finally, the proper distraction screw length is selected [10, 11].

For maxillary widening, the maxilla is expanded anteriorly and posteriorly. The hyrax appliance will expand the maxilla symmetrically, provided that all osteotomies are completed [12–14] (Fig. 5.1). A different scenario occurs in mandibular widening. While the mandible is widened anteriorly, the distance decreases in a posterior direction, for example, from 7 mm widening in the incisor region to only 0.9 mm at the intercondylar level. Postoperatively a transverse crossbite is observed at the level of the canines and premolars that progresses to edge to edge at the first molar region and normal transverse bite at the second molar level. As the orthodontist is closing the anterior gap, the lateral crossbite is corrected (Fig. 5.1). The planning must include all measurements that can be predicted in the models and occlusograms [10–14].

Major mandibular crowding (Brodie bites) requires larger surgical movements. Large mandibular widening must be accompanied with a similar maxillary widening to obtain an optimal transverse maxillomandibular relation to prevent premolar extractions, improve the smile width, and eliminate the "sinking lips" appearance. The latter is observed following orthodontic therapy and premolar extractions. The NiTi arches are widely used in orthodontic therapy and are thermically activated to progressively move the teeth outside the alveolar bone limits. Gingival recession and root resorption can be avoided with proper diagnosis and increasing bone volume by mandibular widening [10–13].

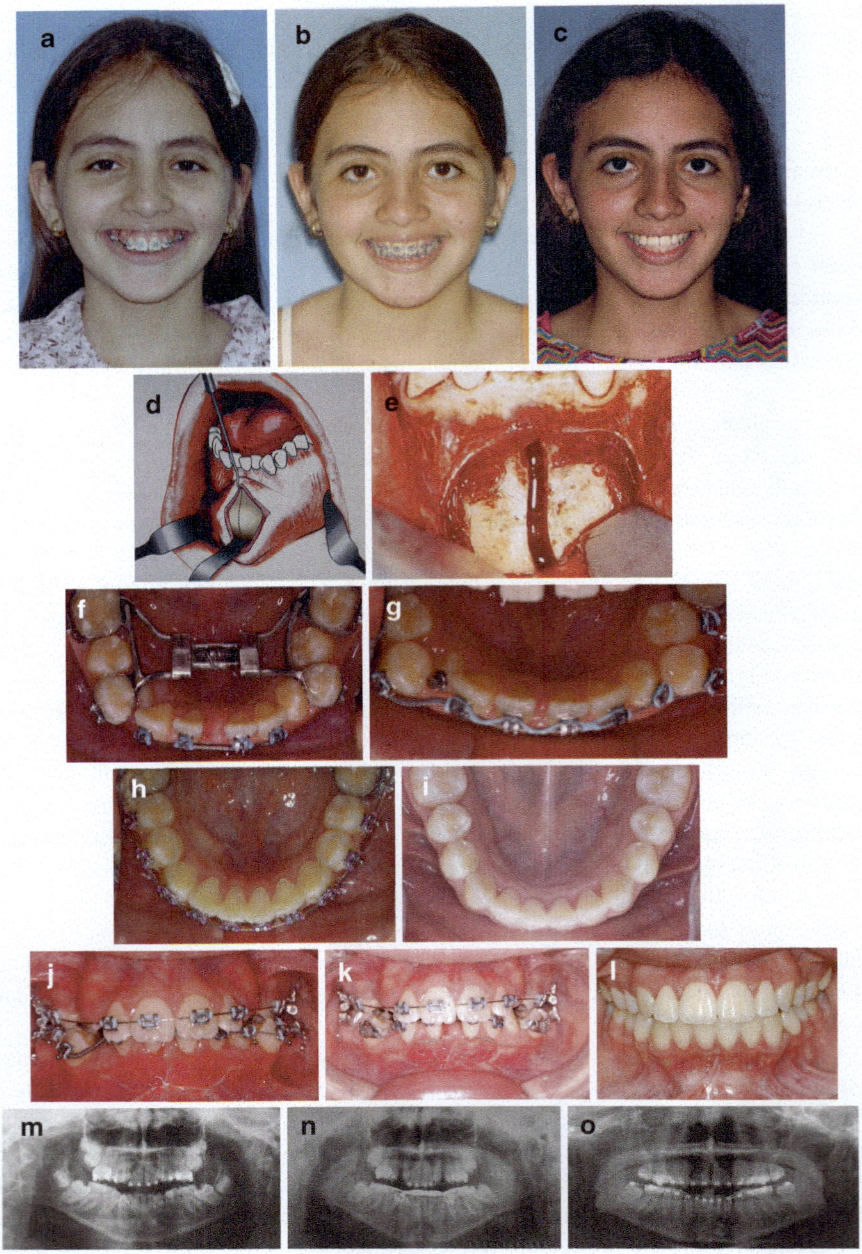

Fig. 5.1 Transverse or horizontal deficiency in a 11-year-old female. Treatment plan included mandibular osteotomy for distraction expansion. Total orthodontic surgical treatment time was 12 months. (**a**) Preoperative. (**b**) Postoperative frontal facial views are shown (**c**) 4 years follow up. (**d–e**) Vertical osteotomy of mandible for mandibular widening. (**f**) Mandibular occlusal view showing transverse deficiency and during activation. (**g**) Orthodontics alignment. (**h**) Mandibular view during orthodontic therapy (**i**) Posttreatment mandibular occlusal view with dental restoration. (**j**) Pretreatment intraoral frontal view. (**k**) Intraoral frontal view during activation. (**l**) Posttreatment intraoral view. (**m**) Pretreatment panoramic radiograph. (**n**) Posttreatment panoramic radiograph. (**o**) Panoramic radiograph 7 years follow-up

5.1.3 Widening the Symphysis or Parasymphyseal Region

The incision is made 4–6 mm labial to the depth of the mandibular vestibule. The periosteum is reflected inferiorly to the lower border of the mandible, and a small channel retractor is placed. It is carefully elevated, keeping in mind that much of the bony generation originates from the periosteum. The soft tissue between the mandibular central incisors is reflected superiorly with a skin hook to the alveolar crest with minimal detachment of the neighboring tissues [8–10] (See Fig. 5.1).

A vertical osteotomy is made in the symphyseal area with a reciprocating saw, starting at the inferior border of the mandible, continuing to the interdental space between the apices of the mandibular incisors, only in the outer cortex, to avoid interdental overheating. A straight hand piece with a surgical bur is used to cut across the labial cortical plate of the mandible to the alveolar crest. No attempt is made to use the saw or the bur between the roots of the teeth. This surgical maneuver emphasizes the importance of proper selection of the distraction site and the need for preoperative orthodontic therapy to open a surgical space. The final sectioning is done with a mallet and a spatula osteotome. The forefinger should be used as a guide to avoid tearing of the lingual soft tissues. An alternative osteotomy site in severe dental crowding is between the lateral incisor and canine. The osteotomy needs to be completed interdentally and continued toward the mandibular midline. A step in the osteotomy design is preferred since a complete vertical lateral osteotomy would create an asymmetric chin as the mandible is widened [8–10] (See Fig. 5.1).

5.1.4 Combined Mandibular Widening and Genioplasty

After the soft tissues have been elevated, a channel retractor is placed through a tunnel under the mental nerve to the level of the first molar. A dental caliper is used to measure the canine from the lateral cephalograms, and the distance plus 5 mm is transposed to the mandible, measuring from the incisal edge to a position under the apex of the canine on either side. Vertical lines are marked to serve as reference lines. A reciprocating saw is used to perform a bicortical osteotomy at the inferior border of the mandible starting at the first or second molar region, continuing anteriorly toward the symphyseal midline and passing by the reference lines. Care must be taken to avoid injury of the alveolar nerve. The osteotomy is completed with the reciprocating saw [8–10] (See Fig. 5.1).

At this point, the inferior segment is attached to the soft tissues. It is important to maintain this pedicle at all times, limiting the periosteal elevation to a minimum. The remainder of the mandibular symphysis is intact at this moment. The reciprocating saw is used to perform a vertical osteotomy at the preselected distraction site. The remainder of the surgical procedure is done as previously described. Genioplasty fixation is accomplished with wires, screws, or plates; a periosteal elevator is used to create a gap at the distraction site between the two bone segments to be distracted. By forcing them open while the wires are tightened or plates are fixated, the site will

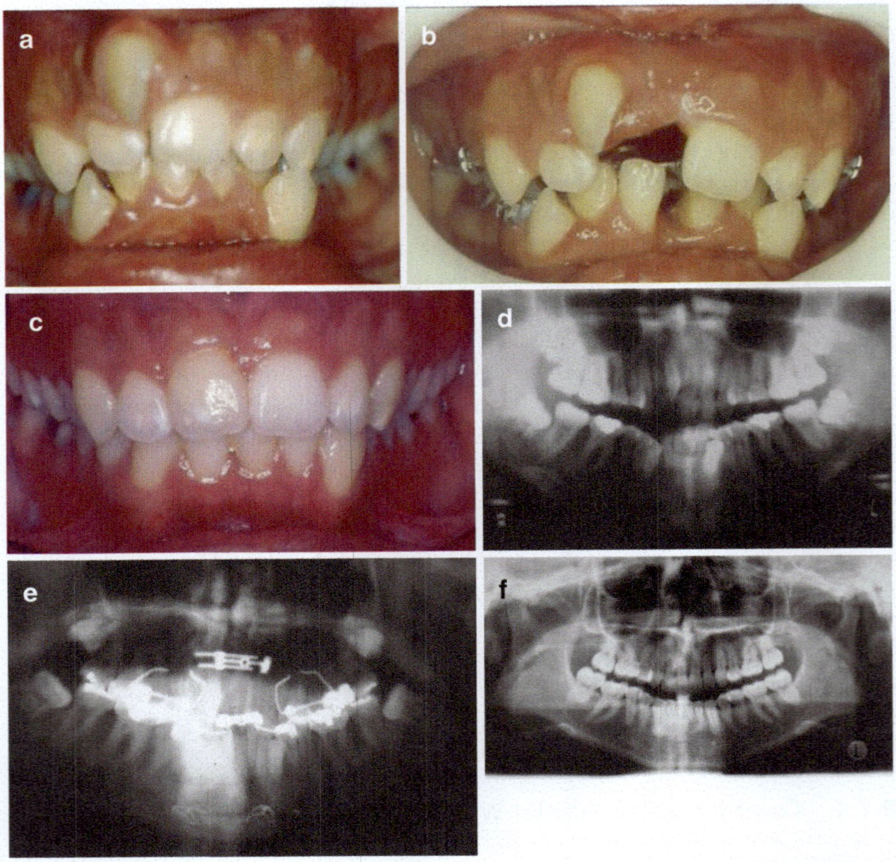

Fig. 5.2 Same patient as in Fig. 5.1. Space was created for descent of the right upper central incisor. Progressive maxillary expansion dictated simultaneous mandibular widening. (**a**) Pretreatment intraoral view. (**b**) Intraoral view during activation. (**c**) Posttreatment intraoral view. Note the satisfactory occlusion; a lower central incisor was removed secondary to Bolton's discrepancy. (**d**) Pretreatment panoramic radiograph. (**e**) Panoramic radiograph during treatment (**f**) Posttreatment panoramic radiograph 25 years later

have a triangular shape at the end of the procedure with an open base at the bottom. After the distraction appliance is activated, the interdental space opens, and the triangular-shaped space transforms into a vertical rectangle (Figs. 5.1 and 5.2).

5.1.5 Distraction Protocol [2, 5, 7–13]

1. Osteotomy: the bone is completely separated either with a reciprocating saw or small fissure bur, under abundant irrigation to avoid overheating. The final separation is done with a small chisel after fixating the distraction device and preventing fragment displacement.
2. Latency period: 7 days after the osteotomy is performed, the distraction device is activated.

3. Rate and rhythm: the device is activated 1 mm a day, or half a millimeter twice a day, until the desired activation is completed.
4. Consolidation: the distraction device remains in place 60 days for each centimeter of distraction.
5. Remodeling: this is the final distraction protocol phase, when function and intermaxillary elastics may mold the regenerate, and the muscles and associated soft tissues settle into the final bone healing stage.

5.1.6 Variables

There are four important variables in distraction osteogenesis: age of the patient, amount of skeletal movement, and quality and quantity of the bone. These variables will influence the distraction protocol; children may require a shorter latency period; an older patient would need an activation rate of half a millimeter per day, and larger movements require much longer consolidation periods, up to 12 months in large movements.

5.1.7 Postoperative Care

At the completion of the distraction process, acrylic is placed over the distraction rod and the wires around the teeth to provide more rigidity and allow the patient to advance to a soft diet. At this time also, the orthodontist adds a cosmetic acrylic tooth in the orthodontic arch to prevent the teeth from "walking" into the immature distraction area. After consolidation is achieved, the appliance is removed, and the clinician evaluates the radiographs for evidence of mineralization. The orthodontist continues the treatment. The interdental incisor distraction gap is filled with a plastic tooth which is reduced 0.5 mm a month from each interproximal surface (1 mm) to progressively close the distraction gap and complete the orthodontic treatment. The orthodontic treatment is resumed 60 days after surgery, and braces are maintained for at least 6 months. The occlusion is carefully finished, and standard retention is indicated. The orthodontist must avoid moving the teeth into the newly formed bone at the distraction zone. The transseptal fibers will pull the adjacent teeth to the distraction zone and could produce periodontal problems and loss of tooth vitality. It is advised to utilize wire ligatures to maintain the teeth in position during the consolidation period. After mineralization is seen in the radiographs, the teeth are moved 1 mm per month to close the interdental space (Fig. 5.2).

5.2 Mandibular Lengthening by Distraction

Virtual analysis, 3-D models, and virtual prediction have become standard tools in making the diagnosis, planning the treatment protocol, and communicating among the orthodontist, surgeon, patient, and family.

In intraoral distraction complex three-dimensional, movements are possible and predictable. Since surgical goals are often multidimensional, more than a single distraction device and vector change may be needed to correct the myriad of clinical presentations of mandibular deficiency. Precise preoperative planning must consider the biomechanical effect of appliance orientation for predictable widening and lengthening of the mandible [15–19].

5.2.1 Clinical Indications

1. Major mandibular 3-D deficiencies
2. TMJ degenerative joint disease
3. Sleep apnea
4. Inadequate mandibular anatomy for bilateral sagittal split osteotomy (BSSO)
5. Secondary mandibular advancements (relapse after conventional BSSO)
6. Children with severe mandibular deformities

5.2.2 Surgical Procedures [19–26]

1. Sagittal split ramus osteotomy
2. Body osteotomy
3. Horizontal ramus osteotomy
4. Combinations (vertical and horizontal lengthening)

5.2.2.1 Ramus Sagittal Split Osteotomy [19–25]

A standard sagittal split osteotomy is performed. An intermediate splint is used, and intermaxillary fixation is applied either to the orthodontic hooks or bone screws. Proximal segment fixation is temporarily achieved with one or two bicortical screws. The wound is closed, and the distraction device is transmucosally fixated. After adequate device stability is obtained, the mandibular provisional bicortical screws fixation are removed (Fig. 5.3). The advantage of having the appliance extramucosal is that the distraction zone will be watertight closed. It is also easier to remove the device at the end of the consolidation period.

For patients requiring bilateral advancement, the distraction device must be parallel to the vector of distraction, as the mandible is wider in the back and narrower in the front. An adjustment is made to the device by creating a step of 5–8 mm to compensate for this important variation in mandibular width. This maneuver is done to avoid placing lateral torque force against the condyle, loosening of the screws, and bending of the appliance (Figs. 5.4 and 5.5).

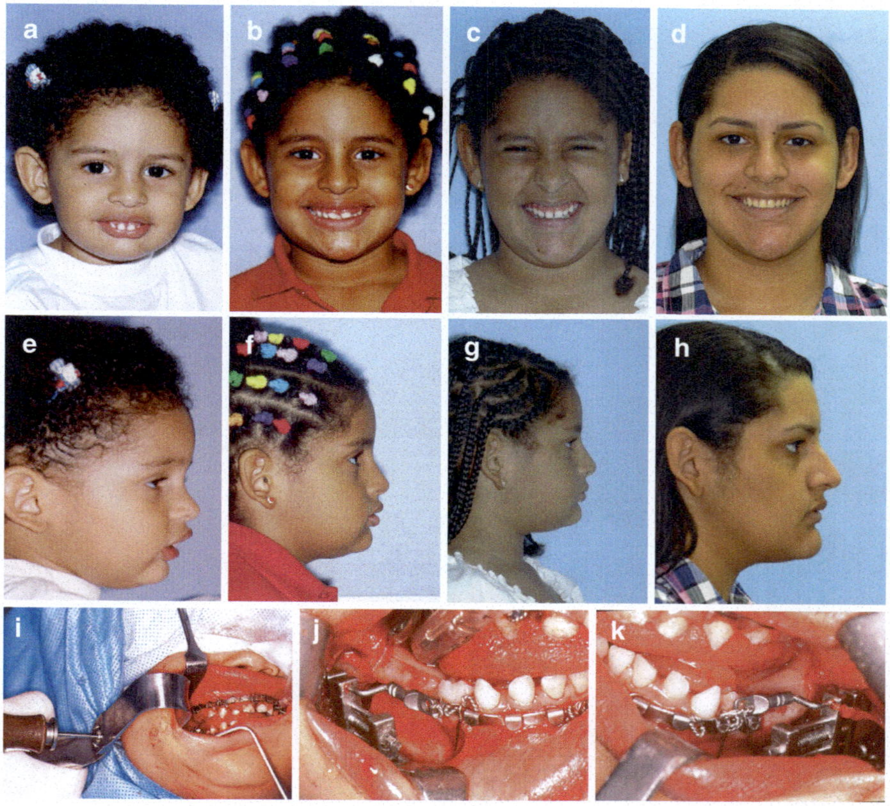

Fig. 5.3 A 2-year-old female with micrognathia and obstructive sleep apnea (OSA) treated by mandibular lengthening via distraction. (**a–d**) Preoperative and postoperative frontal view extending to 17 years follow up. (**e–h**) Preoperative and postoperative Profile view. (**i**) Percutaneous placement of screw in intraoral distraction device. (**j**) Distraction devices in place (*right*). (**k**) Distraction devices in place (*left*)

An anterior open bite could develop during the activation phase because of the lack of parallelism between the occlusal plane and the distractor rod. After the appliance is fully activated, the device arm is released, and the mandible is rotated until the open bite is closed and replaced in the final acceptable occlusal position. This maneuver is performed under IV sedation in the clinic. Lateral cephalograms are essential to plan and evaluate the bony movements (Figs. 5.4 and 5.5).

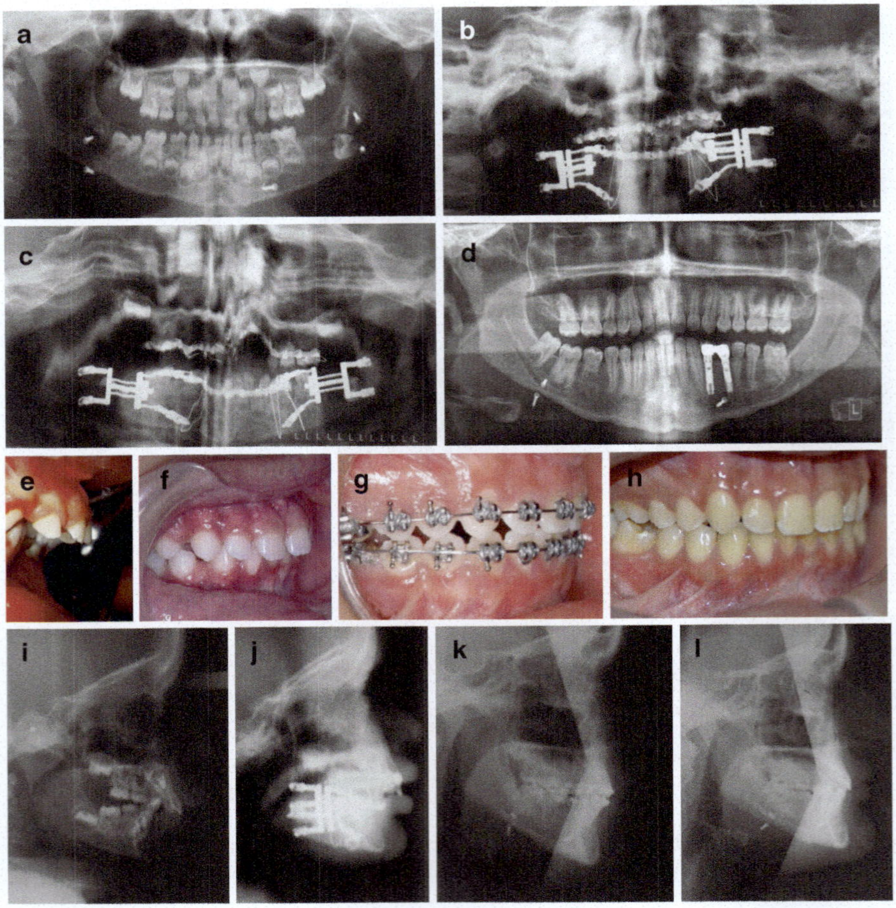

Fig. 5.4 Same patient as in Fig. 5.3. (**a**) Panoramic radiograph preoperative. (**b**) Panoramic radiograph with devices in place and Erich arch fixation by circummandibular wires. (**c**) Panoramic radiograph at the completion of activation. (**d**) Panoramic radiograph 17 years after treatment. (**e**) Intraoral view preoperative. (**f**) Intraoral view at the completion of activation. (**g**) Intraoral view after orthodontic dental alignments. (**h**) Intraoral view 17 years after treatment. (**i**) Lateral cephalogram preoperative. Note the severe micrognathia and retroglossal airway obstruction. (**j**) Lateral cephalogram with distraction devices in place. (**k**) Lateral cephalogram after distraction and during orthodontic therapy. (**l**) Lateral cephalogram final result. Note the lengthening of the mandible and expansion of the airway

5.2.2.2 Body Osteotomy (Anterior to the Mental Nerve) [19–26]

An incision is made in the vestibule, the periosteal layer elevated inferiorly, carefully looking for the mental nerve. A vertical osteotomy anterior to the mental nerve is made between the canine and premolar or between the two premolars (Fig. 5.6). The reciprocating saw is utilized to perform the osteotomy from the inferior border of the mandible, aiming superiorly bicortically with the forefinger on the lingual

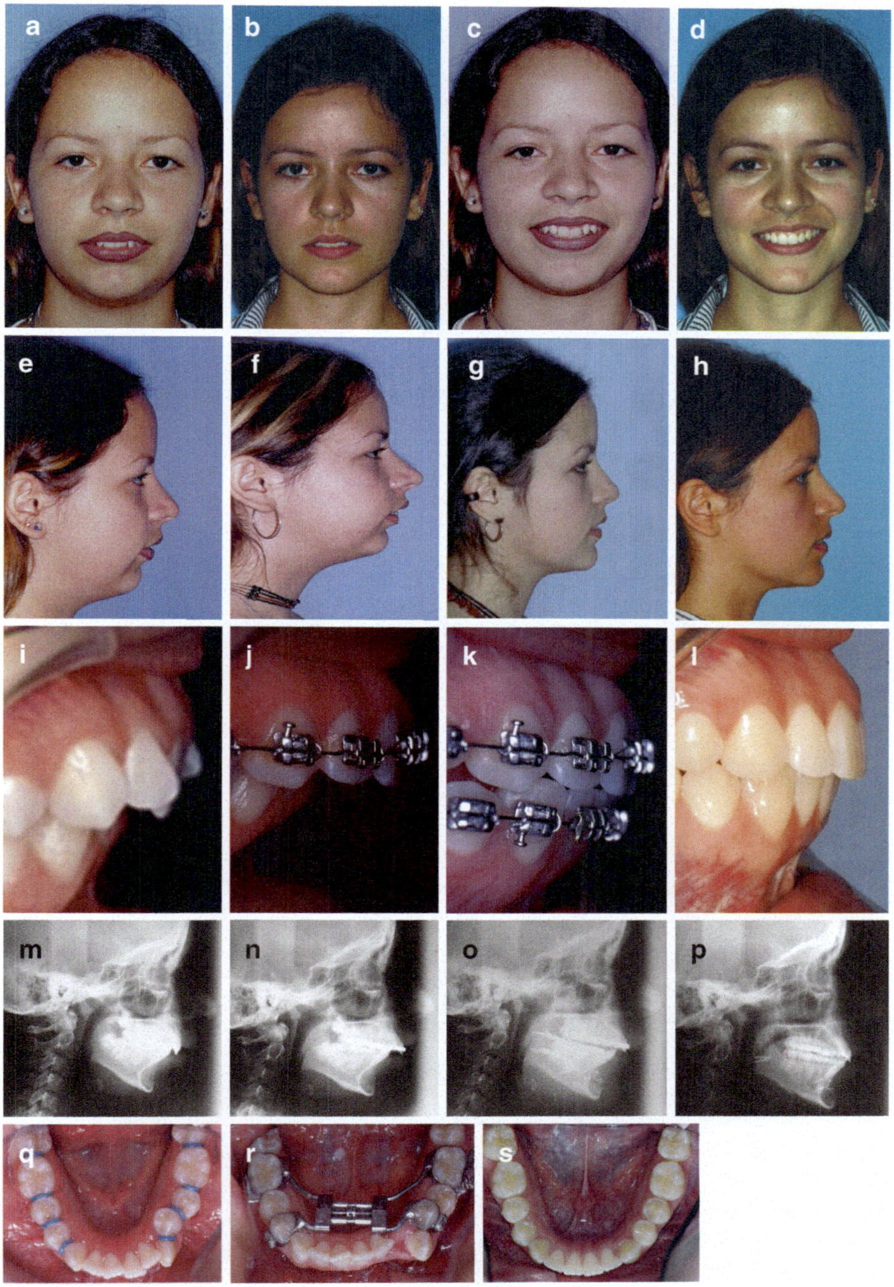

Fig. 5.5 A 17-year-old female with mandibular deficiency and temporomandibular joint degenerative disease treated simultaneously with mandibular lengthening, mandibular widening. and genioplasty. (**a**) Frontal view preoperative. (**b**) Frontal view postoperative. (**c**) Frontal (smiling) view preoperative. (**d**) Frontal (smiling) view postoperative. (**e–h**) Serial profile views. (**i–l**) Serial occlusal views (lateral). (**m–p**) Serial lateral cephalograms. (**q**) Preoperative occlusal view (mandible). (**r**) Occlusal view (mandible) with distraction devices in place. (**s**) Occlusal view (mandible) postoperative

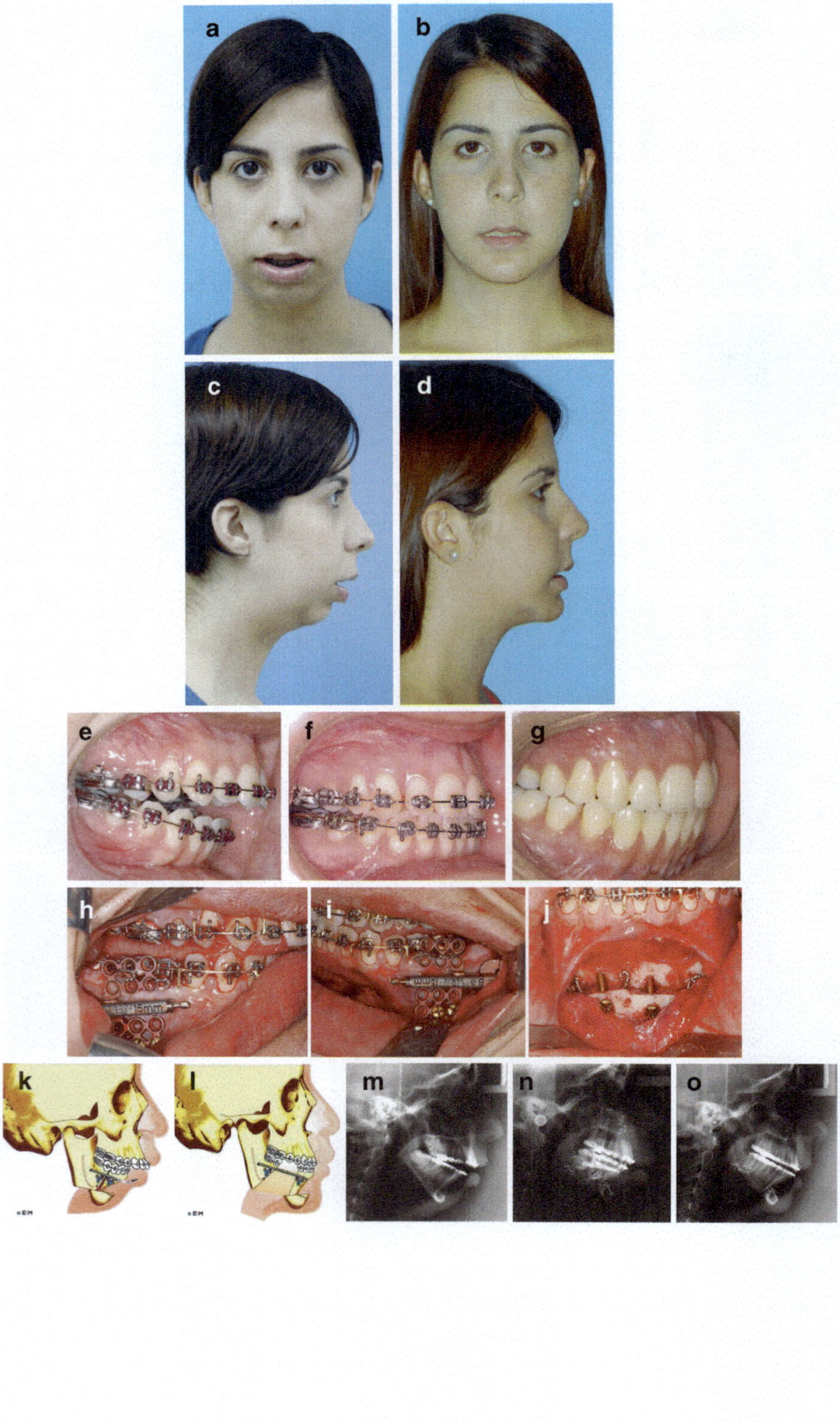
a
b
c
d
e
f
g
h
i
j
k
l
m
n
o
©EM
©EM

side to avoid mucosal perforation, up to the level of the dental roots. A fissure bur is used to make a line of holes between the dental roots, and the holes are united, sectioning the buccal plate under irrigation. A spatula osteotome and a mallet are used to complete the osteotomy. An interdental wire, Bridle wire, around the neck of the teeth, two on either side, is placed for temporary fixation. The wound is closed, and the distraction device is fixed transmucosally with bicortical screws and interdental wires reinforced with acrylic on top for stabilization at the teeth level to avoid dental root damage (Fig. 5.6).

The indication for this technique is major anteroposterior movements, the possibility to obtain a larger movement at the inferior border of the mandible and a smaller movement between the teeth. The mandibular nerve is left intact, and the technique improves the mandibular shape by changing the gonial angle (Fig. 5.6). The new space created between the teeth is closed with orthodontics, either by reciprocal movements or advancement of the posterior teeth anteriorly from mini implants for elastics anchorage at the canine level. The distraction chamber interdental space is closed by orthodontics mechanics (Fig. 5.6).

5.2.3 Postoperative Considerations

The distraction device should be removed only after ossification has been radiographically documented.

5.2.4 Postsurgical Orthodontics

Class II elastics are indicated both during the activation and consolidation phases to prevent reciprocal forces applied to the temporomandibular joints.

After the appliances are removed, the surgical arches are removed, and progressive detailing of the ideal teeth positioning is obtained. It is recommended that the orthodontic appliances are maintained for 12 months after surgery to ensure bone consolidation and stability.

5.2.4.1 Horizontal Ramus Osteotomy [19–26]

A 3 cm incision is made over the mandibular oblique line. The periosteum, muscles, and soft tissues are minimally detached to maintain the best blood supply possible. A Kelley clamp is placed on the anterior border of the ramus as high as

Fig. 5.6 A 21-year-old female with severe mandibular deficiency and obstructive sleep apnea. Bilateral mandibular distraction was performed (body osteotomy anterior to mental nerve). (**a**) Frontal view preoperative. (**b**) Frontal view 5 years after distraction. (**c**) Lateral view preoperative. (**d**) Lateral view after treatment. (**e**) Intraoral view pre-distraction. (**f**) Intraoral view post distraction with orthodontic appliances. (**g**) Intraoral view posttreatment. (**h–j**) Intraoperative view with distraction devices in place. A genioplasty and Le Fort I osteotomy were also performed simultaneously. (**k**, **l**) Schematic outlines of osteotomy and distraction devices before and after activation. (**m**) Lateral cephalogram before treatment. (**n**) Lateral cephalogram during distraction. (**o**) 4 years after distraction

possible, and an inferior border of the mandible retractor is placed just above the inferior alveolar nerve at its entrance just superior to the lingua. A reciprocating saw is used to perform the horizontal osteotomy, protecting the soft tissues working within the periosteal envelope, from the posterior to the anterior border of the mandible. It is an incomplete osteotomy momentarily since the jaw should be in one piece to ease placing the transcutaneous screws that fixate the distraction device. The vertical distraction appliance is secured by bicortical screws through a percutaneous trocar. All distraction devices should be fixated before the osteotomy is completed through. A small straight chisel and the use of a torque movement complete the osteotomy.

5.2.4.2 Combinations

Combining body and ramus distraction allows the formation of the mandibular angle and creates bony regenerate for dental crowding alignment. This is the authors' preferred technique to treat unilateral and bilateral craniofacial microsomia or mandibular deficiency secondary to TMJ ankylosis. In these patients, the surgical goals are to increase mandibular ramus height and mandibular body length and relieve severe dental crowding.

The horizontal osteotomy is completed as previously described, and the wound is closed leaving the distraction device completely buried (Fig. 5.7).

A second osteotomy site is selected, usually between the premolars and a position anterior to the mental nerve. The reciprocating saw is used from the inferior border of the mandible, carefully elevating the soft tissues to visualize the dental roots or space between the premolars. The osteotomy is not completed, but the wound is partially closed, leaving a little gap to exert rotational force with a chisel to complete the osteotomy after placing the distraction device which is fixated with bicortical screws in the inferior arms and usually interdental wires with acrylic for reinforcement. The activation rod must exit at the level of the occlusal plane (Fig. 5.7).

This surgical technique has two objectives: to obtain equal mandibular ramus heights and to correct the severe anterior-posterior deficiency. These allow the orthodontist to align the teeth and correct the dental midline. However, the chin deformity and maxillary vertical issues need to be addressed at the time of distraction device removal. Children during active growth have little trouble treating discrepancies in the maxilla by orthodontic means along, slowly and progressively bringing the maxillary teeth into the new mandibular plane. Adults require a maxillary Le Fort I osteotomy with inferior repositioning, fixation with titanium plates, and vertical bone grafts obtained from the contralateral intact mandibular ramus.

The consolidation period for large movements varies widely. The body osteotomy heals faster than the mandibular ramus distraction. Lengthening the ramus requires a much longer mineralization period. Average time for a neonate is 8 months and up to 18 months in adults. Complex intraoral mandibular distraction is

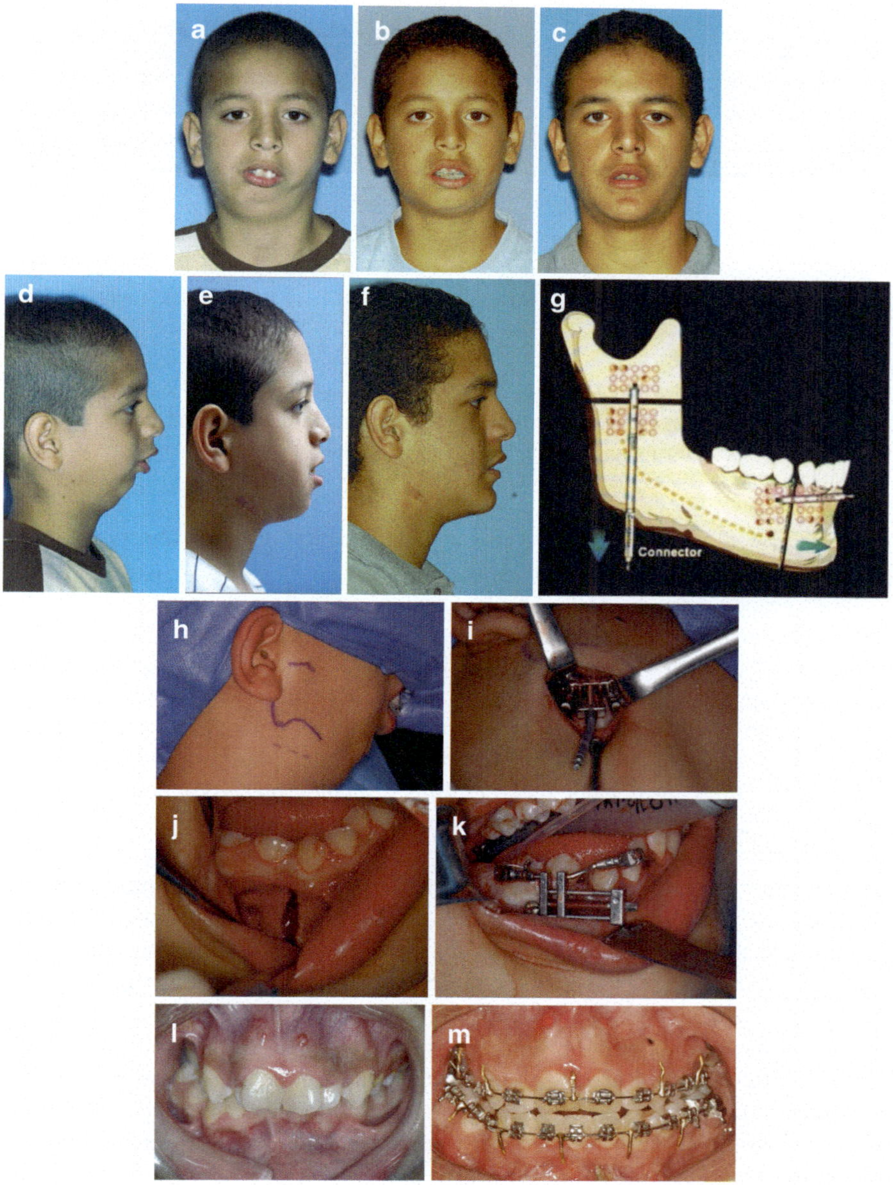

Fig. 5.7 An 8-year-old male patient with TMJ ankylosis treated with unilateral mandibular (ramus and body) distraction. (**a**) Frontal view pretreatment. (**b**) Frontal view immediately post distraction. (**c**) Frontal view 10 years postoperative. (**d**) Lateral view pretreatment. (**e**) Lateral view immediately post distraction and TMJ arthroplasty. (**f**) Lateral view after genioplasty. (**g**) Schematic of osteotomy sites with position of distraction devices. (**h**) Outline of mandible and proposed submandibular incision. (**i**) Distraction device (ramus) inserted through submandibular incision. (**j**) Intraoral view showing activation rod (**k**) Distraction device (body) inserted through intraoral incision. (**l**) Intraoral view preoperative. (**m**) Intraoral view post distraction and during orthodontic therapy

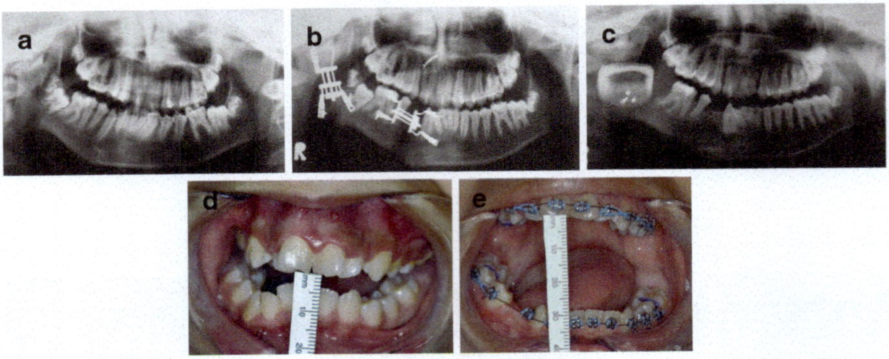

Fig. 5.8 Same patient as in Fig. 5.7. (**a**) Panoramic radiograph preoperative. Note the unilateral TMJ ankylosis. (**b**) Panoramic radiograph following activation of ramus and body distraction devices. (**c**) Panoramic radiograph showing TMJ implant. (**d**) Intraoral view preoperative. (**e**) Intraoral view postoperative. Note the increase in interincisal opening

a stable surgical technique if the complete consolidation period is observed before the distraction devices are removed (Fig. 5.8).

The surgeon must have the ability to change the final position of the distal segment after the activation phase is complete. Large mandibular disharmonies should not be treated by orthodontic therapy alone, since this type of dental movement can result in inadvertent relapse and periodontal defects and tooth loss. Change of the vector during activation or early consolidation period is a safe way to close an anterior or posterior open bite. Increasing the activation unilaterally could correct a deviated midline or mandibular asymmetry. After the activation phase is completed and the patient reaches a class I position with an adequate mandibular projection, the occlusion is carefully evaluated, and a decision to change the distal fragment is taken. The patient is placed under IV sedation, and local anesthetics are injected. Removing selected screws bilaterally disconnects the superior arms of the distraction device, maintaining one single bicortical screw on either side of the inferior arms to maintain the inferior border of the mandible lengthening. After reducing the interdental gap by contracting the segments superiorly, but not inferiorly, following screw removal, the mandible is digitally rotated around the inferior screw, changing the distal segment inclination. The 1 MPa changes from the 100s to the 80s as the segment rotates, and the distraction zone decreases in size between the teeth. The anterior open bite closes, and pogonion position is projected.

Orthodontic therapy is resumed 3 months after surgery, since large distractions require longer consolidation times. Orthodontic micro-implants may be needed to provide anchorage for large anterior movement of the molars to close the created interdental gap by moving the teeth anteriorly. These distraction techniques are predictable and stable, allowing major combined movements of 20–30 mm in each direction. Distraction osteogenesis is indicated for these clinical situations, whereas traditional orthognathic surgery would offer only limited outcomes, relapse, instability, or failures (see Figs. 5.7 and 5.8).

5.3 Bone Transport by Intraoral Distraction

5.3.1 Indications

- Medically compromised patients in whom major bone grafts are not indicated
- As an alternative for secondary surgery after an unsuccessful bone graft reconstruction
- Following removal of benign tumors or malignancies not requiring radiation
- Reconstruction of gunshot wound defects
- Management of osteomyelitis
- Treatment of malunions/nonunions

Bone transport is the concept of creating bone and soft tissues employing the principles of distraction osteogenesis. Osteotomies are made, and distraction devices are applied, following the distraction osteogenesis protocol. Depending on the number of surgical sites for the reconstruction, it could be classified as bifocal, trifocal, tetrafocal, and pentafocal [27–31]. Planning several segments to create an ideal mandibular shape is key to reduce treatment time, to obtain ideal height and width, and to create the optimal implant bone for dental implants.

In order to unite the transplant and receiving bones, the intervening tissue must be removed and either compressed or cancellous bone graft inserted—docking site surgery. An adequate time is required for consolidation and final bone remodeling, approximately 60 days for each centimeter of distraction [32, 33].

The mandible is basically five different straight lines structure, with two rami, two bodies, and one symphysis. Multi-segment bone transport allows the creation of the adequate curves and angles with the height and width necessary for dental implant insertion [31–33].

Serial radiographs are useful to visualize bone formation and mineralization, to remove the distraction appliances, and to insert dental implants for dental rehabilitation [31–35].

5.3.2 Preoperative Planning

Stereolithographic models, CT scans, and panoramic and cephalometric radiographs are used for surgical planning and prediction. The 3-D model is useful for complex reconstructions, and the anatomical model of the defect is essential to provide the exact measurements for pre-bending of the reconstruction plate, application of the devices, distraction vector planning, and location of the screws.

5.3.3 Principles

1. Because the distraction occurs in a linear plane, from point A to point B, the distraction zone will form the bone in a straight line. The elongated collagen fibers progressively mineralize in the months after surgery to convert into calcified bone.
2. The size of the transport disc plays an important role in large reconstructions, especially when the symphysis is involved. Multiple discs can be activated simultaneously, or continuous distraction stages could be performed, having the initial disc subdivided, to be transported in different directions or vectors.
3. The “hourglass” effect is formed if a single-bone disc is traveling over a long distance, or if the original thickness is not sufficient to create adequate volume. The disc must be at least 1.5–2.0 cm in thickness, height, and length.
4. The soft tissues also advance and create soft tissues while the bone is being transported. This is important because it includes the musculature and other soft tissues. Keratinized thick and resistant gingiva are required around the dental implants, and the adjacent gingival tissues are re-created.
5. When bone transport involves the symphyseal bone, a genioplasty must be considered to maintain symmetry of the chin.

5.3.4 Multifocal Distraction [35–37]

The concept of multifocal distraction is based on the use of multiple bone discs to repair the defect and allow rigid fixation to maintain the segments in place.

The reconstruction plate is placed holding the remaining bone segments in the correct position with at least three bicortical screws on each segment. For defects including the body and half or all of the symphyseal area, a complete side-to-side reconstruction plate is indicated. The distraction device travels on top of the plate for vector control, and it is placed supra-periosteally in order to prevent contamination with food and saliva. The biological principles of periosteal nutrition must be maintained. Major angle-to-angle reconstructions are performed in either several stages or using a multi-osteotomies/multidiscs concept.

First stage: the tumor is resected after fixating the reconstruction plate. To avoid segment displacement, the distraction devices are fixated according to the transport discs design, ideally a 15 mm size disc and a 2 mm intraoperative activation. The first disc usually extends from the angle of the mandible or from the most posterior part of the body; this segment will travel to the canine area. To avoid plate exposure in the symphyseal area, a chin prosthesis is temporarily placed and fixed to the most anterior part of the plate, while the two lateral discs (distraction discs) come forward, advancing the associated soft tissues. The chin prosthesis is removed after the transplant segments have been advanced to the parasymphysis area (Fig. 5.9).

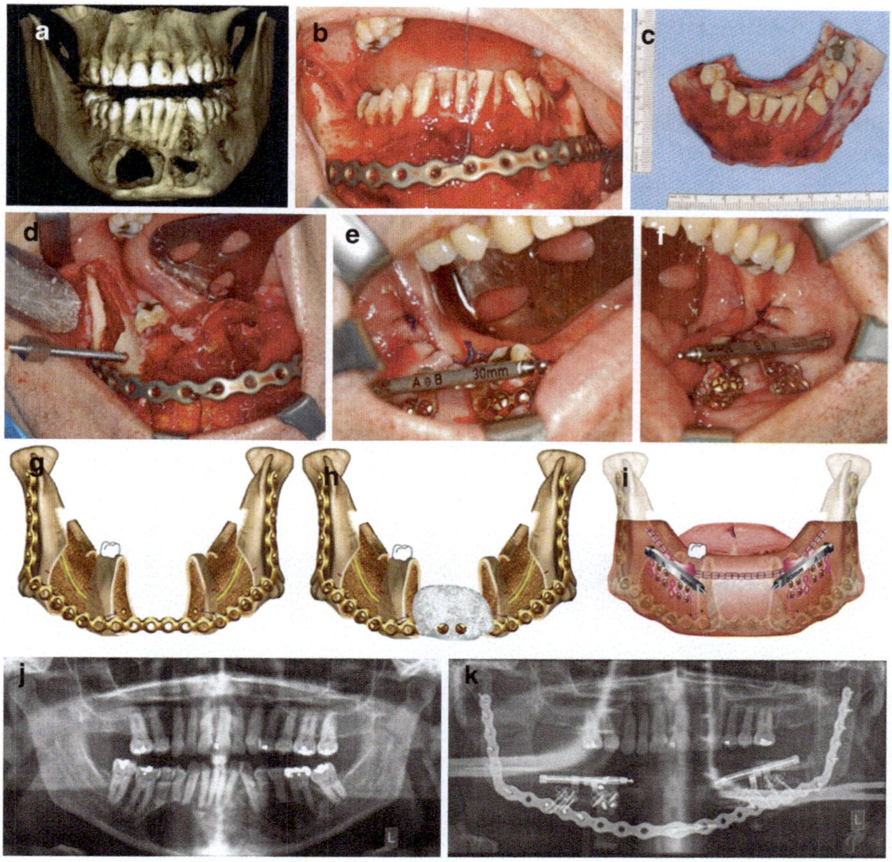

Fig. 5.9 A 45-year-old male with ameloblastic carcinoma who underwent three-dimensional mandibular reconstruction by trifocal transport distraction. (**a**) CT scan of lesion. (**b**) Reconstruction plate fashioned and drill holes made prior to resection. (**c**) Resection specimen. (**d**) Transport segments created by bilateral sagittal split osteotomies. The plate is fixed in position. (**e, f**) Distraction devices in place. Each segment was distracted 35mm. (**g–i**) Schematics illustrating trifocal distraction to reconstruct an anterior mandibular defect. A chin implant was fixed to the reconstruction plate to prevent soft tissue contraction during activation. (**j**) Panoramic radiograph preoperative. (**k**) Panoramic radiograph during bone transport

Second stage: reconstruction of the symphysis. After the first disc reaches the canine area, the traveling disc is sectioned in half, forming two discs. Rigid fixation of the posterior portion of the original disc to the reconstruction plate is accomplished, and the distraction device is removed. The anterior portion of the disc will continue traveling to traverse the symphysis with a new distraction device. It is important to fix the already transported disc to the plate to avoid the spring effect—the contraction of the collagen fibers pulling the segment to its original position before mineralization has been achieved. The consolidation period for major movements is prolonged for many months (Fig. 5.9).

5.3.5 Distraction Protocol

Seven days of latency period are recommended, followed by a 1 or ½ mm activation rate until distraction is completed. The distraction devices remain in place as a fixation system for 2 months for each centimeter of bony gain until they are exchanged for bicortical screws inserted from the reconstruction plate to the bone.

Third stage: at the completion of distraction, docking site surgery is indicated to achieve bony union between the two docking segments. This is a short procedure performed under IV sedation (Fig. 5.10).

5.3.6 Docking Site Surgery [32, 38–44] (Fig. 5.10)

The docking site is the area where the two bone segments meet. At the completion of activation, the leading edges of the two bones are usually hypertrophic and

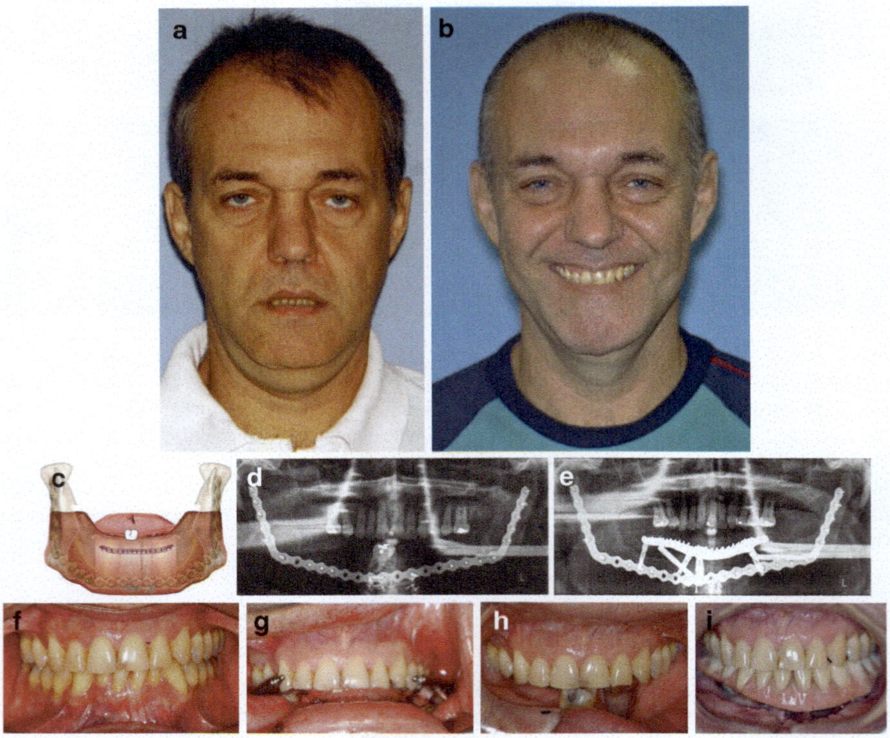

Fig. 5.10 Same patient as in Fig. 5.9. (**a**) Frontal view preoperative. (**b**) Frontal view 2 years postoperative. (**c**) After the consolidation period the fixation plates are *left* in place. (**d**, **e**) During consolidation, zygomatic and dental implants were inserted. (**f**–**i**) Occlusal views: preoperative, during bone transport with devices in place, and during consolidation (note second molar in midline), with final prosthesis on dental implants

sclerotic, covered by fibrous tissue. The two edges should be as close as possible, and the nonvital bone needs to be resected. A mucoperiosteal incision with minimal periosteal elevation is used to expose both edges. It is necessary to obtain a network of neoangiogenesis from the bone marrow and periosteum to enhance bony healing. The bone edges are prepared by making multiple perforations with a bur into the cortical and medullary bone; the distraction device is activated until the two segments meet; bone graft is obtained from the chin and inserted into the defect. Rigid fixation is established between the two bone segments either by the use of the reconstruction plate or by insertion of two miniplates.

The patient is placed on a soft and liquid diet for a prolonged period of time. As masticatory function is diminished, there is mandibular hypomobility and TMJ fibrosis, with interincisal opening reduction. The patient must commence daily functional and physiologic exercises to stimulate masticatory movements.

5.3.7 Dental Implants in Bone Transport

Implant technology allows the use of inclined dental implants and zygoma implants in mandibular areas where the bone of sufficient quality and quantity is available, permitting the prosthodontist to fabricate a fixed or hybrid dental rehabilitation. Most patients have quality bone in the symphysis area where zygoma implants could be inserted and the abutment is based at the level of the mandibular canines or premolars. Most patients are dentally rehabilitated with four dental implants in the anterior mandible with standard fixtures and zygoma implants inserted in the mandible. This protocol allows implant anchorage in the adjacent bone with mucosal penetration at a 45° angle and management parallel to the anterior regular implants.

Pearls and Pitfalls

- Intraoral mandibular distraction can be used for widening, lengthening, and bone transport.
- The techniques are surgeon and orthodontist labor-intensive and require close collaboration.
- Custom-designed distraction devices are often required.

References

1. Ilizarov GA. The tension-stress effect on the genesis and growth of tissues: part I. The influence of stability on fixation and soft tissue preservation. Clin Orthop. 1989;238:249.
2. Guerrero C. Rapid mandibular expansion. Rev Venez Ortod. 1990;48:1–2.
3. Little RM, Riedel RA, Artun J. An evaluation of changes in mandibular anterior alignment from 10 to 20 years post-retention. Am J Orthod Dentofac Orthop. 1988;93:423–8.

4. Karaharju-Suvanto T, Karaharju EO, Ranta R. Mandibular distraction: an experimental study in sheep. J Cranio-Maxillofac Surg. 1990;18:280–2.
5. Guerrero C, Bell WH, Flores A, Modugno VL, Constasti G, Rodriguez AM, et al. Distracción osteogenica mandibular intraoral. Odontol Dia. 1995;11:116–32.
6. Bell WH, Harper RP, Gonzalez M, Cherkashin AM, Samchukov ML. Distraction osteogenesis to widen the mandible. Br J Oral Maxillofac Surg. 1997;35:11–9.
7. Guerrero CA, Bell WH, Contasti GI, Rodriguez AM. Mandibular widening by intraoral distraction osteogenesis. Br J Oral Maxillofac Surg. 1997;35:383–92.
8. Bell WH, Gonzalez M, Guerrero CA, Samchukov ML. Intraoral widening of the mandible by distraction osteogenesis: histologic and radiographic assessment. J Oral Maxillofac Surg. 1997;55:97.
9. Bell WH, Gonzalez M, Samchukov ML, Guerrero CA. Intraoral widening and lengthening the mandible by distraction osteogenesis and histogenesis. J Oral Maxillofac Surg. 1999;57:548–62.
10. Guerrero CA, Bell WH, Contasti GI, Rodriguez AM. Intraoral mandibular distraction osteogenesis. Semin Orthod. 1999;5:35–40.
11. Del Santo M, Guerrero CA, Buschang PH, et al. Long-term skeletal and dental effects of mandibular symphyseal distraction osteogenesis. Am J Orthod Dentofac Orthop. 1999;1–62.
12. Contasti G, Rodriguez A, Guerrero CA. Orthodontic mandibular widening by distraction osteogenesis. Orthod Cyber J. 2001;35:165.
13. Bell WH, Gonzalez M, Guerrero C, Samchukov M. Distraction histogenesis: effect of intraoral widening on gingival and periodontal ligament. In: Arnaud D, editor. 3rd International Congress on Facial distraction processes. Paris and Bologna: Monduzzi editore; 2001. p. 173–178.
14. Bell WH, Epker BN. Surgical-orthodontic expansion of the maxilla. Am J Orthod. 1976;70(5):517–28.
15. McCarthy JG, Schreiber J, Karp N, Thorne CH, Grayson BH. Lengthening the human mandible by gradual distraction. Plast Reconstr Surg. 1992;89:1–8.
16. Chin M, Toth BA. Distraction osteogenesis in maxillofacial surgery using internal devices: review of five cases. J Oral Maxillofac Surg. 1996;54:45–53.
17. Harper RP, Bell WH, Hinton RJ, Browne R, Cherkashin AM, Samchukov ML. Reactive changes in the temporomandibular joint after midline osteodistraction. Br J Oral Maxillofac Surg. 1997;35:20–5.
18. DeDeyne PG, Paley D, Herzenberg JE. Muscle and its connective tissue adaptation to distraction osteogenesis. Abstract #3 ASAMI North America, First International Meeting. New Orleans; 1998.
19. Guerrero CA, Bell WH, Meza LS. Intraoral distraction osteogenesis. Maxillary and mandibular lengthening. Atlas Oral Maxillofac Surg Clin North Am (Distraction Osteogenesis). Suzanne U Stucki-McCormick (Guest Editor). 1999;7(1):111–51.
20. Samchukov ML, Cope JB, Harper RP, Ross JD. Biomechanical considerations for mandibular lengthening and widening by gradual distraction. Am J Oral Maxillofac Surg. 1998;56:51–9.
21. Schendel SA, Wolford LM, Epker BN. Mandibular deficiency syndrome. III. Surgical advancement of the deficient mandible in growing children: treatment results in twelve patients. Oral Surg Oral Med Oral Pathol. 1978;45:364–77.
22. Gonzalez M, Bell WH, Guerrero CA, Buschang PH, Samchukov ML. Positional changes and stability of bone segments during simultaneous bilateral mandibular lengthening and widening by distraction osteogenesis. Br J Oral Maxillofac Surg. 2001;39:169.
23. Trauner R, Obwegeser H. The surgical correction of mandibular prognathism and retrognathia with consideration of genioplasty: part I. Surgical procedures to correct mandibular prognathism and reshaping of the chin. Oral Surg Oral Med Oral Pathol. 1857;10:677–89.
24. Guerrero CA, Bell WH, Gonzalez M, Meza LS. Intraoral distraction osteogenesis. In: Fonseca RJ, editor. Oral and maxillofacial surgery, vol. 2. Philadelphia: W.B. Saunders; 2000. p. 359–402.

25. Guerrero CA, Figueroa F, Bell WH, Olmos-Malave Y, Rojas A, Gonzalez M. Surgical orthodontics in mandibular lengthening. In: Bell W, Guerrero C, editors. Distraction osteogenesis of the facial skeleton. Hamilton: BC Decker; 2007. p. 373–88.
26. Guerrero CA, Bell WH. Intraoral distraction. In: McCarthy JG, editor. Distraction of the craniofacial skeleton. New York: Springer; 1999. p. 219–48.
27. Guerrero CA, Bell WH, Gonzalez M, Figueroa F. Maxillo-mandibular reconstruction by intraoral bone transport. In: Arnaud D, editor. 3rd International Congress on Facial Distraction Processes, vol. 1. Paris and Bologna: Monduzzi; 2001. p. 569–574.
28. Costantino PD, Shybut G, Friedman CD, Pelzer HJ, Masini M, Shindo ML, Sisson GA. Segmental mandibular regeneration by distraction osteogenesis: an experimental study. Arch Otolaryngol Head Neck Surg. 1990;116:535–45.
29. Fonseca RJ, Walker RV. Oral and maxillofacial trauma. Philadelphia: W.B. Saunders; 1991. p. 275.
30. Guerrero CA, Bell WH, Gonzalez M, Rojas A. Intraoral mandibular bone transport: a case report. In: Samchukov M, Cope J, Cherkashin A, editors. Craniofacial distraction osteogenesis. St. Louis: Mosby; 2001. p. 372–5.
31. Gaggl AJ, Schultes GR, Karcher H. Alveolar ridge augmentation with the aid of distraction implants. In: Samchucov ML, Cope JB, Cherkashin AM, editors. Craniofacial distraction osteogenesis. St. Louis: Mosby; 2001. p. 401–13.
32. Gonzalez M, Guerrero CA, Henriquez M, Figueroa F, Domínguez E. Docking site surgery in bone transport. In: Arnaud D, editor. 5th International Congress of Maxillofacial and Craniofacial distraction. Paris and Bologna: Monduzzi editore; 2006. p. 99–104.
33. Guerrero CA, Bell HW, Gonzalez M. Mandibular remodeling: the fifth stage in distraction osteogenesis healing. In: Arnaud E, Diner PA, editors. 3rd International Congress on Cranial and Facial Bone Distraction Processes. Bologna and Paris: Monduzzi Editore; 2001. p. 267–273.
34. Guerrero CA, Bell WH, Gonzalez M, Figueroa F. Maxillo-mandibular reconstruction by intraoral bone transport. In: Arnaud D, editor. 3rd International Congress on Facial distraction processes. Paris and Bologna: Monduzzi Editore; 2001. p. 569–574.
35. Guerrero CA, Rojas A, Figueroa F, Gonzalez M, Bell WH, Boyne P. Radiographic evaluation of traditional versus rhBMP-2 inducted intraoral bone transport in mandibular reconstruction. In: Arnaud D, editor. 4th International Congress of Maxillofacial and Craniofacial distraction. Paris and Bologna: Monduzzi Editore; 2003. p. 391–396.
36. Guerrero CA, Figueroa F, Gonzalez M. 3-D alveolar distraction osteogenesis. In: Diner PA, Arnaud E, editors. Proceedings of the 4th International Congress of Maxillofacial and Craniofacial Distraction. Paris and Bologna: Monduzzi Editore; 2–5 July 2003. p. 37–42.
37. Guerrero CA, Gonzalez M, Dominguez E. Bone transport by distraction osteogenesis for maxillomandibular reconstruction. In: Bell W, Guerrero C, editors. Distraction osteogenesis of the facial skeleton. Hamilton: BC Decker; 2007. p. 501–19.
38. Hidding J, Lazar F, Zoeller JE. Vertical distraction of the alveolar process: a new technique for reconstructing the alveolar ridge. In: Samchucov ML, Cope JB, Cherkashin AM, editors. Craniofacial distraction osteogenesis. St. Louis: Mosby; 2001. p. 393–400.
39. Jensen OT. Alveolar segmental "sandwich" osteotomies for posterior edentulous mandibular sites for dental implants. J Oral Maxillofac Surg. 2006;64:471–5.
40. Oda T, Sawaki Y, Ueda M. Experimental alveolar ridge augmentation by distraction osteogenesis using a simple device that permits secondary implant placement. Int J Oral Maxillofac Implants. 2000;15:95–102.
41. Guerrero CA, Laplana R, Figueredo N, Rojas A. Surgical implant repositioning: a clinical report. Int J Oral Maxillofac Implants. 1999;14:48–54.
42. Guerrero CA, Gonzalez M, Laplana R, Rojas A. Reconstrução do rebordo alveolar mediante distração ostogênica para implantes osseointegrados. In: Dinato JC, Polido W, editors. Implantes osseointegrados: Cirugia e Prótese. Brazil: Artes Mèdicas; 2001. p. 423–39.

43. Razdolsky Y, Dessner S, El-Bialy T. Correction of alveolar ridge deficiency using the ROD-5 distraction device: a case report. In: Samchucov ML, Cope JB, Cherkashin AM, editors. Craniofacial distraction osteogenesis. St. Louis: Mosby; 2001. p. 454–8.
44. Ueda M. Maxillofacial bone distraction processes using osseointegrated implants and an intraoral device. In: Diner PA, Vasquez MP, editors. Proceeding of the International Congress on Cranial and Facial Bone Distraction Processes. Paris and Bologna: Monduzzi Editore; 19–21 June 1997. p. 75–84.

Distraction of the Maxilla (Le Fort I)

6

James P. Bradley

A Le Fort I osteotomy with maxillary advancement can be used to correct Class III malocclusion that is related to congenital or developmental maxillary hypoplasia. A Le Fort I osteotomy *combined with distraction osteogenesis* is a powerful technique that can be used to treat the most severe forms of maxillary hypoplasia [1]. It also offers the benefits of functional airway improvement. Le Fort I distraction advancement may improve obstructive sleep apnea or aid in the removal of a long-standing tracheostomy [2, 3]. It is a technique that may be performed before skeletal maturity or during childhood, after the maxillary canines have erupted. Traditional acute Le Fort I advancement is usually performed after skeletal maturity [4]. Performing a Le Fort I distraction can correct a child's facial deformity and may be important for his/her psychological well-being and self-confidence. Following a Le Fort I distraction during childhood, the subsequent need for a Le Fort I advancement at skeletal maturity may often be avoided. The importance of orthodontic involvement and preciese treatment planning cannot be overemphasized. This chapter will document the indications, techniques, instrumentation, and postoperative care involved with Le Fort I distraction.

6.1 Indications

Le Fort I distraction is used to treat patients with severe maxillary hypoplasia. This may develop in patients with cleft lip and palate deformities from both intrinsic maxillary growth disturbances and surgical scarring. For patients with class III malocclusion and mild to moderate maxillary hypoplasia who have attained skeletal maturity (<10 mm of advancement required), an orthognathic procedure, *acute advancement,* is recommended. However, for patients with class III malocclusion and severe maxillary hypoplasia (>10 mm of advancement required), Le Fort I

J.P. Bradley, M.D.
Temple University, Philadelphia, PA, USA
e-mail: jpbradley4@mac.com

J.G. McCarthy (ed.), *Craniofacial Distraction*,
DOI 10.1007/978-3-319-52564-8_6

distraction offers larger advancements with less evidence of relapse [4, 5]. For patients with alveolar defects, bone graft consolidation must be done prior to a Le Fort I distraction procedure. Cleft patients need to have the dentoalveolar arch unified before a maxillary distraction procedure. If the maxillary segment is not unified and the maxilla is in more than one piece, the distracted segments cannot be controlled and the result will be far from predictable.

Le Fort I osteotomy with an acute advancement allows for correction of a Class III malocclusion in the skeletally mature patient with or without a bilateral sagittal split osteotomy setback and allows for the patient to leave the operating room in optimal occlusion. However, the traditional technique of a Le Fort I osteotomy with an acute advancement has limitations. Alternatively, Le Fort I distraction offers three distinct advantages over the traditional technique for the patient with severe maxillary deficiency: (1) ability to treat younger patients, (2) larger advancements to the maxillary segment, and (3) less relapse. Patients with severe maxillary hypoplasia may have a facial deformity that results in teasing and ridicule by classmates and peers. Rather than waiting until skeletal maturity, younger patients may undergo a maxillary advancement with distraction with the benefit of improvement in facial form. The Le Fort I distraction procedure may be performed provided the maxillary canines have erupted. Prior to eruption of the maxillary canines, the canine roots are in the line of the Le Fort I osteotomy. With an early correction of a maxillary deficiency facial deformity, self-confidence, self-esteem, and social integration may improve. With this in mind, decisions on the timing and technique of the procedure should be tailored to the individual patient.

With traditional techniques, the amount of maxillary advancement is limited by soft tissue recoil and scarring [5]. A Le Fort I acute advancement exceeding 10 mm has been shown to result in more relapse and the need for subsequent corrective surgery [4]. For patients with severe maxillary deficiency, a "compromise procedure" of Le Fort I acute advancement with simultaneous mandibular setback had been offered in the past prior to the introduction of Le Fort I distraction. The outcome of the "compromise procedure" was, however, a compromise in aesthetic improvement. With an optimal sagittal advancement, there is more midface soft tissue fill and a more convex face. Rosen showed that sagittal midfacial fullness, even exceeding normal SNA cephalometric measurements, results in a more pleasing long-term cosmetic outcome: "There is a sense of highlighting, definition, angularity, and refinement when the facial mask is well supported by skeletal foundation. With a lack of skeletal support, the face is devoid of these features and, in the extreme, can be described as amorphous" [6].

6.2 Internal Devices vs. External Devices

The indications for the use of internal devices and external devices are similar. Some practitioners prefer the external device, e.g., a RED device, for Le Fort I distraction procedures [7]. Other practitioners prefer internal device (Zurich device) for Le Fort I distraction procedures [4]. There are advantages and disadvantages for

Table 6.1 Internal vs. external Le Fort I distraction devices advantages and disadvantages

Le Fort I distraction devices		
	Advantages	Disadvantages
External devices	Ease of implantation	Unsightly appearance[a]
	Less periosteal stripping	Cumbersome
	"Pushing" and "pulling" force	Become dislodged, loosen
	3D Control of vectors[b]	Pin site infection
Internal device	Hidden, Concealed[a]	Staged procedures
	Closer to osteotomy	More periosteal stripping
	Earlier return to school/work	More difficult insertion/removal
	Longer consolidation times	Limit to distraction distance

[a]Often cited as the preference for internal devices
[b]Often cited as the preference for external devices

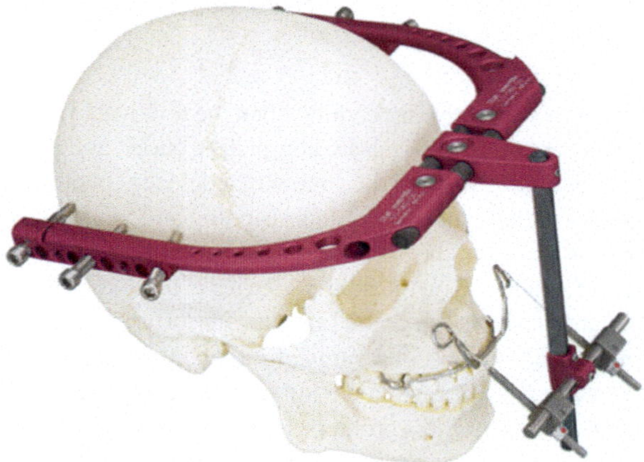

Fig. 6.1 External distraction device placed on a preoperative model showing the halo stabilized to the parietal skull with pins

both (Table 6.1). The osteotomies and down fracture are technically the same for both. The external Le Fort I devices have the theoretic advantage of less periosteal stripping and ease of implantation. An external device allows for both "pulling" and "pushing" of the advancing Le Fort I segment, whereas the internal device only "pushes" the segment forward. An advantage often cited by practitioners who prefer the external Le Fort I device is that it offers better three-dimensional control through the use of external adjustments during the distraction process. However, the external device is more likely to become dislodged or moved during play. This may require a readjustment or a reoperation for replacement. With the external device, pin-site infection is the most common problem and is usually treated with more meticulous pin care and oral antibiotics. The most obvious drawback to the use of external devices for Le Fort I distraction is the appearance of the devices (Fig. 6.1).

There are theoretic and practical advantages to the use of the internal device for Le Fort I distraction. The internal devices are applied closer to the osteotomy site. The devices are concealed (Fig. 6.2). The turning arms may be removed in the office

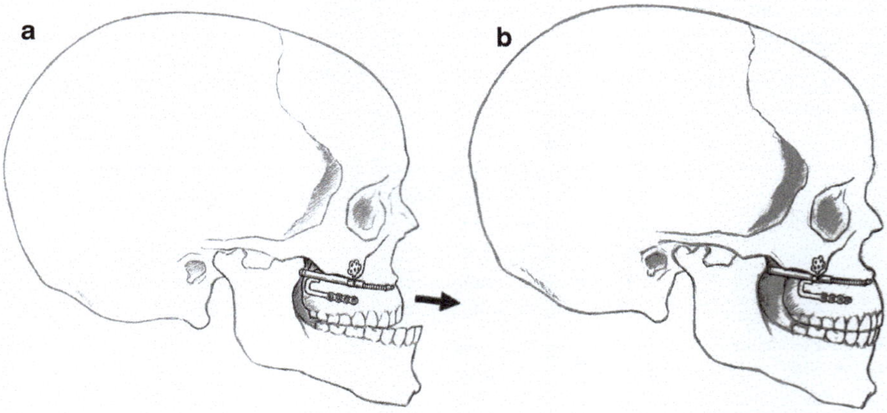

Fig. 6.2 Internal Le Fort I distraction device: (**a**) preactivation maxillary position, (**b**) postactivation maxillary position

without an operative procedure when the removable arms are used. After removal of the turning arms, the devices are completely buried and the patient may return to school or daily activities without the stigma of a device. Theoretical disadvantages of the internal devices include more periosteal stripping and more dissection upon implantation. Also, there is a limit to the distance of distraction with internal devices. The length or size of the activation rod on the internal device is limited by the distance from the plate fixation site anteriorly to the cranial base posteriorly (approximately 20–25 mm). Because of this limitation, a second surgical intervention was necessary in order to "re-zero" the distraction device and gain addition length for severe cases requiring a larger advancement. To alleviate this problem, a new "telescopic" Le Fort I distraction device has been designed to permit greater distraction distances. It has three stages, each of which is 10 mm. At the completion of one stage, the next stage will open. The advantage of the telescopic device is that at the insertion procedure there is a shorter activation rod.

6.3 Preoperative Planning

For any orthognathic surgical procedure, including Le Fort I distraction, preoperative planning is necessary for optimal results. Prior to Le Fort I acute advancement orthognathic procedures, orthodontic removal of dental compensations is necessary. When orthodontically ready, patients undergo preoperative planning including: cephalometric analysis, cephalometric prediction, model surgery, and splint fabrication. Manual cephalometry has been employed for years. More recently, computerized cephalometric prediction has become popular. With the advent of three-dimensional imaging, a Visual Treatment Objective (VTO) may be performed to predict hard and soft tissue changes to achieve facial balance. Likewise, preoperative planning is also useful for Le Fort I distraction. Predicted results presented to the Le Fort I distraction patients prior to the procedure help to assess treatment feasibility, optimize case management, and increase patient understanding.

Virtual Surgical Planning (VSP) has been increasingly used for orthognathic procedures and also has a role in distraction cases. The goals for VSP orthognathic procedures are similar to those of traditional planning for jaw cases with achievement in optimal aesthetic and functional stability with maximum intercuspation. For VSP planning of Le Fort I distraction cases, the following are required: (1) a cone-beam CT scan, (2) maxilla and mandibular impressions, and (3) a bite registration. Planning for the distraction procedure involves location of the osteotomies, cutting guides, vectors, and choice of devices. The procedure can be customized to the patient and treatment plan (Fig. 6.3). In addition, underlying tooth roots are visualized to aid in plate placement.

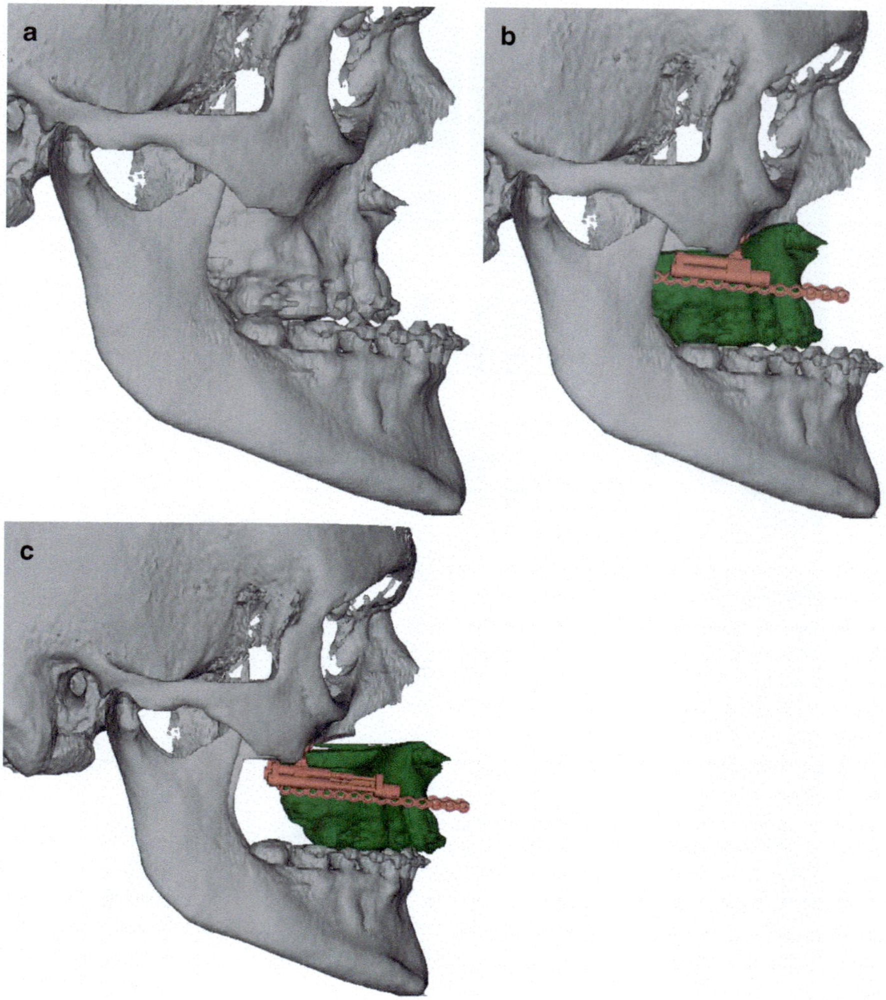

Fig. 6.3 Lateral view of three-dimensional CT scan for visual treatment objective: (**a**) preoperative, (**b**) predistraction position of maxillary segment (*green*) with telescopic device (*pink*), (**c**) postdistraction position of maxillary segment (*green*) with telescopic device (*pink*)

There is a select group of skeletally mature patients who have severe maxillary deficiency (greater than 10 mm) *and* mandibular pathology (prognathism or asymmetry). Rather than a compromise procedure, a staged Le Fort I distraction followed by a mandibular setback/rotation procedure may be done. In this case, the mandibular procedure is often done after the distraction, at the time of device removal (Fig. 6.4).

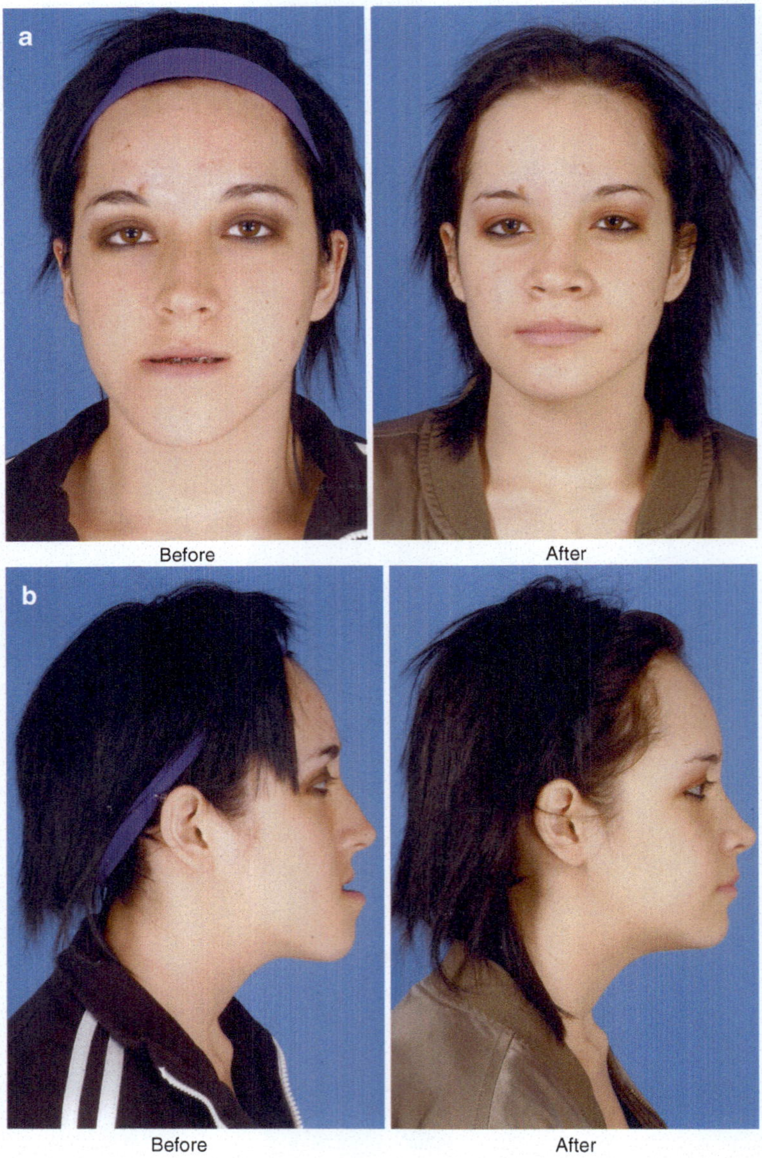

Fig. 6.4 Images of patient who underwent Le Fort I distraction followed by mandibular rotation for correction of asymmetry: (**a**) preoperative and postoperative frontal views, (**b**) preoperative and postoperative lateral views

6.4 Operative Technique

1. A nasoendotracheal tube is suture-secured and a throat pack is placed. The medial canthi are tattooed for vertical measurement to the lateral orthodontic bracket or incisor edge.
2. A gingivobuccal sulcus incision is made with the Colorado tipped bovie. Subperiosteal dissection is performed with a periosteal elevator to deglove the anterior maxilla, piriform aperture, nasal mucosa, and ptergomaxillary region.
3. Osteotomies are performed with the reciprocating saw at the Le Fort I level through the zygomaticomaxillary buttresses, nasomaxillary buttresses, and base of the septum. (A high Le Fort I osteotomy, superiolaterally to the infraorbital foramen, is performed for patients with hypoplastic malar regions.) A Kawamoto osteotome is used to separate the ptergomaxillary junction.
4. Maxillary down fracture is performed. The serrated Kawamoto osteotome is placed within the ptergomaxillary osteotomy site to stretch the soft tissues of the Le Fort I segment.
5. While holding the Le Fort I segment down, posterior bony interferences may be removed with a rongeur.
6. Le Fort I segment is held into position and the vertical height is measured.
7. For the internal devices (Zurich, KLS Martin L.P., Jacksonville, FL), right- and left-side devices are checked for positioning. Plate bending and burring of a notch in the zygomatic body for rod placement are often done at this time. The detachable turning arms are placed and the devices are fixed with monocortical screws.
8. For the external devices (RED device) on table, assembly of the device is required including: the distraction halo with fixation screws, the vertical rod, and horizontal cross bar for wire attachment to the intraoral splint. Alternatively, a bone-borne retention plate to the maxilla may be used and attached by wires to the horizontal bar.
9. Either of the devices should be tested by advancing the distraction device and returning it to the zero position.
10. For the internal devices, elastic bands are placed on hooked brackets or on 4-maxillomandibular fixation (MMF) screws (KLS Martin L.P., Jacksonville, FL). (The elastic bands may be placed either during the primary procedure or at the time of removal of the turning arms following activations. The bands help to guide the Le Fort I segment into appropriate occlusion during activation and prevent an anterior open bite deformity.)
11. Finally, a nasal cinch suture is used to avoid alar base flaring and the gingivobuccal sulcus incision is closed with running locking 4–0 chromic suture.

6.5 Postoperative Care and Orthodontic Manipulation

Activation is commenced the day after the Le Fort I osteotomy (latency = 1 day) at 1 mm per day (rate) for two times per day (rhythm). Patients are followed weekly in the office for progress. During the distraction process, close observation is necessary. The generate bone can be “molded” and the maxillary segment can be guided into proper occlusion or the predicted location. For internal Le Fort I distraction devices, elastic rubber bands are used to guide the maxillary segment. Orthodontic banding and hooks are useful for molding the generate bone. For external Le Fort I distraction (RED) devices, the distraction vector can be altered or adjusted at any time during activation since the device components are external. The horizontal rod(s) can be adjusted up or down along the midline vertical rod. Activation is continued until the proper overjet, overbite, and relatively stable posterior occlusion are achieved (Figs. 6.5 and 6.6). For patients at skeletal maturity, Le Fort I activation is continued until the maxillary segment can be “docked” into an intermediate or final splint.

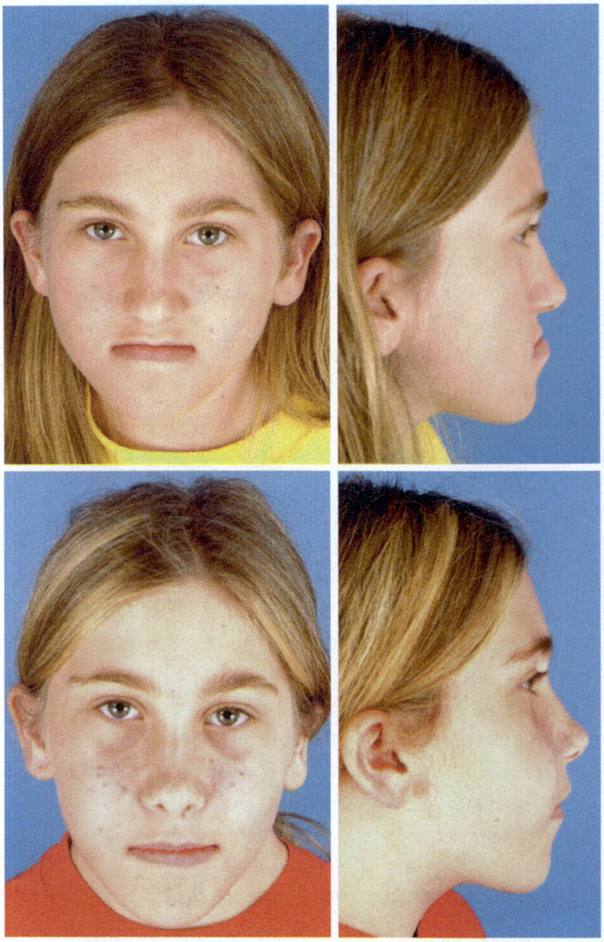

Fig. 6.5 Images of patient before (*upper panel*) and after (*lower panel*) Le Fort I distraction to correct maxillary hypoplasia and obstructive sleep apnea

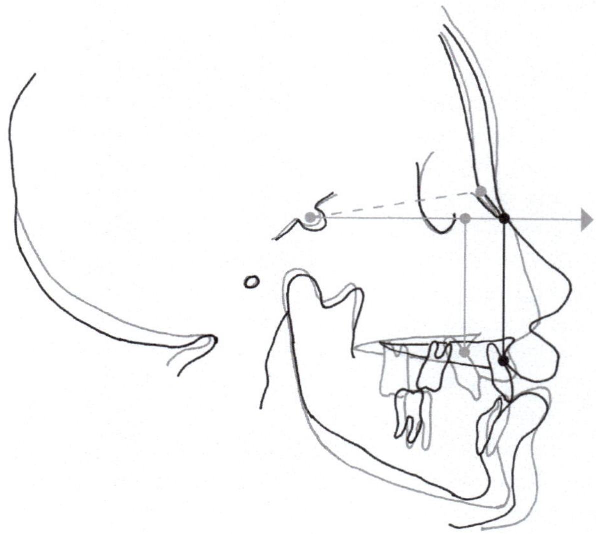

Fig. 6.6 Predistraction lateral cephalometric tracing (*gray*) and postdistraction cephalometric tracing (*black*)

After completion of activation, the Le Fort I distraction device is kept in place during the consolidation period. Follow-up radiographic studies have shown that most consolidation or bony deposition occurs in the ptergomaxillary region [8]. Even when radiolucencies are observed anteriorly, the maxillary segment is typically solid and clinically rigid. When reoperation is necessary after a Le Fort I distraction procedure, down fracture is more difficult because of the substantial bone healing in the ptergomaxillary region.

6.6 Complications

Many of the potential complications to Le Fort I distraction are related to the complications of a Le Fort I osteotomy and down fracture. Complications from a Le Fort I procedure have been estimated to be 6.4% [4]. Patients with cleft lip and palate deformities or patients with major anatomic abnormalities have a higher risk of complications. Reported complications include: malocclusion, septal deviation, hemorrhage, AV fistula, pseudoaneurysm, epistaxis, necrosis of the maxilla, gingival retraction, abscess, sinusitis, eustachian tube dysfunction, and blindness [4].

6.7 Outcomes

The biggest risk for relapse in a Le Fort I procedure is the length of advancement [9]. A subset of cleft patients with severe maxillary deficiency (>10 mm) were studied to compare traditional Le Fort I acute advancement to Le Fort I distraction [5].

The distraction group underwent a greater mean length of advancement (25 mm vs. 11 mm). The traditional group of patients had more relapse (63% developed relapse and 55% required reoperation). The distraction group had only 15% relapse. Soft tissue constriction was thought to contribute to the higher rate of relapse in the traditional group of patients. The gradual stretch of soft tissues probably accounted for the improved outcome in the distraction group of patients.

It is known that velopharyngeal insufficiency (VPI) may develop after Le Fort I advancement in cleft patients [10]. As the maxilla moves forward, the palate moves with it. Enlargement of the velopharyngeal space may impede closure of the sphincter. Le Fort I distraction has been shown to be protective against speech problems even in severe maxillary deficiency cases. In the study above, none of the severe maxillary deficiency patients had velopharyngeal insufficiency (VPI) preoperatively [5]. Postoperatively, VPI was found in 42% more patients in the traditional or acute Le Fort I advancement group as compared to the Le Fort I distraction group.

For syndromic patients with craniofacial dysostosis who require a midface advancement, the degree of advancement required for the midface and maxilla are usually not the same. Often, the advancement needed to correct the midface is less than the advancement needed for the maxilla. The midface advancement should be aimed at correcting orbital deficiencies. The maxillary advancement should be aimed at obtaining optimal final occlusion with acceptable aesthetics. The same indications for a Le Fort I distraction should be used with these patients as previously outlined in this chapter. If a Le Fort III distraction is performed in midchildhood, the Le Fort I advancement can be delayed until skeletal maturity. Decisions on the timing and technique are on a case-by-case basis with the help of orthodontist input.

Pearls and Pitfalls

- For the management of facial skeletal deformities, Le Fort I distraction offers the ability to correct a wider range of malocclusions by movement of the maxilla in all three planes of space.
- Le Fort I distraction allows for movement of the maxilla a *greater distance* with *less relapse*.
- Clinical outcomes after Le Fort I distraction have shown the added benefit of functional airway improvement (resolution of sleep apnea).
- Clinical outcomes for Le Fort I distraction also suggest protection of speech problems (less VPI).
- An emphasis should be placed on precise orthodontic preparation, presurgical planning, choice of devices, operative techniques, and postoperative adjustments for predictable and stable results.
- Recent advances in technology are aiding surgeons with virtual surgical planning and more precise outcomes.

References

1. Bradley JP. Craniofacial distraction osteogenesis. In: Thaller S, Bradley CP, Gari JI, editors. Craniofacial surgery. New York: CRC Press; 2007.
2. Taylor BA, Brace M, Hong P. Upper airway outcomes following midface distraction osteogenesis: a systemic review. J Plast Reconstr Aesthet Surg. 2014;67:891–9.
3. Gokce SM, Gorgulu S, Karacayli U, Gokce HS, Battal B. Three-dimensional evaluation of nasal and pharyngeal airway after Le Fort I maxillary distraction osteogenesis. Int J Oral Maxillofac Surg. 2015;44:455–61.
4. Buchanan EP, Hyman CH, Le Fort I. Osteotomy. Semin Plast Surg. 2013;27:149–54.
5. Kumar A, Gabbay JS, Nikjoo R, Heller JB, O'Hara CM, Sisodia M, Garri JI, Wilson LS, Kawamoto Jr HK, Bradley JP. Improved outcomes in cleft patients with severe maxillary deficiency after Le Fort I internal distraction. Plast Reconstr Surg. 2006;117:1499.
6. Rosen HM, Treatment planning: the role of facial disproportion. In: Rosen HM, editors. Aesthetic perspectives in jaw surgery, New York, Springer, 1997.
7. Polley JW, Figueroa AA. Management of severe maxillary deficiency in childhood and adolescence through distraction osteogenesis with an external, adjustable, rigid distraction device. J Craniofac Surg. 1997;8:181.
8. Dua G, Navin Kumar A, Roy ID, Roy SK. Maxillary distraction osteogenesis in cleft lip and palate cases with midface hypoplasia using rigid external distractor: an alternative technique. J Craniofac Surg. 2014;25(3):746–51.
9. Proffit WR, Phillips C, Turvey TA. Stability following superior repositioning of the maxilla by Le Fort I osteotomy. Am J Orthod Dentofac Orthop. 1987;92:151.
10. Witzel MA, Munro IR. Velopharyngeal insufficiency after maxillary advancement. Cleft Palate J. 1977;14:176.

Distraction of the Midface: Le Fort III and Monobloc

7

Joseph G. McCarthy and Roberto L. Flores

Gillies and Harrison [1] reported the first Le Fort III advancement osteotomy, which underwent relapse, and Gillies vowed never to repeat the procedure. The technique was later refined and popularized by Tessier [2] who placed iliac bone graft between the separated bony segments and performed the intraorbital osteotomy posterior to the medial canthus. The technique was eventually promoted and practiced in the younger patient [3]. The monobloc acute advancement was reported and popularized by Ortiz-Monasterio et al. [4]. However, in the Le Fort III/monobloc acute advancement osteotomy, there were multiple problems. Bone grafts had to be harvested, and there was a hardware burden, including maxillomandibular fixation (MMF). The infection rate was relatively high, especially in the monobloc procedure. Overall, these procedures had a high morbidity rate with a prolonged operating time and hospital stay.

After the clinical success with mandibular distraction, preliminary lab work was focused on midface distraction in animals by several groups around the world [5, 6]. At the same time, two types of midface distraction devices were developed. Buried devices were designed to be secured to the mobilized midface segment and the temporal bone [7], whereas an external halo frame was developed by Polley and Figueroa [8].

The development of midface and monobloc distraction represented a major paradigm shift. When applied to younger patients, it was a simpler procedure, and in all patients, it obviated the need to harvest bone grafts and to use complicated fixation systems. The amount of blood transfusion was reduced, a greater degree of stable midface advancement was achieved, and there was less morbidity, as well as reduced operative times and shorter lengths of hospital stay [9–11].

J.G. McCarthy, M.D. (✉) • R.L. Flores, M.D.
Wyss Department of Plastic Surgery, NYU Langone Medical Center, New York, NY, USA
e-mail: Joseph.mccarthy@nyumc.org

J.G. McCarthy (ed.), *Craniofacial Distraction*,
DOI 10.1007/978-3-319-52564-8_7

7.1 Pathology

The most common diagnosis of the patient undergoing midface distraction is syndromic craniosynostosis such as Crouzon, Apert, and Pfeiffer syndromes, although Le Fort III reconstruction can be used in patients with a cleft and infraorbital hypoplasia [12].

In syndromic craniosynostosis, there are a variety of cranial vault abnormalities, the most common of which is a brachycephaly with a reduction in the anteroposterior dimension of the cranial vault. This can be associated with increased intracranial pressure, an important finding leading to the recommendation of monobloc distraction. The supraorbital rims can also be recessed, resulting in exorbitism. These midface anomalies are characterized by exorbitism, downward slanting of the palpebral fissures, recession of the nasomaxillary and zygomatic complexes accompanied by a Class III malocclusion (anterior crossbite), and nasopharyngeal respiratory obstruction. The midline of the midface can be vertically foreshortened in the patient with Apert syndrome, and the convexity of the face is commonly lost due to bony hypoplasia in this area. While the mandible is of normal size and position, there is usually retrusion of the bony chin.

7.2 Indications

The usual indications for midface or monobloc distraction are increased intracranial pressure (ICP), exorbitism, airway obstruction, midface hypoplasia with malocclusion, and craniofacial dysmorphism.

The cranial vault abnormality is usually characterized by frontal bone retrusion or brachycephaly with or without evidence of increased intracranial pressure.

The exorbitism can result in exposure of the cornea with threat of blindness. One must define the skeletal pathology contributing to the exorbitism. If there is supraorbital retrusion, as characterized by an A-Cor value of −5 mm [13], the planned exorbitism correction must include monobloc distraction. If the supraorbital rims are not retruded, a subcranial Le Fort III distraction should adequately advance the recessed inferior orbital rims and obviate the need for a transcranial approach.

Airway obstruction is another indication for midface distraction. The usual anatomic site for the obstruction is in the nasopharyngeal space, but it should be noted that patients with syndromic craniosynostosis commonly have a multilevel obstruction pattern [14–17]. Pfeiffer syndrome, in particular, has a high incidence of tracheobronchial anomalies [18, 19] which would not be corrected by a midface distraction. Therefore, comprehensive airway analysis is recommended in all patients experiencing airway obstruction.

Midface hypoplasia with malocclusion is a prominent feature of the patient with syndromic craniosynostosis. The "dishpan facies" is associated with a Class III malocclusion, anterior crossbite, obstructive sleep apnea, and significant dysmorphism, all of which can be corrected by midface distraction.

Absolute indications for midface distraction in the *growing child* are:

(a) Increased intracranial pressure/brachycephaly
(b) Exorbitism/corneal exposure
(c) Severe airway obstruction
(d) Severe dysmorphism with malocclusion

Absolute indications in the *adult patient* are:

(a) Severe exorbitism
A-Cor of −5 mm. This finding tilts the decision in favor of a monobloc distraction because of the retrofrontal infection threat with the monobloc acute osteotomy advancement.
(b) Midface hypoplasia with an anterior crossbite greater than 13 mm.
(c) History of previously unsuccessful midface advancement.

Controversial indications for midface distraction in the *growing child* are:

(a) Mild dysmorphism without evidence of increased ICP, OSA, and corneal exposure
(b) Severe OSA in the background of a second and significant airway anomaly

Controversial indications for the *adult patient* are:

(a) Midface hypoplasia with an anterior crossbite less than 13 mm and no evidence of airway obstruction. One must recognize that in the skeletally mature patient there must be a functioning Class I occlusion at the completion of the treatment process.

7.3 Preoperative Assessment

Preoperative assessment is conducted with the appropriate members of the craniofacial clinical team.

7.3.1 Physical Examination

Examination is carefully done. The forehead and supraorbital rim are examined to detect retrusion of these anatomic elements. The Mulliken A-Cor value [13] must be recorded. The nasomaxillary complex as well as the orbitozygomatic areas are usually recessed. The exorbitism must be assessed by recording the retrusion of the supraorbital and inferior orbital rims. Scleral show usually accompanies retrusion of the inferior orbital rims (negative vector). There can be scarring of the cornea secondary to corneal exposure, and the support (or lack of support) for the lower eyelids must be recorded.

The occlusion is assessed and the crossbite recorded in millimeters. The maxillary arch is constricted and there can be dental crowding. An unusually long velum is usually noted. The details of the dental/orthodontic assessment are presented in more detail in Chapter 9.

7.3.2 Ophthalmology Assessment

As there is a significant incidence of increased intracranial pressure in patients with syndromic craniosynostosis, ophthalmologic assessment should be pursued prior to surgical intervention. The presence of papilledema may affect the surgical plan as well as the timing of surgery. Although craniocerebral disproportion, hydrocephalus, and CO_2 retention resulting from obstructive sleep apnea are known causes of increased intracranial pressure and progressive visual loss, there are other eye disorders that are common to this patient population. Strabismus, anisometropia, astigmatism, and ametropia should be identified and treated to prevent the subsequent development of amblyopia. Finally, regular evaluation of the cornea with fluorescein stain will identify corneal exposure. Ironically, many cases of corneal exposure are related to iatrogenic injury during surgery. Therefore, it is important to protect the cornea by lubricating the eyes during and after surgical intervention.

7.3.3 Respiratory Evaluation

Patients affected by syndromic craniosynostosis commonly have airway obstruction at the level of the nasopharynx (see [14]); however, a multilevel pattern of airway obstruction is common in this patient population (see [15]). Therefore, any patient with clinical evidence of airway obstruction should undergo nasoendoscopic evaluation by an otolaryngologist and a sleep study evaluation to quantify the severity of airway obstruction and rule out central sleep apnea. The functional outcome of midface distraction on breathing should be followed by a postoperative sleep study.

7.3.4 Photography

Medical quality photographs are a critical component of documentation and are also used in preoperative planning. The following views are obtained: frontal, three-quarters, profile, submental vertex, bird's eye, occlusal, and oculomotor. Three dimensional photography has the benefit of creating a digital moulage of the face in which linear and volumetric values may be recorded for surgical planning and serial follow-up.

7.3.5 Cephalograms

Cephalograms (posteroanterior, lateral, and basilar views) are easily obtained in the patient over 3–4 years of age. They are invaluable in documenting skeletal integrity, the dental and occlusal status, and retropharyngeal airway. These images, which expose the growing patient to less radiation than a CT scan, allow linear and angular measures to be plotted to define the pathology and to plan the surgical procedure with software programs. Follow-up cephalograms are particularly indicated in the postoperative period and long-term follow-up. Panoramic radiographs (panorex) are also obtained.

7.3.6 CT Scans

CT scans are mandatory prior to surgical intervention, and the introduction of the ICAT has simplified this aspect of the preoperative evaluation. The CT scans document the quality and volume of the affected bone and the dimensions/volume of the airway and orbits and provide insight into the pathology of the cranial vault. Particular attention should be paid to the integrity of the lateral orbital rims if a fronto-orbital advancement had been performed in infancy. Cranial defects should also be assessed in terms of pin placement for positioning of the distraction devices.

7.3.7 Other Key Variables

7.3.7.1 Age of Patient

It is difficult to perform midface distraction in the patient 1–3 years of age because patient cooperation can be challenging. It is also important to establish that family cooperation will also be available through the entire treatment course. These decisions are best made with the nurse practitioner and psychologist, especially in the pediatric patient. In the adolescent patient (13–17 years of age), elective midface distraction is delayed until skeletal maturity is achieved, provided there is no need for intervention because of the dangers of increased ICP, corneal exposure, or obstructive airway. Although there are case reports of neonatal midface distraction, long-term analysis is lacking to support this type of intervention.

7.3.7.2 General Health

As in any preoperative assessment, it is important that the patient enjoy optimal health, especially when one considers neurologic, respiratory, and cardiac problems. Cardiac clearance should be obtained from patients with congenital heart anomalies. Respiratory dysfunction should be assessed by a pediatric otolaryngologist and pulmonologist.

7.3.7.3 Bone Volume/Quality

Bone of adequate volume is essential for application of the distraction devices, and a fundamental principle of distraction osteogenesis is that the osteotomy is made through healthy, well-vascularized bone of adequate volume for optimal generation of bone. The cranial vault should be assessed for any defects resulting from previous surgical procedures that could interfere with the application of distraction devices. The lateral orbital walls can be hypoplastic because of previous

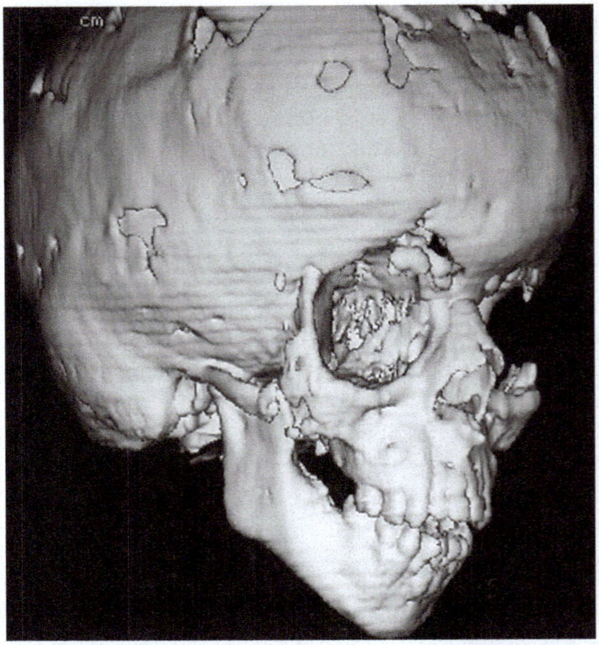

Fig. 7.1 Absence of lateral orbital wall following fronto-orbital advancement and cranial vault remodeling in infancy

fronto-orbital advancements (Fig. 7.1). If previous surgery has rendered the lateral orbital walls severely hypoplastic, the surgeon should consider a first-stage autogenous bone grafting procedure.

7.4 Orthodontic Assessment

See Chapter 9.

7.5 Preoperative Surgical Planning

As mentioned earlier, appropriate cardiac clearance, airway analysis, and ophthalmologic evaluation are required prior to surgery. The team anesthesiologist's input and planning are likewise important. Complete blood count and a type and crossmatch should be obtained. History of all previous craniofacial, neurological, ophthalmologic, and airway interventions are carefully documented. Presence of a VP shunt or Chiari malformation should warrant a neurosurgical assessment prior to surgery. If there is history of airway obstruction, an endoscopic evaluation of the airway and sleep study should be obtained. Physical exam should include palpation for cranial defects, position of the supraorbital and infraorbital rim in relation to the anterior cornea (A-cor), vertical position of the lateral and medial canthus, the anterior/posterior position of the malar eminence, the degree of anterior crossbite, and a detailed dental evaluation.

Photographs, cephalograms, and CT scans, as previously mentioned, are mandatory in the preoperative period. If the patient has had a previous midface advancement, the quality of the bony volume at the lateral orbital rim, the zygoma, and the pterygomaxillary suture is carefully evaluated. The vertical position of the cribriform plate and crista galli are likewise noted.

Planning the vector of distraction is critical, and the details are discussed later in the chapter.

The choices of osteotomy are as follows:

- Monobloc (frontofacial)
- Le Fort III (subcranial)
- Le Fort III and Le Fort I
- Bipartition/monobloc (see Chapter 8)
- Le Fort II and orbitozygomatic advancement

In the selection of the distraction device, the surgeon should consider several variables, but rigidity, as in all distraction procedures, is an absolute requirement to achieve adequate advancement and bony consolidation at the osteotomy sites. The buried devices, usually fixated between the temporal bone and the osteotomized midface segment, are less conspicuous and less vulnerable to postoperative trauma (Fig. 7.2). However, they are restricted to a single vector, and, if there is device

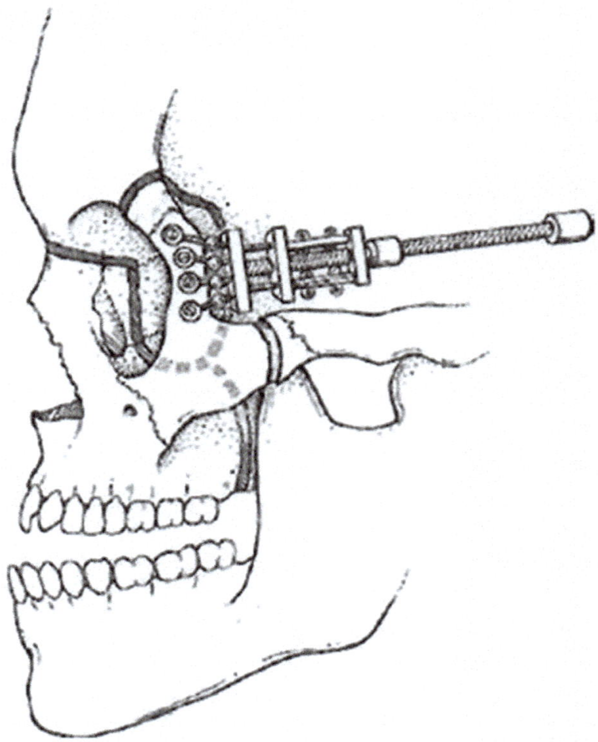

Fig. 7.2 Example of an internal midface distraction device (Reprinted from Mathes ed. Plastic Surgery 2nd edition, Saunders, Philadelpia, PA; December 23, 2005)

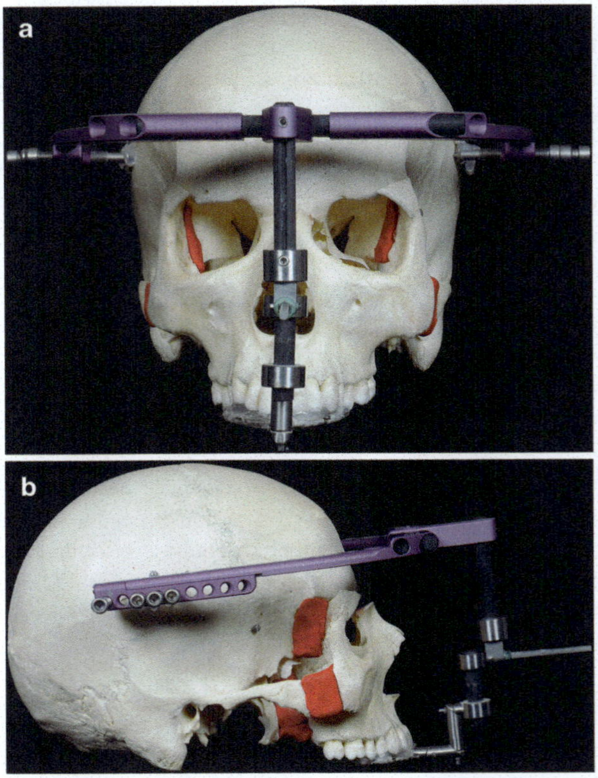

Fig. 7.3 External halo or RED® device. (**a**) Frontal view. (**b**) Lateral view showing the rigid distraction splint (occlusal). *Red* designates the zones of bone generation

malfunction, the repair requires a surgical intervention with anesthesia. The external halo frame (Fig. 7.3) is obtrusive and noticeable. However, it provides the greatest stability and rigidity. Moreover, if there is a device problem, it can often be solved in the clinic without the need for surgical intervention. In addition, modifications can be made to the device during activation to change the vector or rotate the central rod.

Virtual planning, reported by some authors, is currently in its early stages of application to this specific craniofacial technique and has yet to prove particularly helpful.

7.6 Operative Technique

More detailed description of surgical technique, complemented by 3D simulation, is available at: www.myface3D.com.

7.6.1 Monobloc Distraction (Fig. 7.4)

Oroendotracheal intubation is preferred. After lubrication is applied to the corneas, lid occlusal sutures are inserted. Packed red blood cells (PRBC) should be

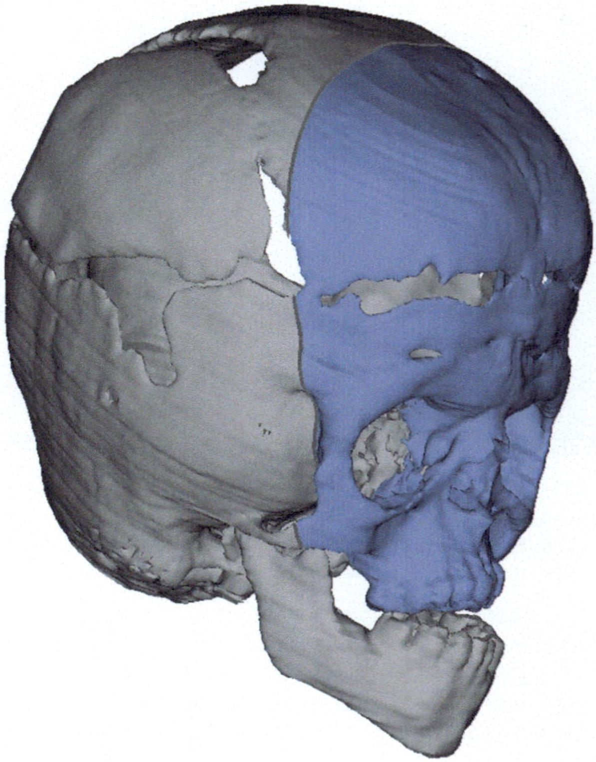

Fig. 7.4 Monobloc osteotomy as depicted in virtual surgical planning

available in the room prior to the start of the surgery. A coronal zigzag incision is made across the skull from ear to ear. Subperiosteal exposure includes the superior aspect of the nasal bones, the medial orbital wall posterior to the medial canthus, the superior and lateral orbital rim, the malar eminence to the zygomaticofacial foramen, the lateral orbital wall, and the lateral aspect of the orbital floor. The anterior attachments of the temporalis to the posterior aspect of the lateral orbital rim are separated. Using the coronal exposure, a subperiosteal pocket is made in the pterygomaxillary fissure. The neurosurgeon performs an anterior craniotomy with removal of the frontal bone.

Through the coronal incision, anterior cranial fossa osteotomies are made 1 cm posterior to the frontal bone with a power-driven saw on both sides (Fig. 7.5). Malleable retractors are used to protect both the frontal lobe and the orbital contents. The saw is then used to perform full-thickness lateral orbital wall osteotomies at the junction with the temporal bone, care being taken to avoid injury to the temporal lobes of the brain and the orbital contents. This osteotomy is then extended medially across the orbital floor. The infraorbital rim should be directly visualized during this portion of the procedure to avoid inadvertent fracture. An osteotomy is made through the body of the zygoma (not the arch), so that there is adequate bone volume for bone generation (Fig. 7.5).

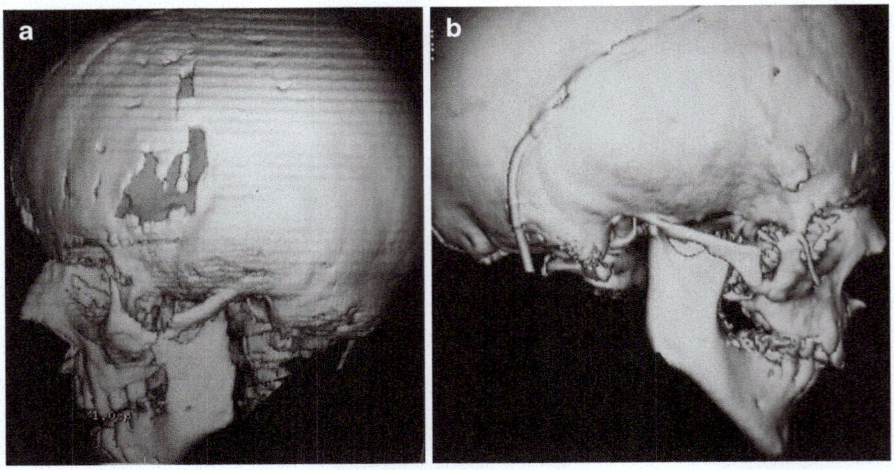

Fig. 7.5 Value of making the osteotomy through the body of the zygoma. (**a**) Absence of bone generation following osteotomy through the thin arch of the zygoma. (**b**) Bone generation following osteotomy through the thicker body of the zygoma

Through the coronal incision, an osteotomy is made through the pterygomaxillary fissure. The index finger of the non-dominant hand is placed intraorally to palpate the tip of the osteotome along the lingual aspect of the maxillary tubercle as the osteotomy is completed. This osteotomy is then extended superiorly and anteriorly to join the osteotomy of the lateral orbital rim. Note in patients with a maxillary sinus that has not been pneumatized, this osteotomy must be extended medially for complete bony separation.

An osteotomy is made with a fine tapered osteotome anterior to the foramen caecum. The osteotomy is carried bilaterally down the medial orbital wall behind the posterior lacrimal crest to join the osteotomy made across the orbital floor. Exposure for these osteotomies can be complemented with bilateral eyelid incisions, if required.

With the surgeon's fingers in the mouth as a guide, the septum is sectioned through the cranial base osteotomy. The osteotome is directed posteriorly and inferiorly toward the posterior nasal spine. As the osteotomy extends deeper toward the base of the nose, the monobloc segment can be rocked anteriorly to better position the osteotome in a posterior trajectory.

The monobloc segment can now be fully separated from the skull base if all osteotomies are complete. The mobilization of the segment can be confirmed by inserting Rowe-Kiley forceps and the monobloc segment advanced. Common locations for an incomplete osteotomy are the pterygomaxillary fissure and the junction of the lateral orbital rim osteotomy with the pterygomaxillary fissure osteotomy. Once complete monobloc separation has been confirmed, the mobilized segment should be placed back in position, and drill holes can be placed between the lateral orbital wall and temporal bone for the insertion of chromic catgut sutures, which will be broken during the activation process.

It is at this time in the procedure that internal distraction devices can be applied, usually between the temporal bone and zygomatic process (see Fig. 7.2).

The coronal incision is closed over Jackson-Pratt catheters, and, after the closure is complete, the halo device can be applied. The main frame is applied parallel to Frankfort horizontal, and the horizontal component should be at least 2 cm above the supraorbital rims. The craniofacial CT should be carefully inspected to avoid placing the screws into cranial skeletal defects.

Pillars are usually applied with intermaxillary fixation (IMF) screws at the lateral aspect of the supraorbital rims prior to closure of the coronal incision. Small stab-like incisions allow penetration of the pillars through the skin. A rigid occlusal splint [10, 11] is secured to the teeth, but double wires are also used in the younger patient to secure the splint circumferentially to drill holes in the body of the zygoma. Alternatively wires can be passed between the splint outrigger to the halo sidearms. Wires are also passed from the supraorbital pillars through the lateral eyebrows to the sidearm of the external halo splint. The rigid occlusal splint is also inserted to the central pole of the halo device (see Fig. 7.3).

7.6.2 Le Fort III Distraction (Subcranial) (Fig. 7.6)

Oroendotracheal anesthesia is preferred and lid occlusal sutures are inserted. Packed red blood cells are available in the room prior to the start of the

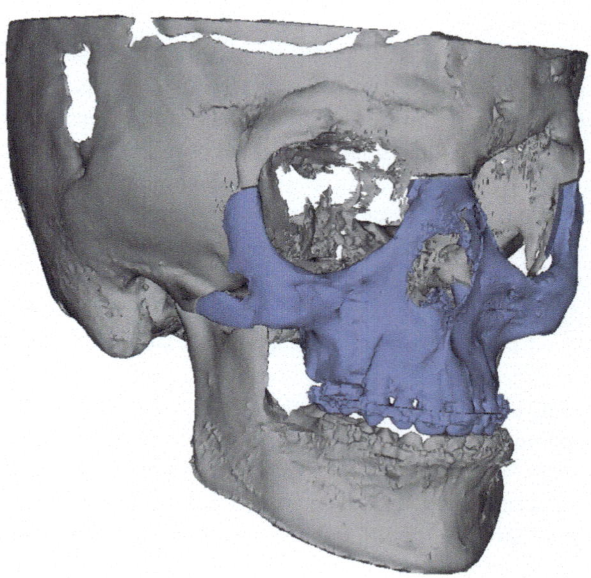

Fig. 7.6 Subcranial Le Fort III osteotomy as depicted in virtual surgical planning

procedure. A coronal zigzag incision is made on both sides and the scalp flap is reflected. Subperiosteal exposure includes the superior aspect of the nasal bones, the medial orbital wall posterior to the medial canthus, the superior and lateral orbital rim, the malar eminence to the zygomaticofacial foramen, the lateral orbital wall and lateral aspect of the orbital floor. The anterior attachments of the temporalis to the posterior aspect of the lateral orbital rim are separated. Using the coronal exposure, a subperiosteal pocket is made in the pterygomaxillary suture. Lateral orbital wall osteotomies are made at the temporal bone on both sides with care to protect the orbital contents. This osteotomy is extended medially across the orbital floor. The infraorbital rim should be directly visualized throughout this portion of the procedure to avoid inadvertent fracture. An osteotomy is made through the body of the zygoma (not the arch), so that there is adequate bone volume for bone generation.

Through the coronal incision, the osteotomy is made through the pterygomaxillary fissure. As the osteotomy is made through the fissure, the index finger of the non-dominant hand is placed intraorally to palpate the tip of the osteotome on the lingual surface of the maxillary tubercle as the osteotomy is completed. This osteotomy is then extended superiorly and anteriorly to join the osteotomy of the lateral orbital rim. Note that in patients with a maxillary sinus that has not been pneumatized, this osteotomy must be extended medially for complete bony separation.

The nasofrontal junction osteotomy is made with a sagittal saw. It is important to review the posteroanterior cephalogram to ensure that the osteotomy is made below the cribriform plate. Medial orbital wall osteotomies are made with an osteotome posterior to the posterior lacrimal crest to join the osteotomy made across the orbital floor. Exposure can be supplemented, if required, with bilateral eyelid incisions.

The septum is sectioned with an osteotome inserted through the nasofrontal osteotomy. With the surgeon's fingers in the mouth as a guide, the osteotome is directed posteriorly and inferiorly toward the posterior nasal spine. As part of the septum is cartilaginous, this separation may be completed with a curved Mayo scissors. Rowe-Kiley forceps can assist in separating the last bony bridges from the skull base. One must be careful to avoid injury to the palate in the younger patient at this stage. Common locations for an incomplete osteotomy are the pterygomaxillary fissure and the junction of the lateral orbital rim osteotomy with the pterygomaxillary fissure osteotomy. The Le Fort III segment can be rocked with the fingers placed behind the zygomatic complexes once all osteotomies are complete. After complete midface separation has been confirmed, the mobilized segment should be placed back in position, and drill holes can be placed between the lateral orbital wall and temporal bone for the insertion of chromic catgut sutures, which will be broken during the activation process.

Internal distraction devices can be inserted at this time, the plates of which are fixated to the temporal bone and zygomatic complex (see Fig. 7.2).

The coronal incision is closed over Jackson-Pratt catheters.

The external halo frame is applied, care being taken to ensure that screws are not passed through a cranial defect. This can be avoided by careful inspection of the craniofacial CT prior to application of the frame. The horizontal component of the halo should be at least 2 cm above the supraorbital rims. The central (carbon) rod should be in the craniofacial midline. A rigid occlusal splint is inserted to the central rod, and, if desired, pillars can be inserted and penetrated through the bilateral alar creases. Wires can also be passed from the IMF screws through the alar creases to the sidearm of the central rod of the external halo device. In the younger patient without adequate dentition for retention, double wires are passed from the splint and secured to drill holes in the zygomas.

7.6.3 Vector Control

Vector control is critical. The midface transport segment, if uncontrolled, can:

(a) Translate forward without rotation
(b) Rotate clockwise and show downward displacement
(c) Displace forward and rotate counterclockwise
(d) Translate forward and downward [20]

Measures have been designed to ensure that the desired vector and distraction trajectory are achieved [20]. Havlik et al. [21], in order to control yaw, pitch, and roll of the midface segment during activation, proposed a "cat's cradle" maneuver based on circumferential suspension of the midface transport segment passed through the palate. The NYU team [10, 11] developed a rigid occlusal distraction splint, attached to the central rod of the halo device, to control the vertical plane of the osteotomized midface segment (Fig. 7.7) and to avoid inferior movement of the posterior nasal spine (counterclockwise rotation).

Studies have been conducted to establish the site of the *centers of mass* (free body) for the various osteotomized segments: monobloc at a point 43.5% of the

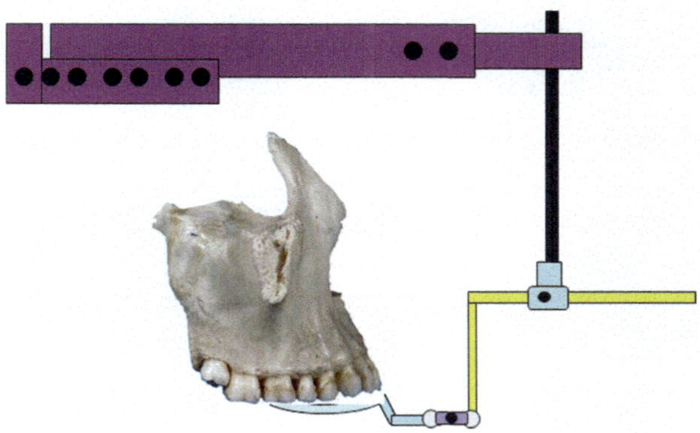

Fig. 7.7 Attachment of the rigid occlusal splint to the vertical rod of the RED® device

total height from the occlusal plane to the supraorbital osteotomy and Le Fort III at a point 38% of the total height from the occlusal plane to the osteotomy at the nasofrontal junction [22]. Shetye and the NYU group [20] recommended forward translation of the Le Fort III segment without rotation when the distraction force is applied 55% of the distance between the occlusal plane and the nasion and the vector is parallel to the maxillary occlusal plane. Another group proposed orthodontic micro-implants to anchor inter-arch Class III elastics to prevent midface counterclockwise rotation [23].

7.6.4 Variations in Technique

Several techniques of differential distraction have been designed to address the variables in retrusion of the individual components of the craniofacial skeleton. Hopper et al. [24] employed "nasal passages grafts" in patients whose nasal bone hypoplasia exceeded that of the midface. Wire cerclage swing advancement was used to provide more advancement on the more severely retruded side, and the same group [25] recommended Le Fort II midface distraction and simultaneous zygomatic repositioning to normalize craniofacial ratios in Apert patients (Figs. 7.8 and 7.9).

Another group [26] presented an Apert patient who underwent a monobloc distraction with internal distraction devices anchored temporally, combined with a Le Fort II distraction fixated by an external halo device.

In another effort to achieve differential midface distraction, especially between the upper and lower portions of the midface, the two transport segments were

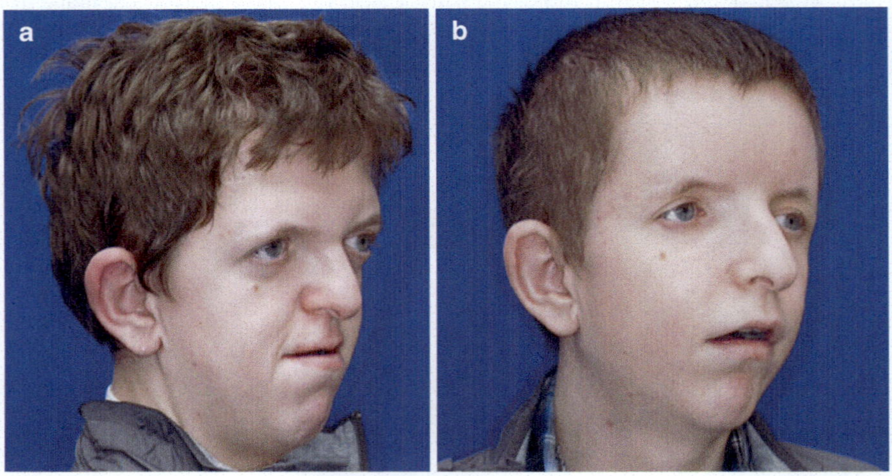

Fig. 7.8 Le Fort II distraction combined with zygomatic repositioning. (**a**) Preoperative view. (**b**) Postoperative view (Images courtesy of Dr. Richard Hopper)

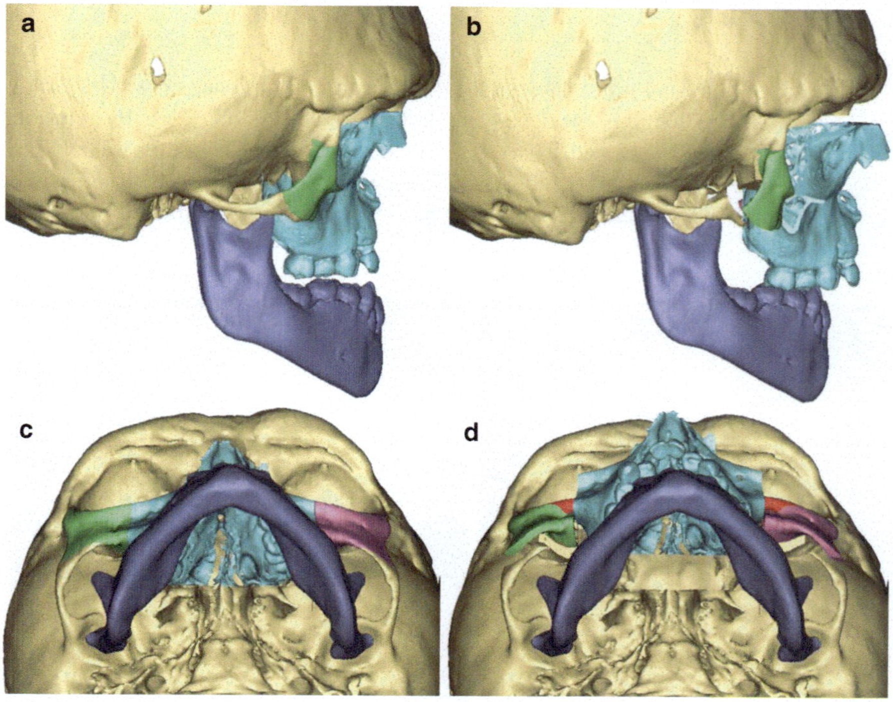

Fig. 7.9 Virtual surgery planning images of Le Fort II and zygomatic repositioning. (**a**) Preoperative profile view. (**b**) Postoperative profile view. (**c**) Preoperative basilar view. (**d**) Postoperative view following Le Fort II distraction and before zygomatic repositioning (Images courtesy of Dr. Richard Hopper)

distracted differentially [27]. The upper midface (lower orbits and nose) distraction was performed via single vector buried devices, and the lower segment (Le Fort I segment) was distracted via an external halo device which permits adjustments to control occlusal position.

Another approach in the Apert patient combines a bipartition procedure with monobloc distraction [16, 17] (see Chapter 8).

7.7 Postoperative Period

7.7.1 Latency

The latency period lasts approximately 5–7 days. This time length is especially important in monobloc distraction to allow time to establish some type of seal at the anterior cranial base osteotomy site. Attempts at reducing the length of the latency period can result in an increased infection rate.

7.7.2 Activation

The rate of activation is 1 mm a day, and the rhythm can either be once or twice (0.5 mm b.i.d.) a day. The endpoint is age dependent. In the growing child, a Class II occlusion or overjet should be achieved as long as it does not create a nonfunctional bite (Fig. 7.10). The cephalogram (lateral view) is especially helpful in monitoring movement of the midface segment. In the growing patient, the zygomatic-orbital form, rather

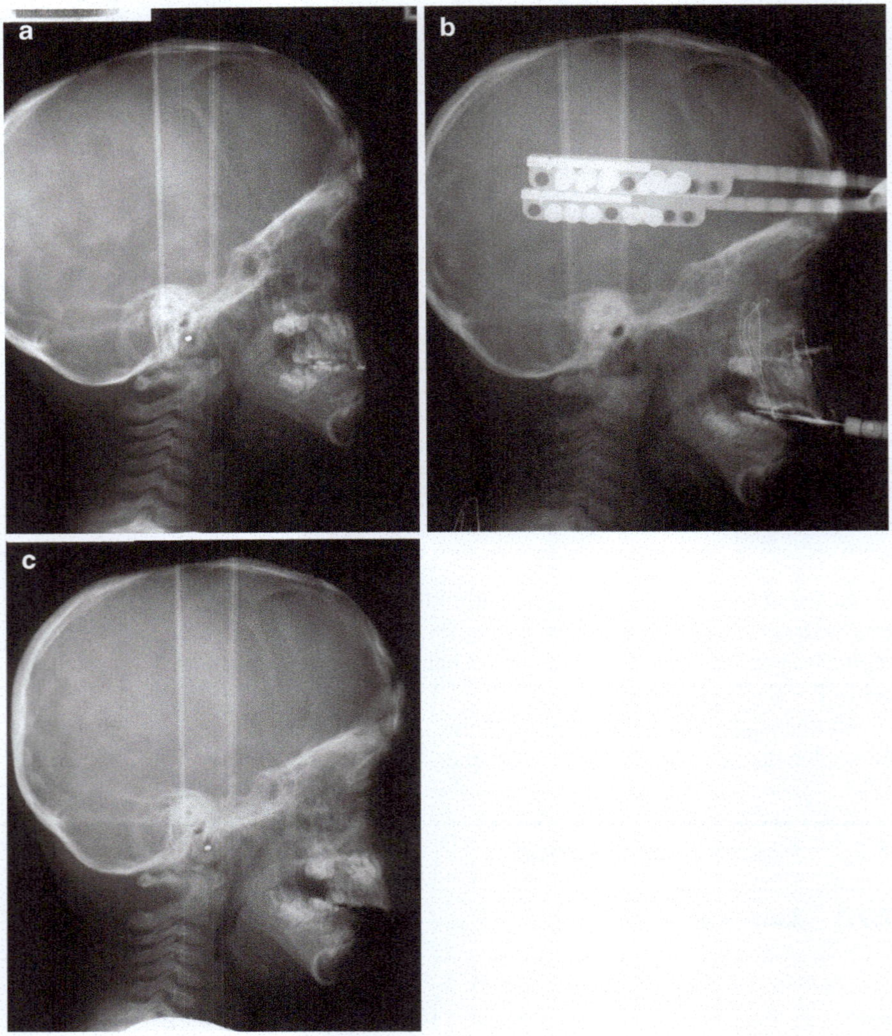

Fig. 7.10 Class II occlusion or overjet as the desired endpoint after Le Fort III distraction in the growing child. (**a**) Preoperative lateral cephalogram. (**b**) At the conclusion of activation with the external halo and rigid occlusal splint in place. (**c**) Following removal of the distraction device

than the occlusion, is the primary decision-making metric in discontinuing activation. Zygomatic "over-projection" is essential, consisting of creating mild enophthalmos and advancement of the infraorbital rim to a supercorrected position (Fig. 7.11).

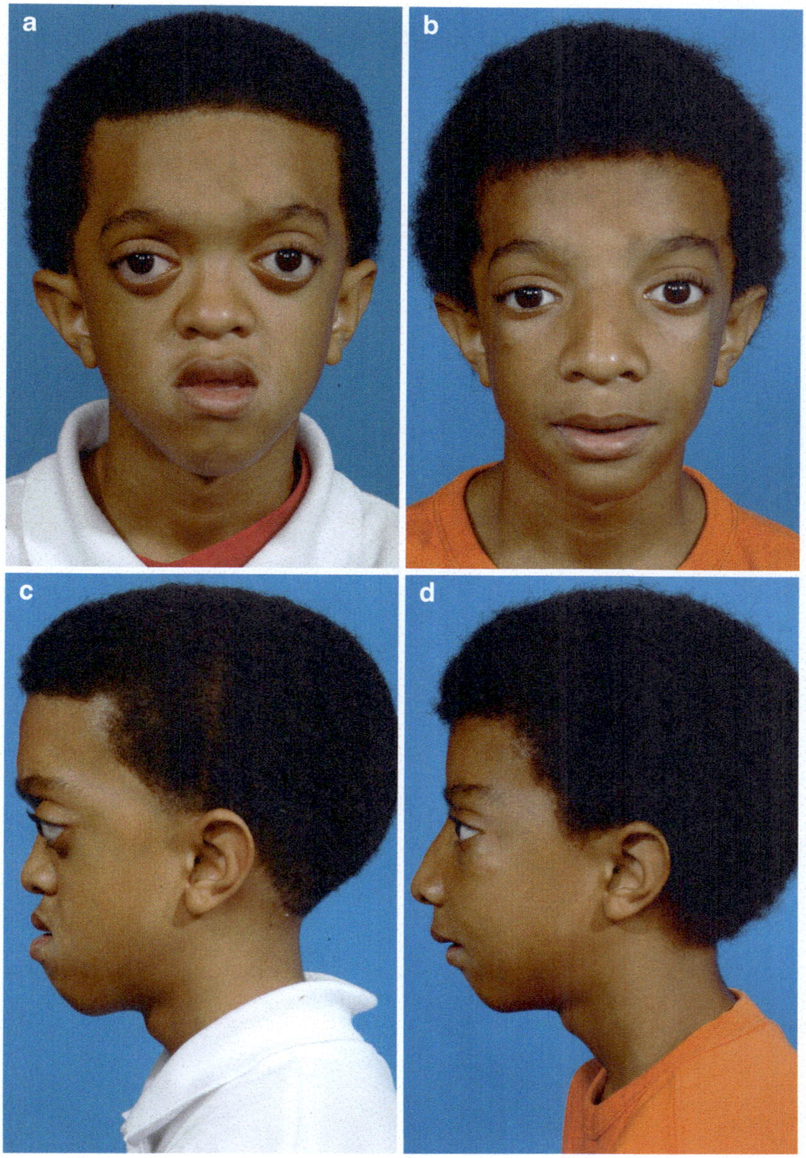

Fig. 7.11 Zygomatic overprojection as the desired endpoint after Le Fort III distraction in the growing child. (**a**, **c**) Preoperative views at 9 years of age. (**b**, **d**) Postoperative views at one year showing correction of the exorbitism and projection of the orbitozygomatic complex

7.7.3 Consolidation

The consolidation period is 2 months in length to allow adequate bone generation at the distracted osteotomy sites [28–30] and reduce the relapse rate.

7.7.4 Orthodontic Management/Molding of Generate

See Chapter 9

7.8 Le Fort III Case Reports (Figs. 7.12, 7.13, 7.14, 7.15, 7.16, 7.17, 7.18, 7.19, 7.20, 7.21 and 7.22)

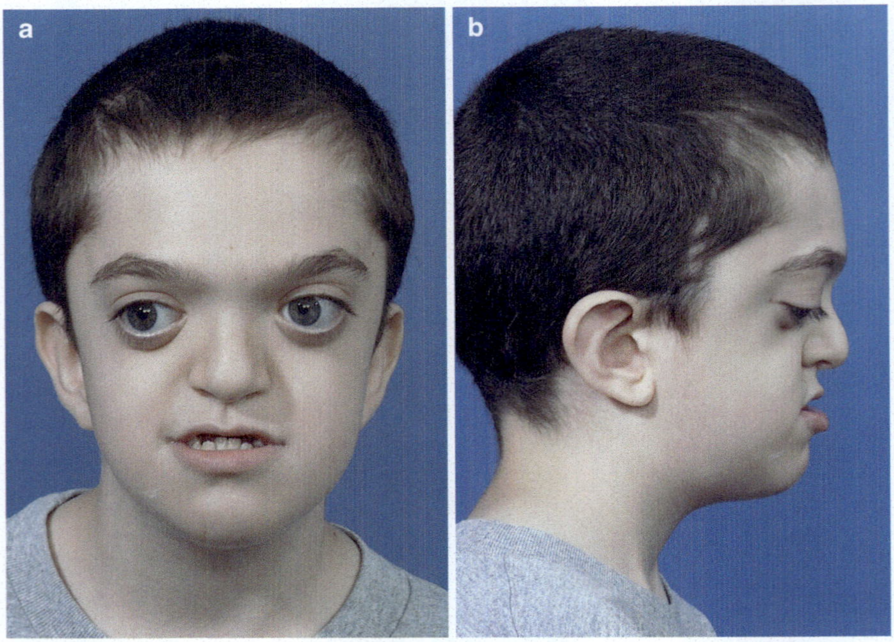

Fig. 7.12 A 5-year-old boy with Crouzon syndrome who underwent Le Fort III distraction. He had previously had fronto-orbital advancement in infancy. (**a**, **b**) Preoperative views. (**c**, **d**) Postoperative views at one year

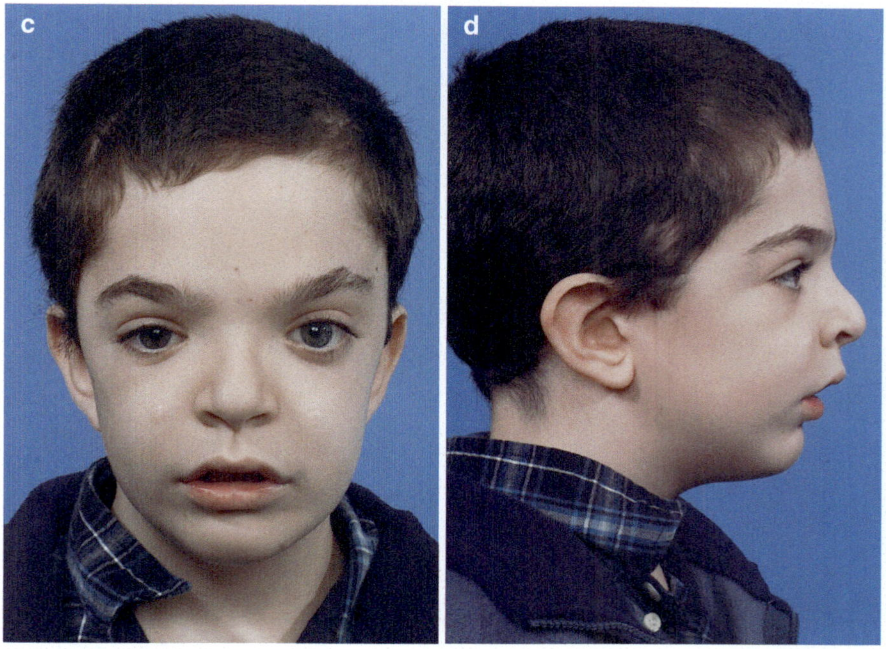

Fig. 7.12 (continued)

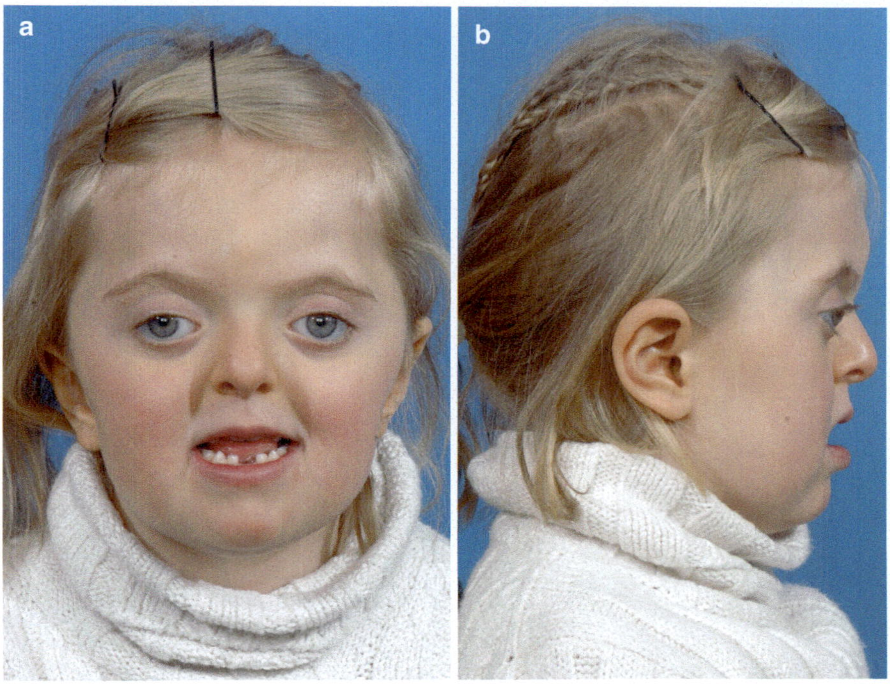

Fig. 7.13 A 6-year-old girl with Apert syndrome who underwent Le Fort III distraction. She had previously had fronto-orbital advancement in infancy. (**a, b**) Preoperative views. (**c, d**) Postoperative views at one year. (**e, f**) Five years postoperative

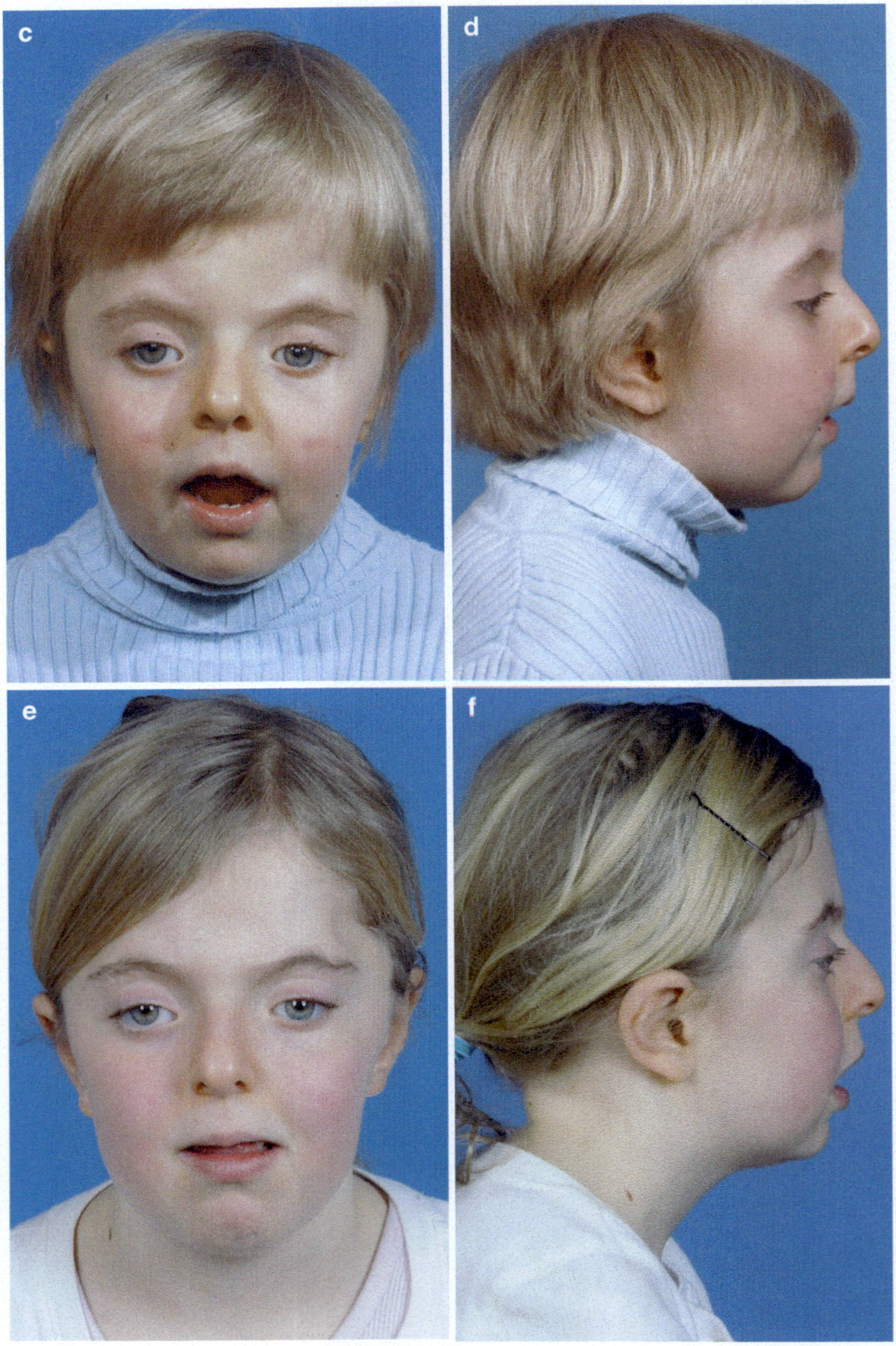

Fig. 7.13 (continued)

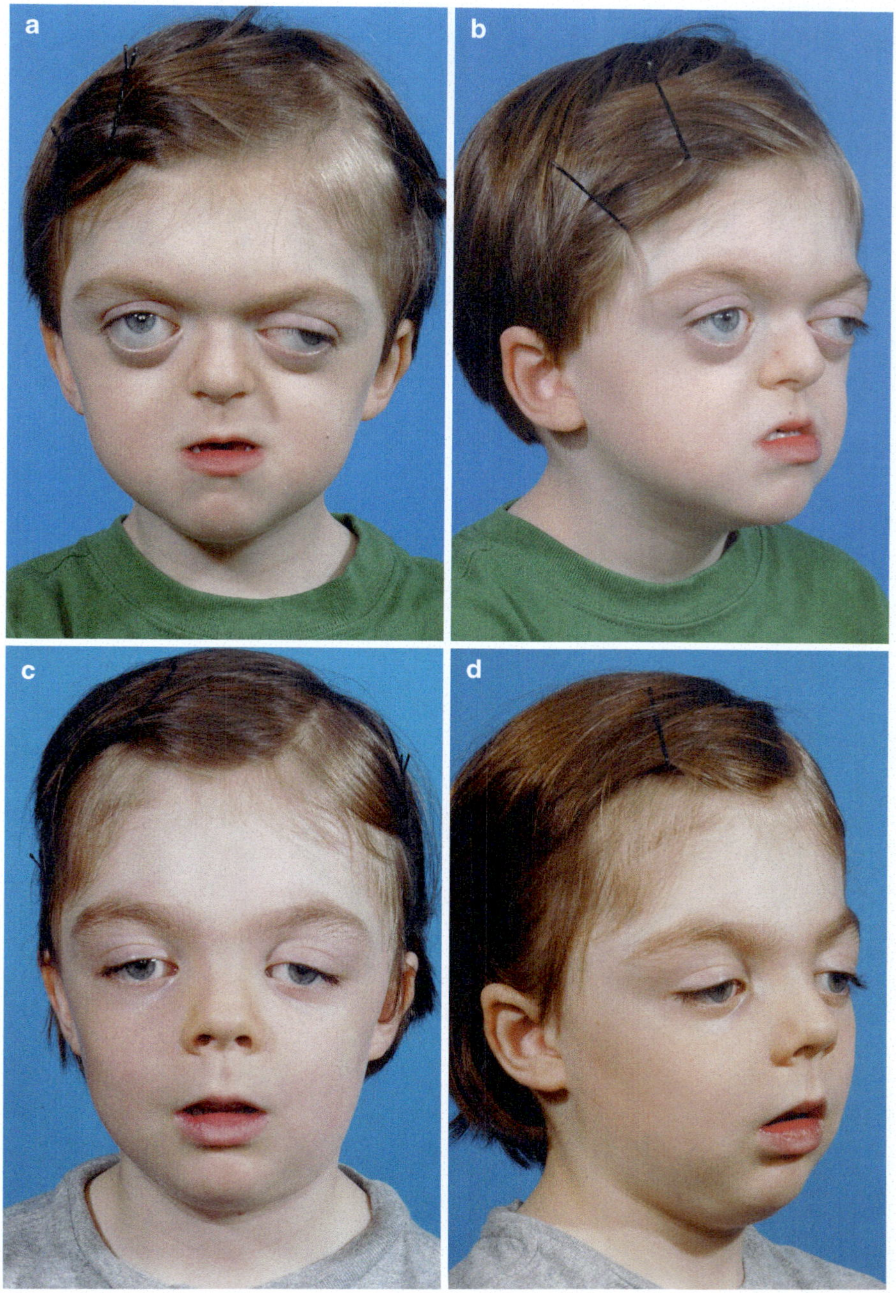

Fig. 7.14 A 4-year-old boy with Crouzon syndrome who underwent Le Fort III distraction. He had previously had fronto-orbital advancement in infancy. (**a**, **b**) Preoperative appearance with significant exorbitism. (**c**, **d**) Postoperative views at one year. (**e**, **f**) Six years postoperative

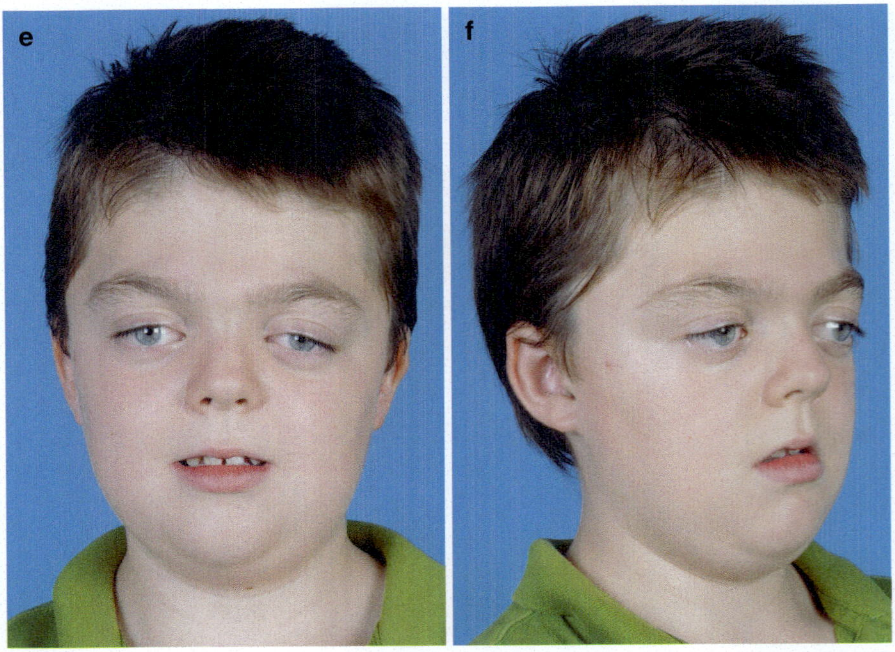

Fig. 7.14 (continued)

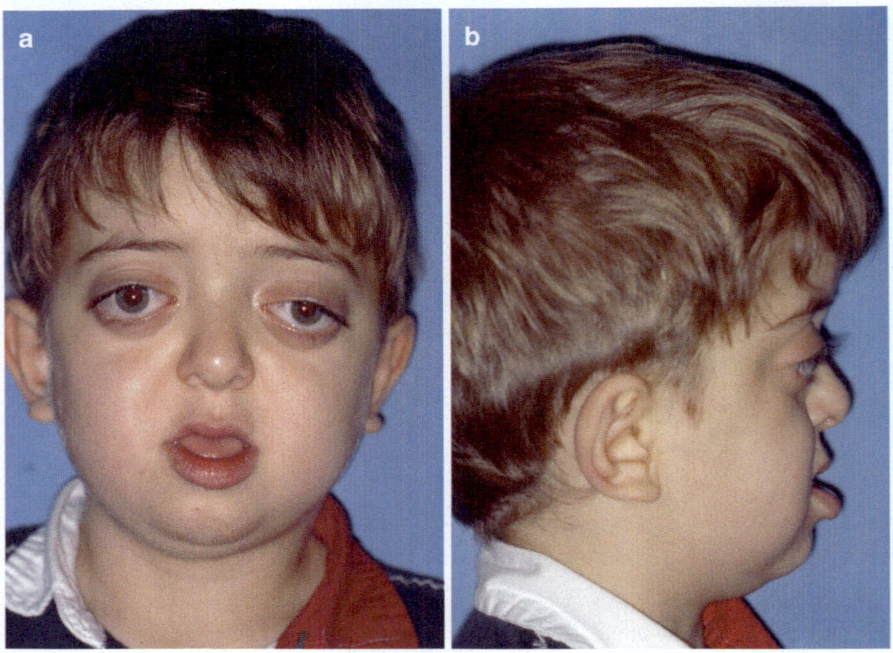

Fig. 7.15 A 5-year-old boy with Crouzon syndrome who underwent Le Fort III distraction. He had previously had fronto-orbital advancement in infancy. (**a**, **b**) Preoperative views. (**c**, **d**) Postoperative views at 1 year. (**e**, **f**) Appearance at 4 years postoperative

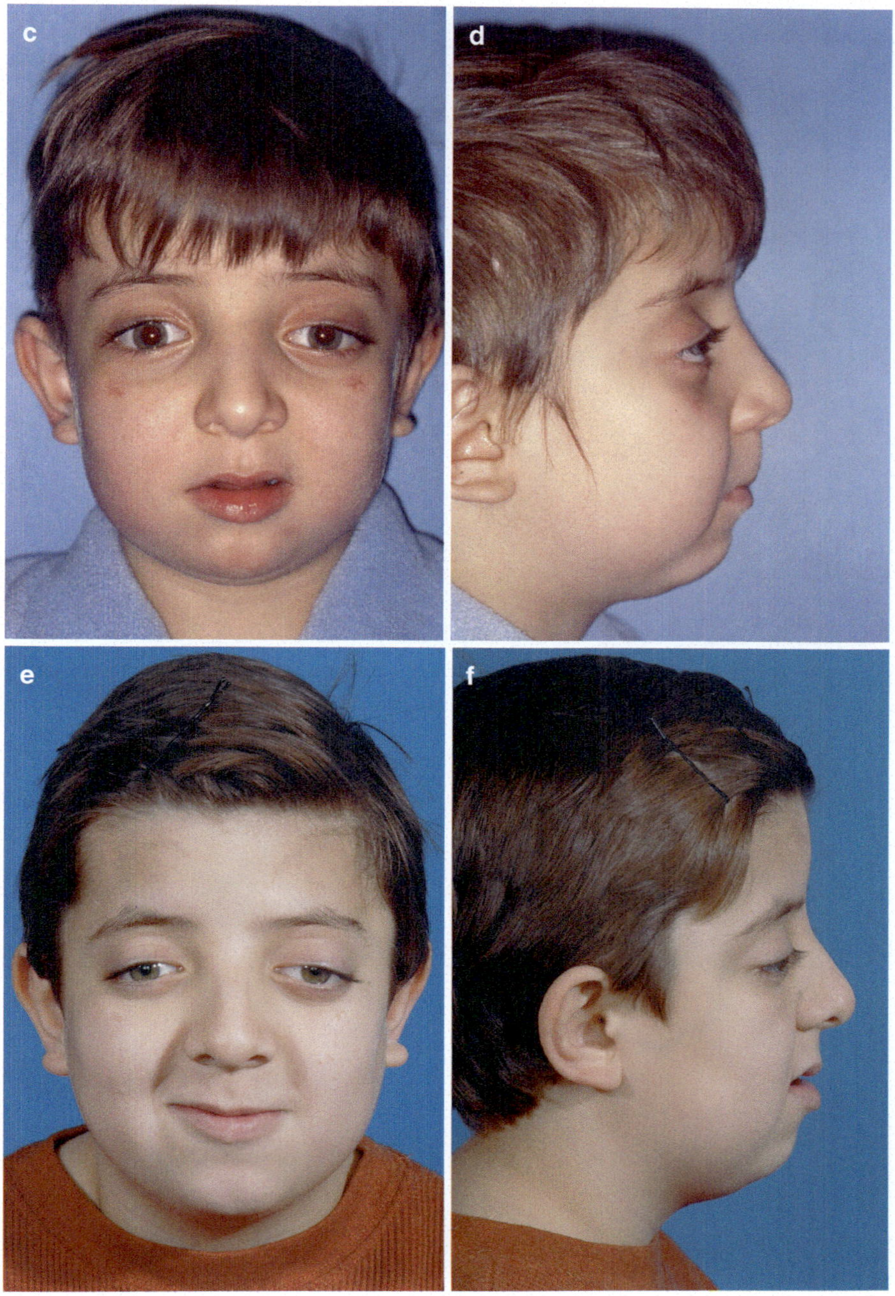

Fig. 7.15 (continued)

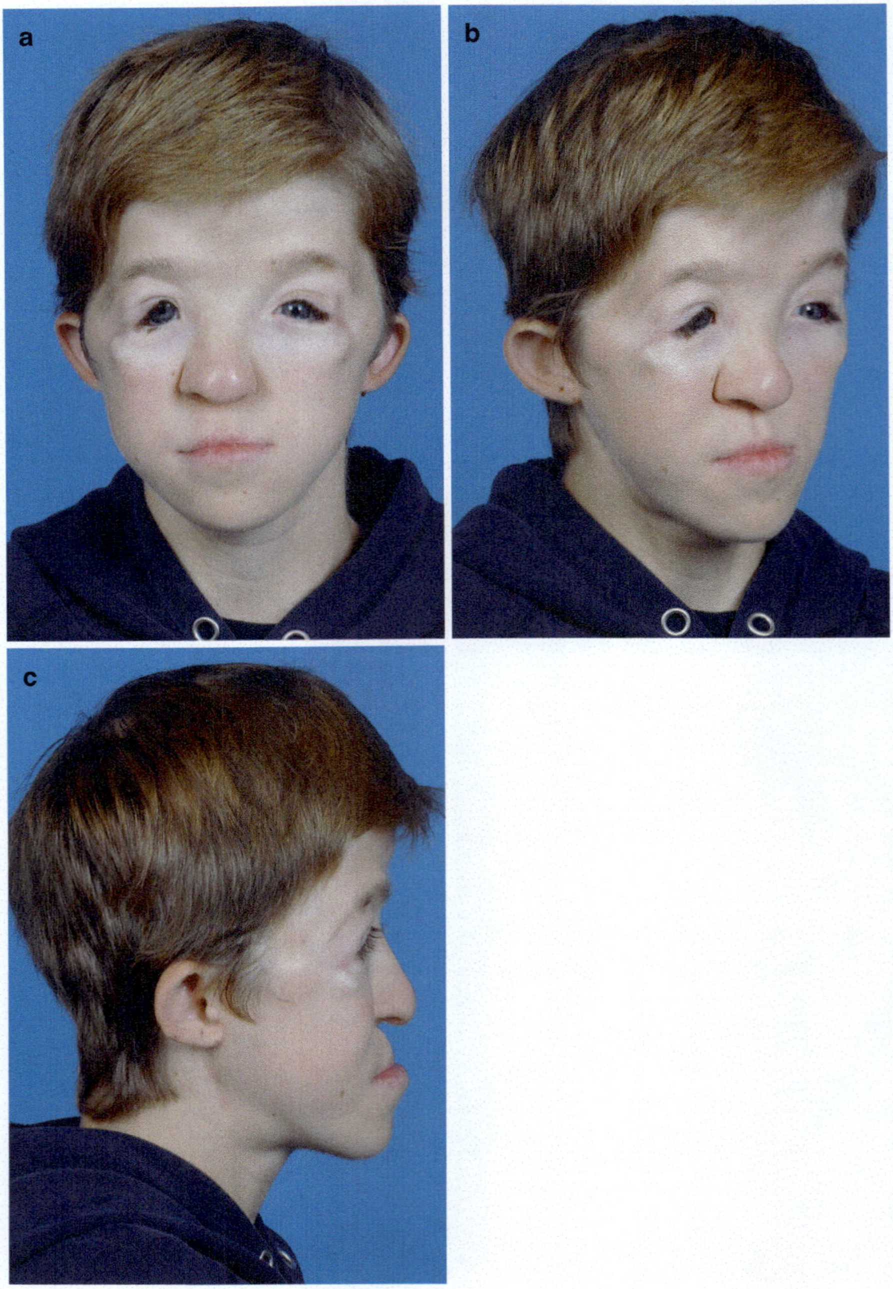

Fig. 7.16 A 13-year-old boy with Antley-Bixler syndrome who had undergone Le Fort III distraction at another institution. There had been inadvertent fracture at the zygomatico-maxillary sutures with inferolateral displacement of the orbitozygomatic complexes and lateral canthal mechanisms. The nasomaxillary segment was displaced laterally with inadequate sagittal projection. (**a**) Frontal view. (**b**) Oblique view. (**c**) Profile view

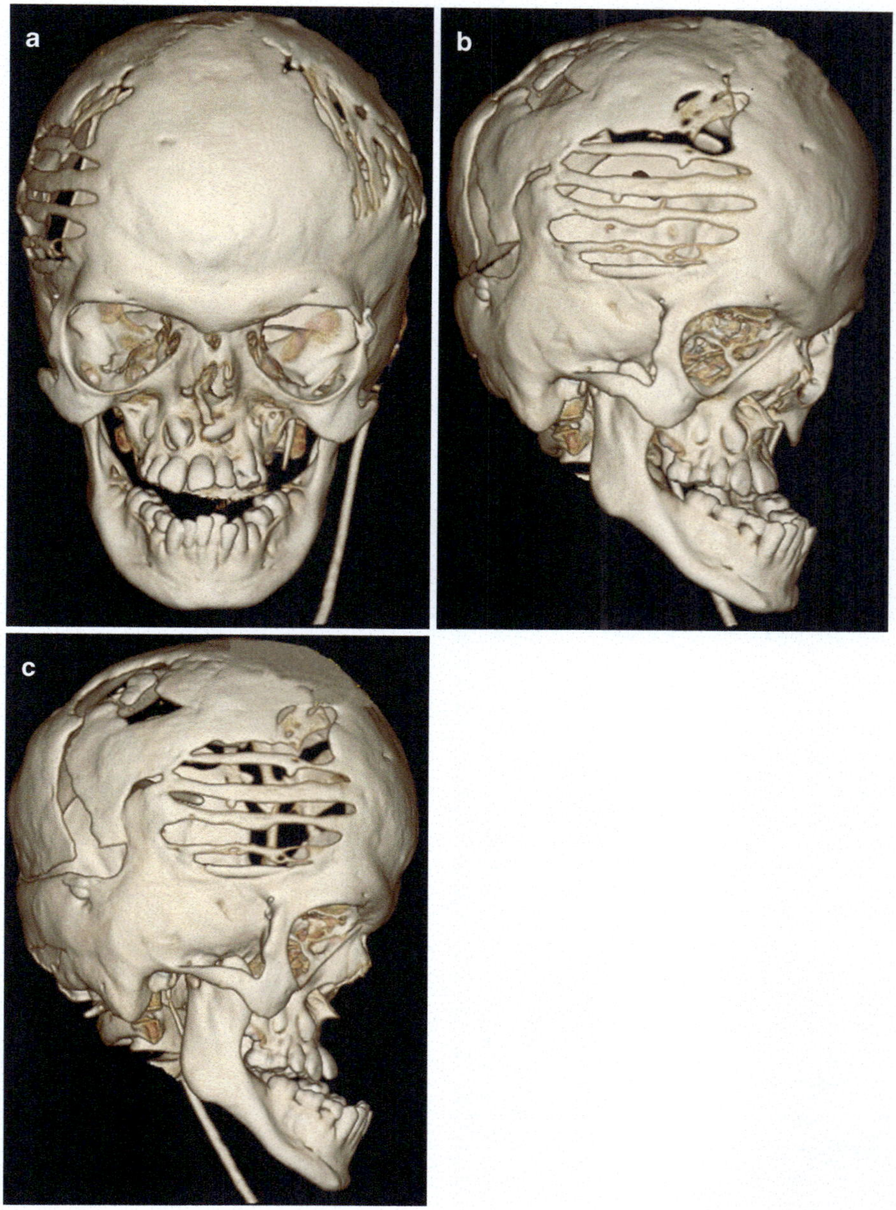

Fig. 7.17 CT scans corresponding to Fig. 7.16. Note the inferolateral displacement of the orbito-zygomatic complexes and the lateral displacement and the absence of sagittal projection of the nasomaxillary segment. He had previously undergone a cranioplasty

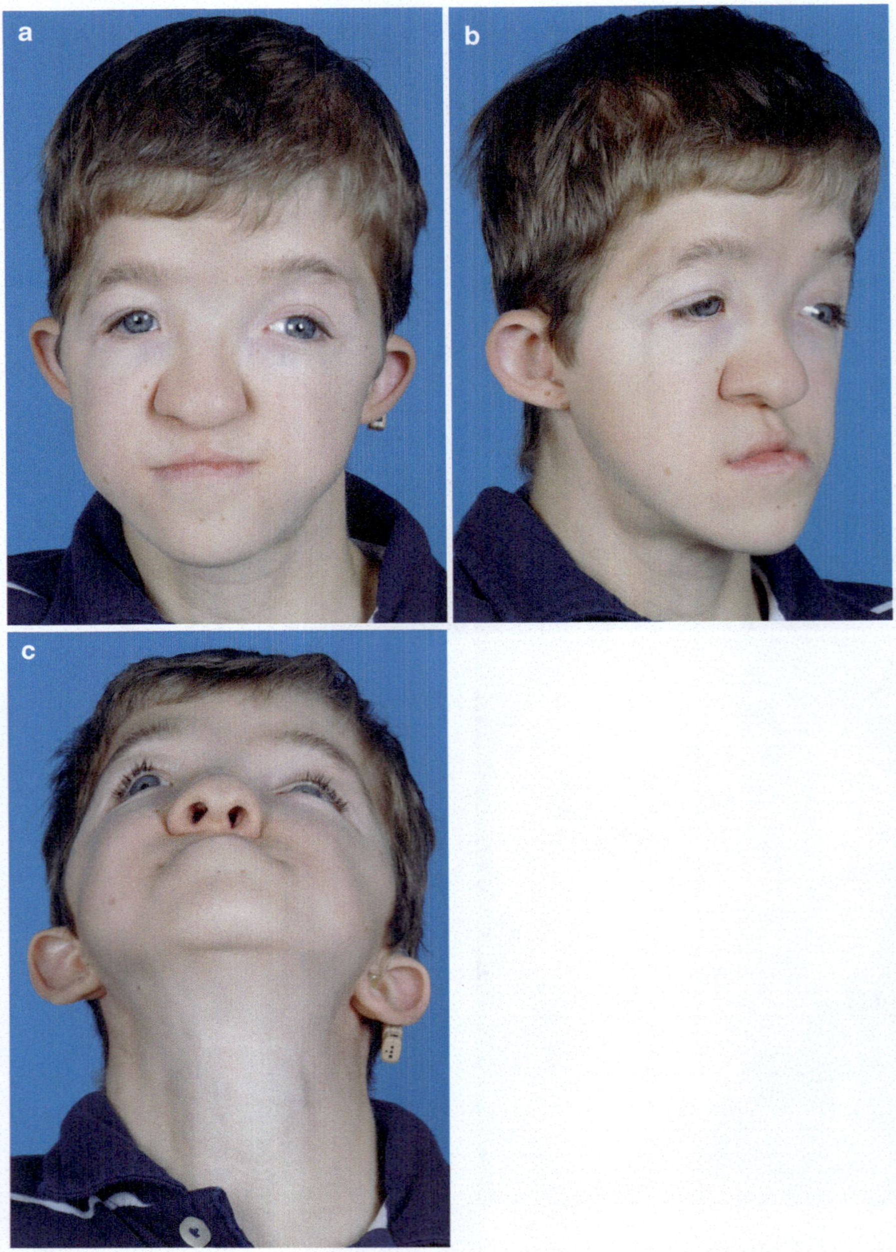

Fig. 7.18 In a primary procedure, the areas of fibrous union in the orbitozygomatic areas were resected and bone grafted after skeletal repositioning. (**a–c**) Patient appearance following this procedure. (**d–f**) Corresponding CT images

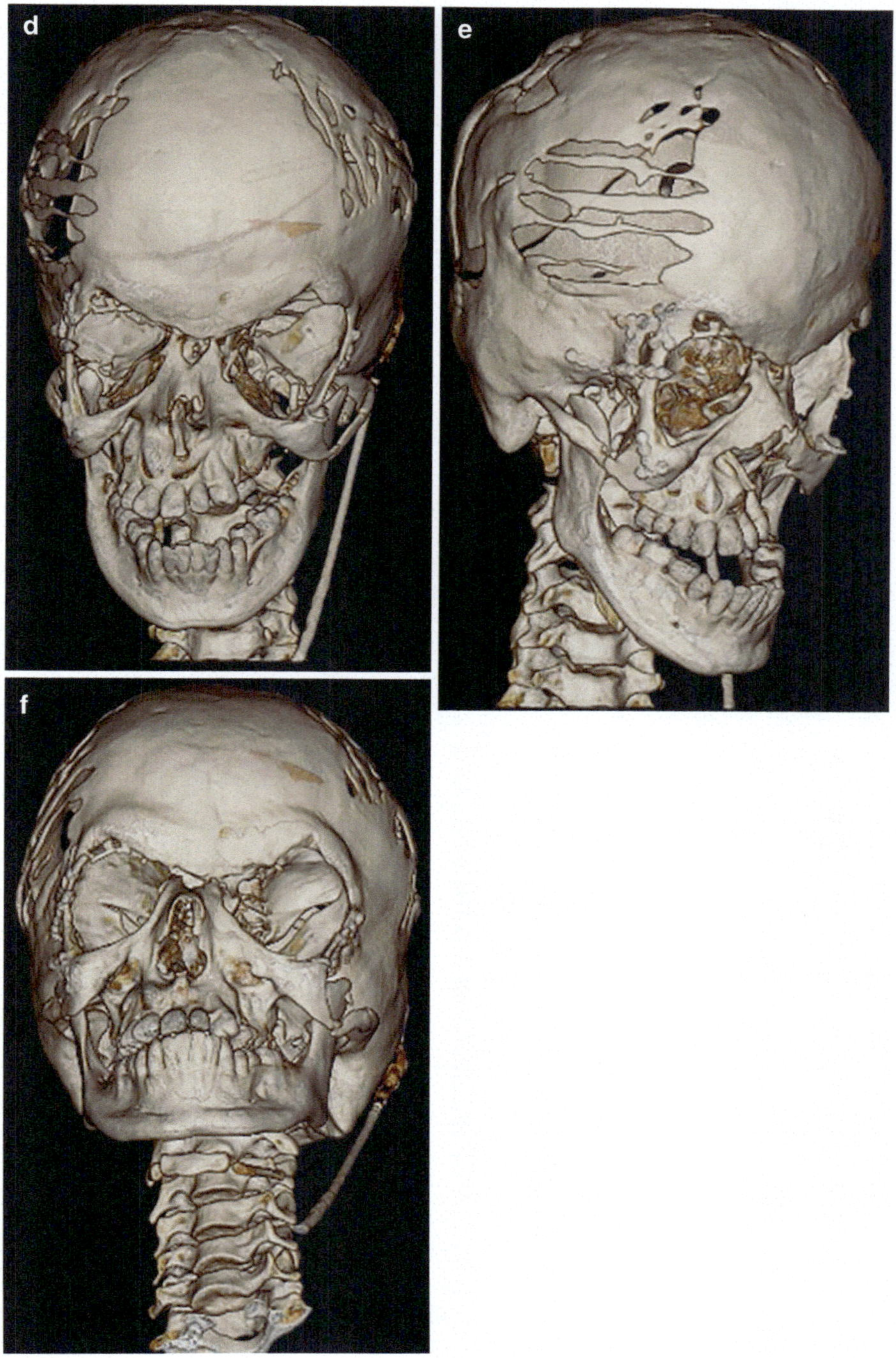

Fig. 7.18 (continued)

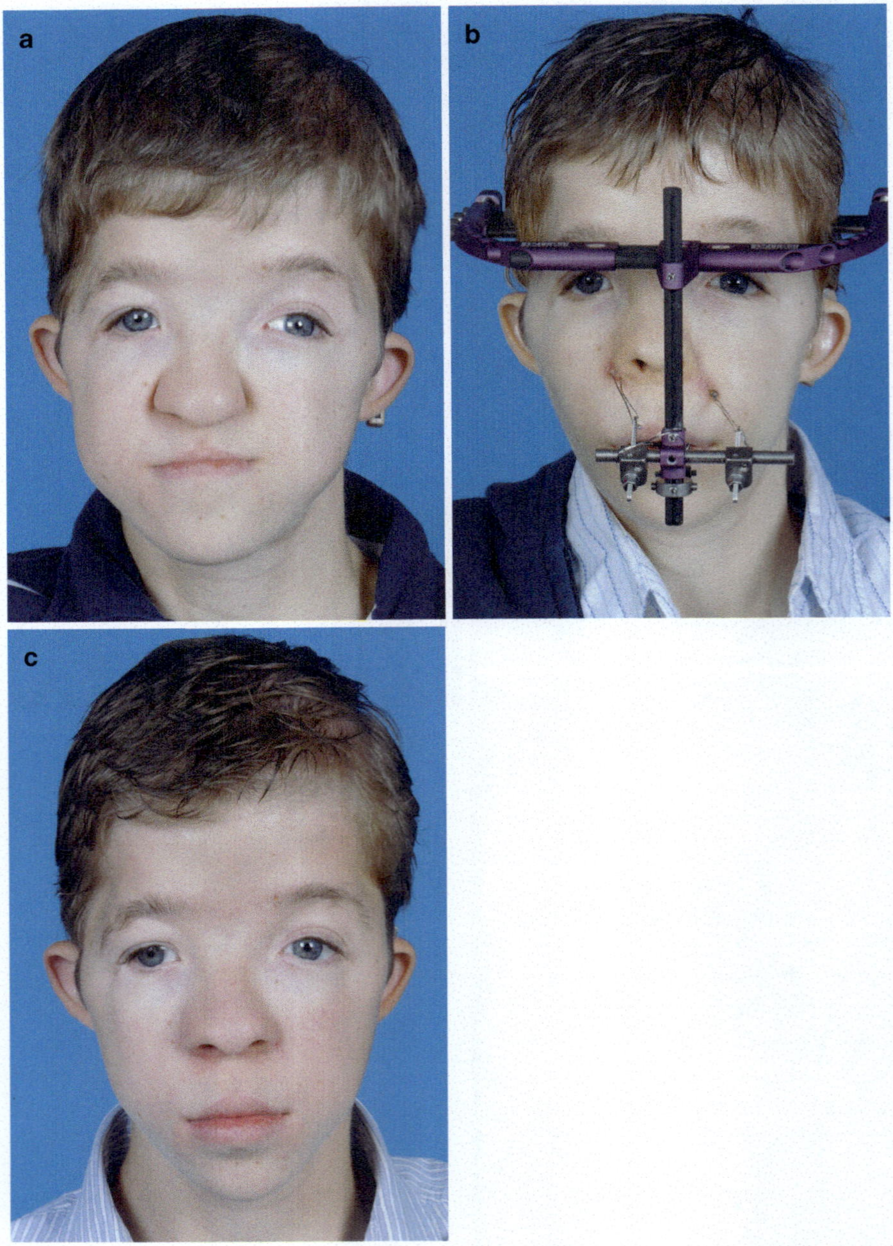

Fig. 7.19 In a second procedure 6 months later, the patient underwent Le Fort III distraction. After 10 days of activation, the outrigger connecting the wires to the pyriform apertures was displaced to the patient's left side, and the activation resumed (molding of the generate). (**a**) Predistraction appearance. (**b**) In the activation period, the outrigger/wires attached to the central rod were moved laterally and activation resumed. (**c**) Appearance following removal of the halo frame. Note the movement of the nasomaxillary complex to the midline and the midface fullness

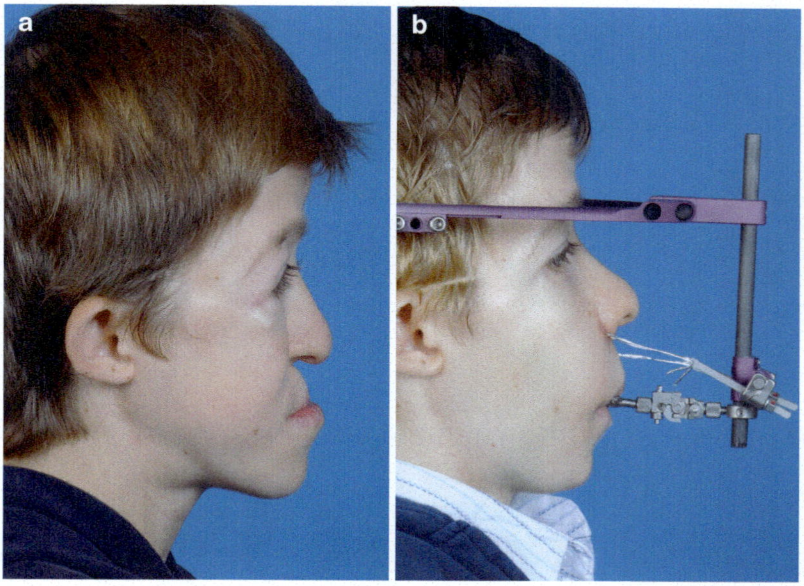

Fig. 7.20 (**a**) Profile view before Le Fort III distraction. (**b**) Profile view at the conclusion of the consolidation period. Note the improvement in midface projection and upper lip position

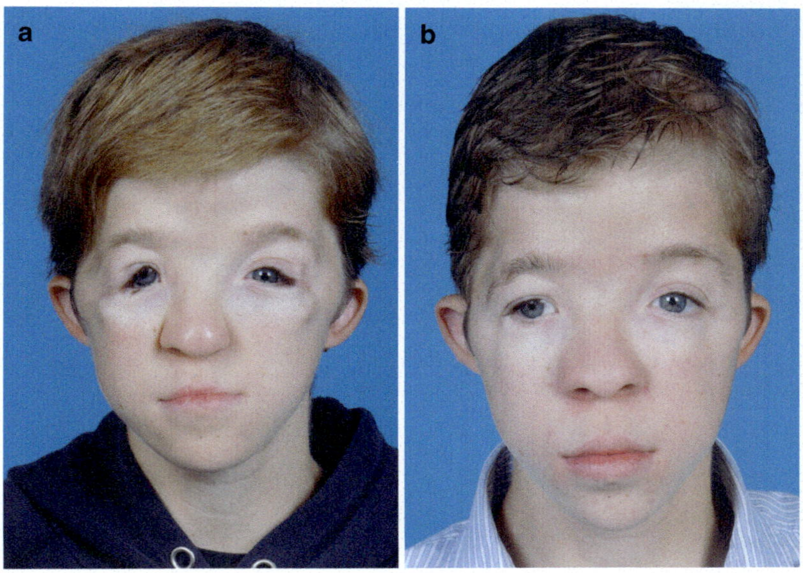

Fig. 7.21 (**a**) Preoperative frontal view on arrival at the NYU unit. (**b**) Frontal view after the two procedures described above. Note the improvement in orbitozygomatic position, repositioning of the nasomaxillary segment in the midline and midface projection. (**c**) Original occlusal view. (**d**) Occlusal view after the two surgical procedures. Note the movement of the maxillary midincisor line toward the midline

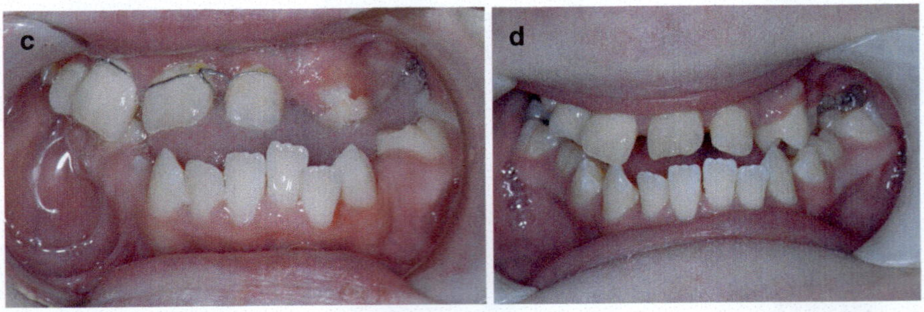

Fig. 7.21 (continued)

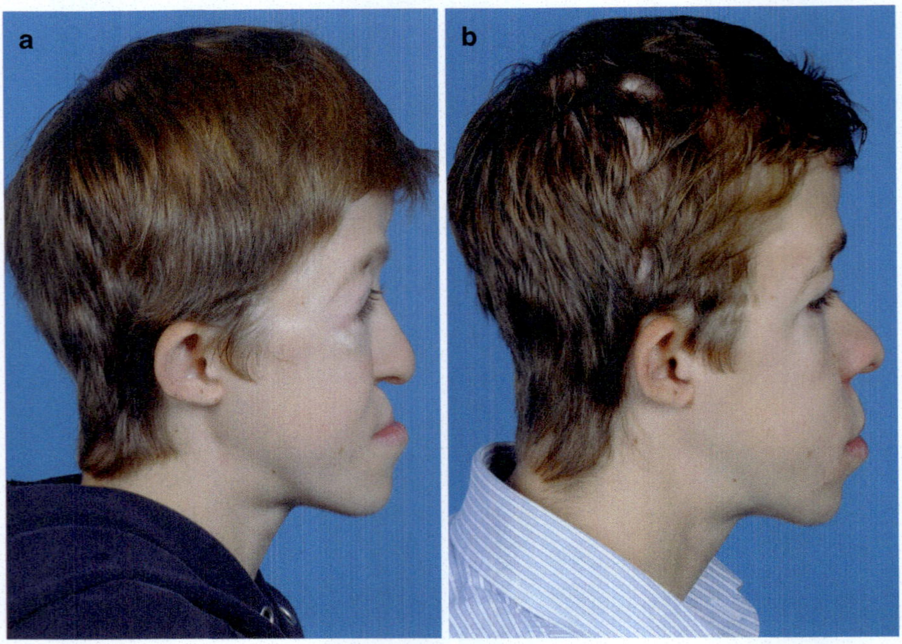

Fig. 7.22 (**a**) Preoperative profile on arrival at the NYU unit. (**b**) Profile after the two procedures described above. Note the projection of the midface and upper lip

7.9 Monobloc Case Reports (Figs. 7.23 and 7.24)

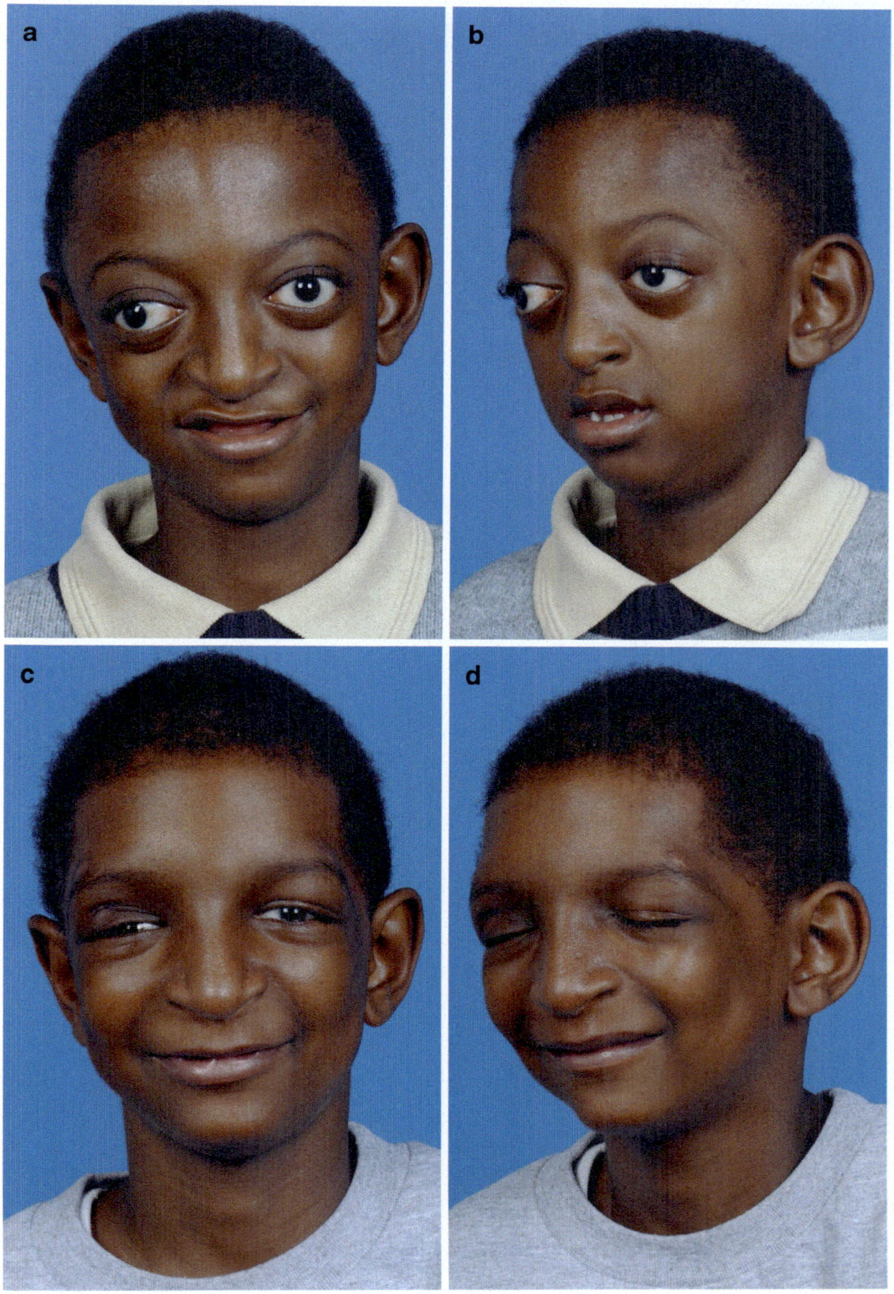

Fig. 7.23 A 7-year-old male with Crouzon syndrome, exorbitism, corneal ulceration, and obstructive sleep apnea. He underwent a monobloc distraction. (**a**, **b**) Preoperative views. (**c**, **d**) Postoperative views at 1 year

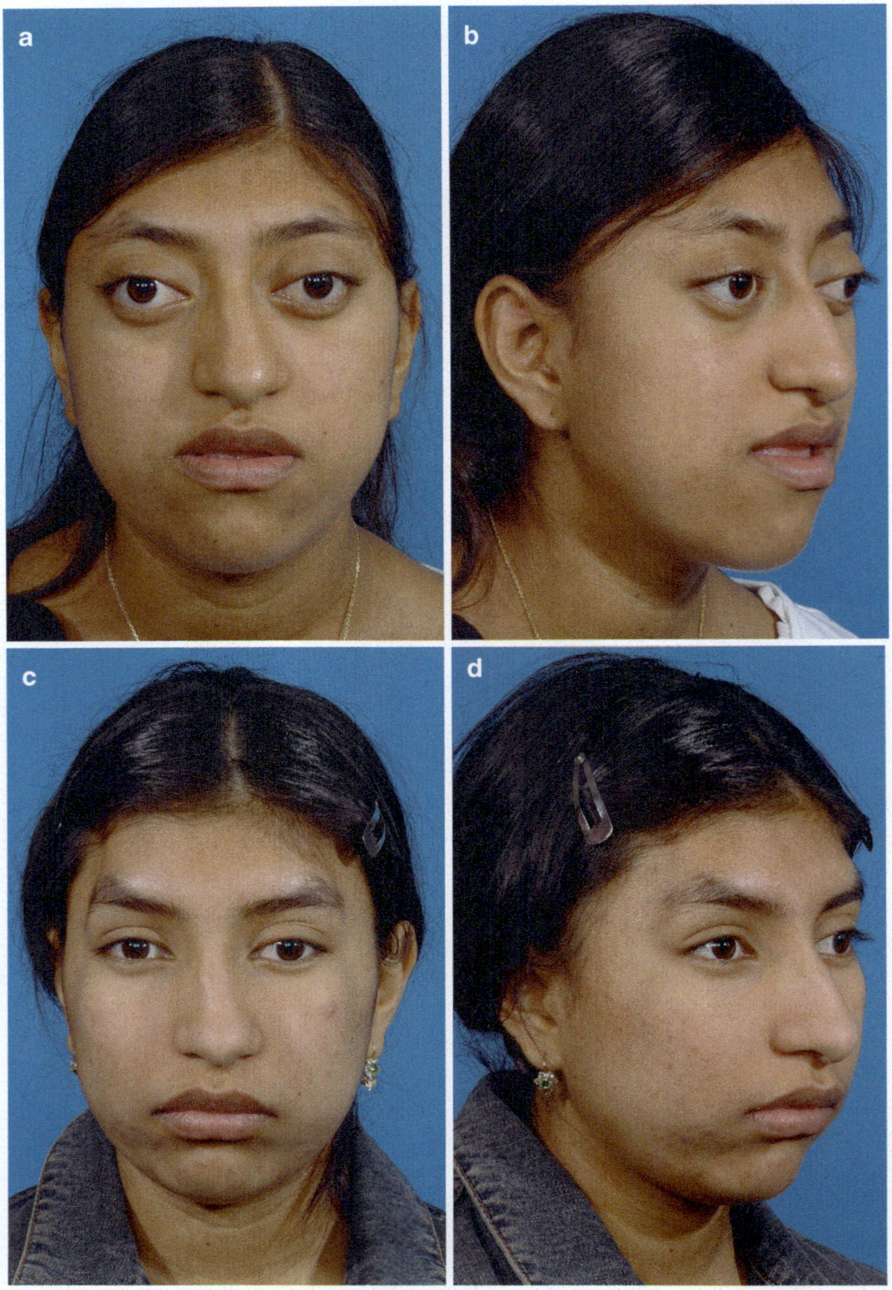

Fig. 7.24 A 17-year-old female with Crouzon syndrome, exorbitism, and increased intracranial pressure who underwent monobloc distraction. (**a**, **b**) Preoperative views. (**c**, **d**) Postoperative views at one year. (**e**, **f**) Postoperative views at four years

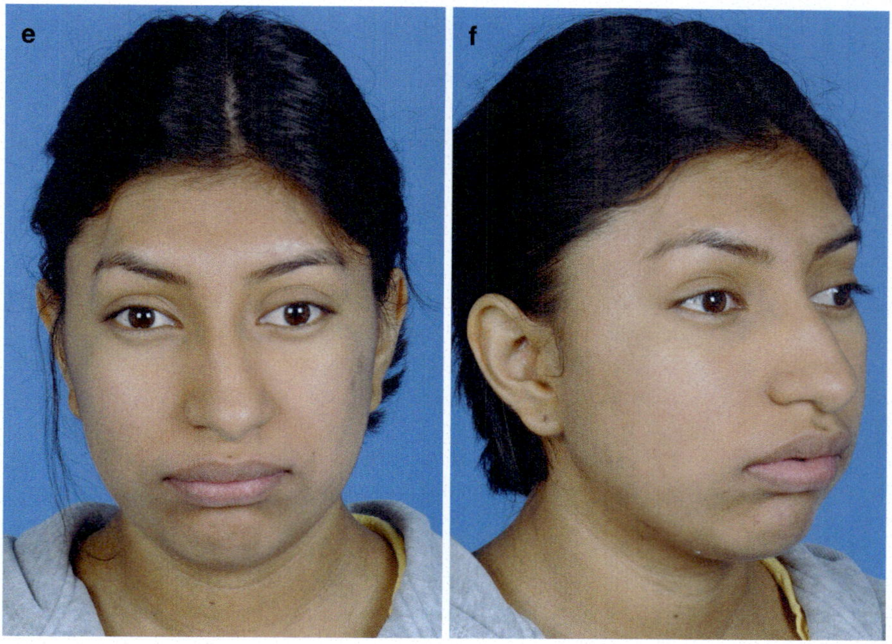

Fig. 7.24 (continued)

7.9.1 Complications

The more common complications following midface or monobloc distraction include hardware-related problems, infection, inadequate osteotomy with inability to apply distraction forces, fractures, dural tears/brain damage, and injury of the permanent molars. Complications can be classified as major (surgical intervention required) or minor (complication resolved by medication alone).

It can be stated that the morbidity rate associated with midface and especially monobloc distraction is much lower than that reported after traditional Le Fort III or monobloc osteotomy/acute advancement (see [9–11, 31]). This is primarily due to decreased operative time, avoidance of nonvascularized bone grafts, and the absence of significant intracranial to nasal communication.

Distraction device or hardware problems can be attributed to imprecise device application or to postoperative trauma (falls, etc.). In a review of 53 subcranial Le Fort III or monobloc distractions, the hardware-related complications associated with the external halo (29) and buried (24) cases were compared, and the complication rate was similar (18.2% vs. 16.4%), as was the percentage of patients requiring a separate surgical intervention for correction of the problem (9.1% vs. 10.1%) [32]. It should be noted that repair of hardware problems in the external halo can occasionally be made without return to the operating room. In a comparison of the external and buried distraction devices, it was reported that the infection rate was significantly lower in the former group [32]. Most postoperative infections can be resolved without surgical intervention.

With the introduction of the distraction technique, the most striking reduction in infection has been noted in the monobloc group of patients. In the traditional monobloc osteotomy/acute advancement, there is immediate expansion of the retrofrontal space or anterior cranial cavity with direct communication established into the nasal cavity. In contrast, in monobloc distraction, there is no advancement of the mobilized frontal bone until the completion of the latency period (5–7 days), during which time, a seal has formed at the cranial base osteotomy between the bone segments. This seal may be reinforced by a galeal-pericranial flap over the osteotomy. Moreover, during the activation period, the frontofacial or monobloc segment is advanced at the rate of only 1 mm/day. The latter stands in contrast to the acute expansion of the retrofrontal space in the traditional monobloc advancement. However, in the patient with a functioning V-P shunt, there is still the risk of retrofrontal infection with monobloc distraction, as the V-P shunt prevents expansion of the frontal lobes to fill the space as the frontal bone is moved forward in the distraction process (Fig. 7.25).

While in midface/monobloc distraction there is not an acute advancement, the osteotomized segment, however, must be mobile. If this goal is not realized, initiation of the distraction forces can result in inadvertent fractures at the sites of incomplete osteotomy. Reports of "early consolidation" of the distraction sites likely represent incomplete osteotomies which were not recognized at the time of surgery. Care should be taken to ensure all osteotomies are complete. The

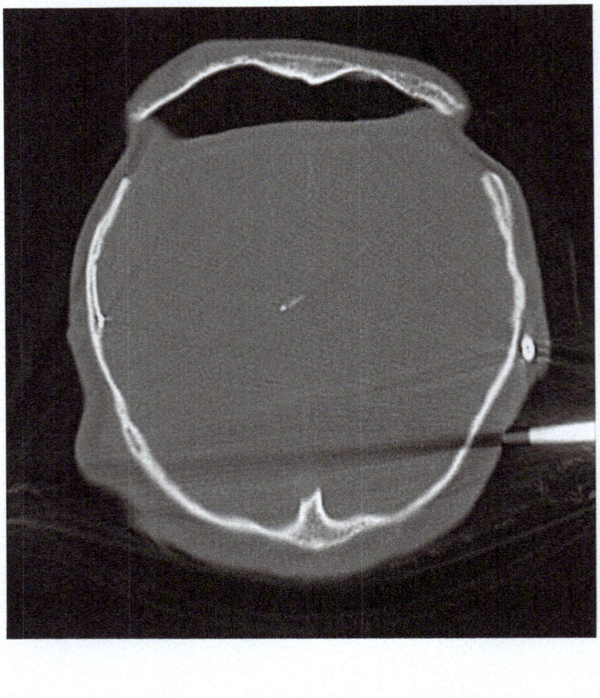

Fig. 7.25 CT scan demonstrating retrofrontal dead space after monobloc distraction with a functioning V-P shunt

zygomatic-maxillary suture, if it is mobile as in the young patient, can also be the site of an inadvertent displaced "fracture" during the activation phase [33]. This can also occur if the orbital floor osteotomy is made too close to the inferior orbital rim. If a zygomatic fracture is suspected, a plate/screw should be applied across the zygomatic-maxillary suture at the time of the osteotomy.

The maxillary permanent molars are at risk, especially in the growing child, when a Le Fort III or monobloc osteotomy is performed [34, 35]. Midface distraction results in a lengthening of the posterior maxillary arch with horizontal movement of the first and second molars. In young patients, disruption of the development of the first, second, and third molars can be observed. Special care and attention are important in performing pterygomaxillary disjunction with the osteotome.

Other possible complications include dural tears, brain injury, cerebrospinal fistula, corneal exposure, eyelid problems, and other complications associated with any type of surgical procedure.

7.10 Clinical Outcomes/Longitudinal Follow-Up

Midface/monobloc distraction is usually performed in patients with syndromic craniosynostosis. The goals of the procedure are to correct elevated ICP (monobloc), to protect the globes in exorbitism, to relieve an obstructed airway, to improve occlusion, and to lessen craniofacial dysmorphism. As the experience with midface/monobloc distraction increased over the past two decades, protocols have been designed to study various aspects/results of the technique in the short and intermediate term.

As the distracted midface has been shown to be stable over the short or intermediate terms (see [10, 11]), as well as 5 years postoperative [36], studies were conducted to document bony deposition/generation at the osteotomy sites. A CT study of ten patients conducted approximately 6 months after distraction showed that bone deposition was found more consistently at the nasofrontal junction and pterygomaxillary buttresses (see [28]). Bone deposition was more consistent at the medial rather than the lateral orbital walls (probably because of previous fronto-orbital advancement surgery). In addition, if the osteotomy is made through the thicker zygomatic body rather than the thinner arch, there was greater volume of bone generate (see Fig. 7.5). In another CT study of 15 pediatric patients undergoing Le Fort III distraction at 1 year follow-up, there was again noted variability of bone deposition in the pterygomaxillary region with clinical stability of the Le Fort III segment and evidence of generation of a minimal amount (25th percentile) of bone formation as early as 4 weeks into consolidation (see [29]). Bone scintigraphy (see [30]) is an alternative technique to study new bone formation after distraction. In all cases of clinically successful distraction, radiotracer uptake rose to the maximum during the consolidation period.

The increase in orbital volume after monobloc and Le Fort III distraction has also been studied by serial CT scans using software programs [37]. As expected, the orbital volume increase was greater after the monobloc or circumferential (360°)

orbital expansion. It all cases, postoperative volumes were within normal range. Two study programs (haptic-aided semiautomatic segmentation and manual 3D slicer segmentation) can provide reproducible documentation of orbital expansion after distraction [38].

Syndromic craniosynostosis patients can have dramatic relief of obstructive sleep apnea after midface distraction. A combined cephalometric and CT study (three-dimensional airway casts) showed significant expansion in the nasopharyngeal and velopharyngeal airways, especially enlarged in those patients showing preoperative airway compromise (see [14]). Cephalometric analysis also showed an increase in the velar angle [39]. In another study [40] of patients before and after Le Fort III distraction, quantitative CT scans and polysomnographic analysis noted that a post-distraction angular increase in the sella-nasion-point A angle was more important than the linear or horizontal change in maxillary position alone for optimal treatment of obstructive sleep apnea. As stated, improvement in respiratory function has a direct correlation with airway volume expansion [41].

The relationship or correlation of soft tissue change to skeletal increase has also been studied. It has been reported that for every 1 cm of skeletal gain after monobloc distraction, there was 0.78 cm gain in the overlying soft tissue [42]. These findings were confirmed in another study of the horizontal relationship from nasal dorsum to orbitale, nasal tip to anterior nasal spine, soft tissue point A to skeletal point A, and upper lip to maxillary incisor [43]. However, as in the vertical dimensional changes, there was a nonlinear relationship. After monobloc distraction and orbital expansion/correction of exorbitism, there is a decrease in the distance between the margins of the upper and lower eyelids, but the downward slant of the palpebral fissure is increased [44] (lowering of the external canthus), hence, the frequent need for an external canthopexy at the time of device removal.

Often, additional surgery is required after midface/monobloc distraction. As mentioned above, external canthopexy is often done at the time of device removal. Ptosis correction may be required after the exorbitism is relieved. Tonsillectomy and adenoidectomy may be indicated to increase the airway space. Secondary distraction may be required if there is inadequate "overcorrection" at the first midface distraction. Definitive orthognathic jaw surgery is usually required at the time of skeletal maturity in the patient with syndromic craniofacial synostosis. Because the chin point is recessed in the syndromic craniosynostosis patient, genioplasty is usually part of the orthognathic surgical procedure at the time of skeletal maturity.

In a review extending back to 1977, the NYU team (see [10, 11]) reviewed 60 patients who underwent Le Fort III advancement stratified into the following time groups: Group I (1977–1987)—Traditional Le Fort III acute advancement with fixation by interosseous wiring and MMF; Group II (1987–1996)—Traditional Le Fort III acute advancement with fixation by only rigid plates/screws, and Group III (2000–2005)—Le Fort III distraction by external halo device. Analysis of the Group III (midface distraction) data showed a statistically significant larger advancement at cephalometric orbitale, Point A, and upper incisal edge in the Group III versus

Groups I and II [10, 11]. Again in comparison to Groups I and II, the distraction group had a lower morbidity rate and reduced operation time and length of hospital stay. In all groups, there was stability of the advanced segment at 1 year follow-up. The surgical trend toward midface distraction is historically reflected in a case report of a Crouzon family whose members underwent midface advancement over a three-decade period, including a mother who had a monobloc osteotomy with acute advancement and rigid fixation/bone grafting, followed years later by her son and daughter treated by monobloc distraction alone [45].

Another study comparing the traditional or acute monobloc advancement with bone grafts and rigid skeletal fixation to the monobloc distraction with buried devices noted that the distraction group had a much greater advancement with less relapse, as well as a lower morbidity rate (see [9]). A similar comparative study at another institution noted improved respiratory status in the Le Fort III distraction group probably because they also had greater horizontal skeletal advancement (19 mm vs. 6 mm in the non-distraction group); moreover, superior aesthetic results in the facial midline were obtained in the external halo versus the buried distraction device [46].

Many studies have documented that the mobilized midface segment is stable at 1 year and also at 5 years postoperative (see [36]), but additional midfacial growth cannot be expected [47–50]. It should also be remembered that midface or maxillary growth is also limited in the unoperated syndromic craniosynostosis patient [51], a reflection of the innate biology of the syndrome. Consequently, when midface/monobloc distraction is performed in the growing child, activation should not be discontinued unless there is a resulting overjet to a degree that does not cause occlusal dysfunction (overcorrection). The family should be forewarned that some type of maxillary advancement may be required at the time of skeletal maturity.

In a series of follow-up reports of patients who underwent monobloc distraction at the Great Ormond Street Hospital, it was noted that the distracted segment remained stable, especially when a latency period of 7 days and an activation rate of 1 mm/day were employed. It was again noted that anterior growth of the midface did not occur after monobloc distraction. It was noteworthy that long-term follow-up (mean of 10.2 years) showed a deterioration of respiratory function in the patients undergoing monobloc distraction at a younger age, and the authors recommended regular follow-up of such patients for this reason [52, 53]. The same institution reported a series of 12 young patients who underwent monobloc distraction under 30 months of age with acceptable morbidity and satisfactory functional results (increased intracranial pressure, corneal exposure, airway obstruction, and feeding problems) as well as improvement in craniofacial appearance [54].

In a unique long-term study of patients [55] who underwent acute Le Fort III advancement and were followed to skeletal maturity, it was noted that most required a repeat Le Fort III advancement (including the orbitozygomatic complex). However, this was not always possible because of skeletal deficiency and the burden of extensive hardware. Many were treated at skeletal maturity with Le Fort I advancement, bilateral sagittal split osteotomy, and genioplasty.

Pearls and Pitfalls

- Midface/monobloc distraction should be undertaken only under the auspices of an experienced multidisciplinary craniofacial team.
- Continuation of the surgeon-orthodontic relationship is critical in the postoperative period for decision-making (vector change, activation endpoint, length of consolidation period).
- Decision of device selection. While the buried devices are less conspicuous and less subject to childhood trauma, the external halo device provides more stability (and less chance for relapse) and allows for postoperative vector manipulation or rotation (swing) of the central rod.
- A posterior descent of the mobilized midface segment during activation is best avoided by a rigid occlusal splint connected to the central rod of the external halo device.
- A latency period of 5–7 days should be practiced to avoid relapse and to allow a seal at the anterior cranial base osteotomy in the monobloc patient. The preferred activation rate is 1 mm/day.
- Beware the presence of a functional V-P shunt in the monobloc distraction patient, as it prevents or lessens expansion of the brain into the enlarged retrofrontal space.
- Endpoints for discontinuation of activation in the growing child include an exaggerated overjet, provided there is no occlusal dysfunction. In the growing child, the more critical endpoint is an overly projected orbitozygomatic complex.
- The distracted midface should be stable, but there will be no post-distraction maxillary growth. Some type of midface advancement will most likely be required at skeletal maturity.
- External or lateral canthopexy is recommended at the time of device removal.

References

1. Gillies H, Harrison SH. Operative correction by osteotomy of recessed malar maxillary compound in a case of oxycephaly. Br J Plast Surg. 1950;3:123.
2. Tessier P. Total facial osteotomy: Crouzon's syndrome, Apert's syndrome, oxycephaly, scaphocephaly, turricephaly. Ann Chir Plast. 1967;12:273.
3. McCarthy JG, Grayson B, Bookstein F, Vickery C, Zide B. Le Fort III advancement osteotomy in the growing child. Plast Reconstr Surg. 1984;74:343.
4. Ortiz-Montasterio F, del Campo AF, Carillo A. Advancement of the orbits and the midface in one piece, combined with frontal repositioning, for the correction of Crouzon's deformities. Plast Reconstr Surg. 1978;61:507.
5. Rachmiel A, Jackson IT, Potparic Z, Laufer D. Midface advancement in sheep by gradual distraction: a 1-year follow-up study. J Oral Maxillofac Surg. 1995;53(5):525–9.
6. Staffenberg DA, Wood RJ, McCarthy JG, Grayson BH, Glasberg SB. Midface distraction advancement in the canine without osteotomies. Ann Plast Surg. 1995;34(5):512–7.
7. Cedars MG, Linck II DL, Chin M, Toth BA. Advancement of the midface using distraction techniques. Plast Reconstr Surg. 1999;103(2):429–41.

8. Polley JW, Figueroa AA. Management of severe maxillary deficiency in childhood and adolescence through distraction osteogenesis with an external, adjustable, rigid distraction device. J Craniofac Surg. 1997;8(3):181–5. Discussion 186
9. Bradley JP, Gabbay JS, Taub PJ, et al. Monobloc advancement by distraction osteogenesis decreases morbidity and relapse. Plast Reconstr Surg. 2006;118(7):1585–97.
10. Shetye PR, Davidson EH, Sorkin M, Grayson BH, McCarthy JG. Evaluation of three surgical techniques for advancement of the midface in growing children with syndromic craniosynostosis. Plast Reconstr Surg. 2010;126(3):982–94.
11. Shetye PR, Grayson BH, McCarthy JG. Le Fort III distraction: controlling position and path of the osteotomized midface segment on a rigid platform. J Craniofac Surg. 2010;21(4):1118–21.
12. Hettinger PC, Hanson PR, Denny AD. Le Fort III distraction using rotation advancement of the midface in patients with cleft lip and palate. Plast Reconstr Surg. 2013;132(6):1532–41.
13. Mulliken JB, Godwin SL, Pracharktam N, Altobelli DE. The concept of the sagittal orbital-globe relationship in craniofacial surgery. Plast Reconstr Surg. 1996;97(4):700–6.
14. Flores RL, Shetye PR, Zeitler D, et al. Airway changes following Le Fort III distraction osteogenesis for syndromic craniosynostosis: a clinical and cephalometric study. Plast Reconstr Surg. 2009;124(2):590–601.
15. Doerga PN, Spruijt B, Mathijssen IM, Wolvius EB, Joosten KF, van der Schroeff MP. Upper airway endoscopy to optimize obstructive sleep apnea treatment in Apert and Crouzon syndromes. Craniomaxillofac Surg. 2016;44(2):191–6.
16. Greig AV, Wagner J, Warren SM, Grayson B, McCarthy JG. Pfeiffer syndrome: analysis of a clinical series and development of a classification system. Craniofac Surg. 2013;24(1):204–1.
17. Greig AV, Britto JA, Abela C, et al. Correcting the typical Apert face: combining bipartition with monobloc distraction. Plast Reconstr Surg. 2013;131(2):219e–30e.
18. Fearon JA, Rhodes J. Pfeiffer syndrome: a treatment evaluation. Plast Reconstr Surg. 2009;123(5):1560–9.
19. Fujimoto T, Imai K, Matsumoto H, Sakamoto H, Nakano T. Tracheobronchial anomalies in syndromic craniosynostosis with 3-dimensional CT image and bronchoscopy. Craniofac Surg. 2011;22(5):1579–83.
20. Shetye PR, Giannoutsos E, Grayson BH, McCarthy JG. Le Fort III distraction: part I. Controlling position and vectors of the midface segment. Plast Reconstr Surg. 2009;124(3):871–8.
21. Havlik RJ, Seelinger MJ, Fashemo DV, Hathaway R. "Cat's cradle" midfacial fixation in distraction osteogenesis after Le Fort III osteotomy. J Craniofac Surg. 2004;15(6):946–52.
22. Figueroa AA, Polley JW, Figueroa AD. Biomechanical considerations for distraction of the monobloc, Le Fort III, and Le Fort I segments. Plast Reconstr Surg. 2010;126(3):1005–13.
23. Francis C, Rommer E, Mancho S, Carey J, Hammoudeh JA, Urata MM. Vector control in internal midface distraction using temporary anchorage devices. J Craniofac Surg. 2012;23(7 Suppl):2000–3.
24. Hopper RA, Prucz RB, Iamphongsai S. Achieving differential facial changes with Le Fort III distraction osteogenesis: the use of nasal passenger grafts, cerclage hinges, and segmental movements. Plast Reconstr Surg. 2012;130(6):1281–8.
25. Hopper RA, Kapadia H, Morton T. Normalizing facial ratios in Apert syndrome patients with Le Fort II midface distraction and simultaneous zygomatic repositioning. Plast Reconstr Surg. 2013;132(1):129–40.
26. Paliga JT, Goldstein JS, Storm PB, Taylor JA. Monobloc minus Le Fort II for single-stage treatment of the Apert phenotype. J Craniofac Surg. 2013;24(4):1380–2.
27. Satoh K, Mitsukawa N, Hosaka Y. Dual midfacial distraction osteogenesis: Le Fort III minus I and Le Fort I for syndromic craniosynostosis. Plast Reconstr Surg. 2003;111(3):1019–28.
28. Jensen JN, McCarthy JG, Grayson BH, Nusbaum AO, Eski M. Bone deposition/generation with Le Fort III (midface) distraction. Plast Reconstr Surg. 2007;119(1):298–307.
29. Hopper RA, Sandercoe G, Woo A, Watts R, Kelley P, Ettinger RE, Saltzman B. Computed tomographic analysis of temporal maxillary stability and pterygomaxillary generate formation following pediatric Le Fort III distraction and advancement. Plast Reconstr Surg. 2010;126(5):1665–74.

30. Rojvachiranonda N, Tepmongkol S, Mahatumarat C. Quantitative study of new bone formation in distraction osteogenesis of craniofacial bones by bone scintigraphy. J Craniofac Surg. 2007;18(5):1236–41.
31. Dunaway DJ, Britto JA, Abela C, Evans RD, Jeelani NU. Complications of frontofacial advancement. Childs Nerv Syst. 2012;28(9):1571–6.
32. Goldstein JA, Paliga JT, Taylor JA, Bartlett SP. Complications in 54 frontofacial distraction procedures in patients with syndromic craniosynostosis. J Craniofac Surg. 2015;26(1):124–8.
33. Gosain AK, Santoro TD, Havlik RJ, Cohen SR, Holmes RE. Midface distraction following Le Fort III and monobloc osteotomies: problems and solutions. Plast Reconstr Surg. 2002;109(6):1797–808.
34. Sant'Anna EF, de A Cury-Saramago A, Figueroa AA, Polley JW. Evaluation of maxillary permanent molars in patients with syndromic craniosynostosis after monobloc osteotomy and midface advancement with rigid external distraction (RED). Cleft Palate Craniofac J. 2010;47(2):109–15.
35. Santiago PE, Grayson BH, Degan M, Brecht LE, Singh GD, McCarthy JG. The effect of early Le Fort III surgery on permanent molar eruption. Plast Reconstr Surg. 2005;115:423.
36. Patel PA, Shetye P, Warren SM, Grayson BH, McCarthy JG. Five year follow-up of midface distraction in growing children with syndromic craniosynostosis. Accepted: Plast Reconstr Surg. 2016.
37. Antunes RB, Camilo AA, da Silva AM, da Silva JV, Alonso N. Assessment of orbital volume in frontofacial advancements. J Craniofac Surg. 2015;26(3):843–8.
38. Smektala T, Nysjo J, Thor A, et al. Three-dimensional eyeball and orbit volume modification after Le Fort III midface distraction. J Craniofac Surg. 2015;26(5):1652–5.
39. McCarthy JG, Coccaro PJ, Schwartz M, Wood-Smith D, Converse JM. Velopharyngeal function following maxillary advancement. Plast Reconstr Surg. 1979;64:180.
40. Ettinger RE, Hopper RA, Sandercoe G, et al. Quantitative computed tomographic scan and polysomnographic analysis of patient with syndromic midface hypoplasia before and after Le Fort III distraction advancement. Plast Reconstr Surg. 2011;127(4):1612–9.
41. Nout E, Bannink N, Koudstaal MJ, et al. Upper airway changes in syndromic craniosynostosis patients following midface or monobloc advancement: correlation between volume changes and respiratory outcome. J Craniomaxillofac Surg. 2012;40(3):209–14.
42. Chan FC, Kawamoto HK, Federico C, Bradley JP. Soft-tissue volumetric changes following monobloc distraction procedure: analysis using digital three-dimensional photogrammetry system (3dMD). J Craniofac Surg. 2013;24(2):416–20.
43. Shetye PR, Caterson EJ, Grayson BH, McCarthy JG. Soft-tissue profile changes following early Le Fort III distraction in growing children with syndromic craniosynostosis. Plast Reconstr Surg. 2013;132(4):945–54.
44. Cruz AA, Akaishi PM, Arnaud E, Marchas D, Renier D. Palpebral fissure changes after monobloc frontofacial advancement in faciocraniosynostosis. J Craniofac Surg. 2008;19(1):106–9.
45. Raposo-Amaral CE, Denadai R, Ghizoni E, Buzzo CL, Raposo-Amaral CA. Family of Crouzon syndrome represents the evolution of the frontofacial monobloc advancement technique: from immediate movement to monobloc distraction to monobloc bipartition distraction. J Craniofac Surg. 2015;26(6):1940–3.
46. Fearon JA. The Le Fort III osteotomy: to distract or not to distract? Plast Reconstr Surg. 2001;107(5):1104–6.
47. Shetye PR, Boutros S, Grayson BH, McCarthy JG. Midterm follow-up of midface distraction for syndromic craniosynostosis: a clinical and cephalometric study. Plast Reconstr Surg. 2007;120(6):1621–32.
48. Patel N, Fearon JA. Treatment of the syndromic midface: a long-term assessment at skeletal maturity. Plast Reconstr Surg. 2015;135(4):731e–42e.
49. Reitsma JH, Ongkosuwito EM, Buschang PH, Adrichem LN, Prahl-Andersen B. Craniofacial stability in patients with Crouzon or Apert syndrome after Le Fort III distraction osteogenesis. Cleft Palate Craniofac J. 2013;50(5):561–9.

50. Ianetti G, Raamieri V, Pagnoni M, Fadda MT, Cascone P. Le Fort III external midface distraction: surgical outcomes and skeletal stability. J Craniofac Surg. 2012;23(3):896–900.
51. Coccaro PJ, McCarthy JG, Epstein F, Wood-Smith D, Converse JM. Early and late surgery in craniofacial dysostosis. A longitudinal cephalometric study. Am J Orthodont. 1980;77:421.
52. Witherow H, Thiessen F, Evans R, Jones BM, Hayward R, Dunaway D. Relapse following frontofacial advancement using the rigid external distractor. J Craniofac Surg. 2008;19(1):113–20.
53. Gwanmesia I, Jeelani O, Hayward R, Dunaway D. Frontofacial advancement by distraction osteogenesis: a long-term review. Plast Reconstr Surg. 2015;135(2):553–60.
54. Ahmad F, Cobb AR, Mills C, Jones BM, Hayward RD, Dunaway DJ. Frontofacial monobloc distraction in the very young: a review of 12 consecutive cases. Plast Reconstr Surg. 2012;129(3):488e–97e.
55. Caterson EJ, Shetye P, Grayson BH, McCarthy JG. Surgical management of patients with an early Le Fort III advancement after they have attained skeletal maturity. Plast Reconstr Surg. 2013;132:592e.

Facial Bipartition Distraction

8

Aina V.H. Greig and David J. Dunaway

8.1 Introduction

There is a specific group of patients with syndromic craniofacial dysostosis, who have a biconcave facial morphology, including the majority of Apert patients and some Pfeiffer patients. The midface is hypoplastic and 'short' in both sagittal and axial planes leading to midfacial retrusion and reduced midfacial height. Midface hypoplasia is more pronounced in the central face, resulting in a biconcave appearance in the midsagittal (vertical) and axial (horizontal) planes [1]. Until recently these findings were thought to be due to a true hypoplasia of the midface. However, 3D CT analysis indicates that there is no volume loss to the midface structures but rather the maxilla and sphenoid are deformed [2]. The midface retrusion in Apert syndrome is a result of an increased angle of divergence of the greater wings of the sphenoid, a posterior rotation of the pterygoid plates, and a shortened maxilla [2]. The occlusal plane is rotated counterclockwise, so that the patients often have an anterior open bite.

In the Apert patient, there is a decreased midface to orbital vertical height ratio and a foreshortened nasal dorsum with prominent nasojugal grooves [3].This finding means that the central part of the face is often much more hypoplastic than the lateral orbital walls and malar prominences, such that the position of the lateral orbital walls is often relatively normal. These anatomical features make the conventional monobloc or Le Fort III osteotomy unsuitable for midface advancement in these patients. Traditional monobloc or Le Fort III advancement, sufficient to

A.V.H. Greig, M.D., Ph.D. F.R.C.S. (Plast.)
Consultant Plastic Surgeon, Guy's and St Thomas' NHS Trust, London SE1 7EH, UK
e-mail: aina.greig@gstt.nhs.uk

D.J. Dunaway, F.D.S.R.C.S., F.R.C.S. (Plast.) (✉)
Consultant Plastic Surgeon, Department of Craniofacial Surgery, Great Ormond Street Hospital, London, WC1N 3JH, UK
e-mail: david.dunaway@gosh.nhs.uk

J.G. McCarthy (ed.), *Craniofacial Distraction*,
DOI 10.1007/978-3-319-52564-8_8

adequately reposition the central part of the face, will lead to over advancement of the lateral orbital walls, resulting in enophthalmos.

In patients with Apert syndrome, there may also be true orbital hypertelorism, characterised by a negative canthal axis and counter-rotated orbits. The periorbital morphology in Apert syndrome is characterised by a downward slant of the palpebral aperture, a compressed supratarsal crease, proptosis and hypertelorism [4]. These aesthetic concerns are often accompanied by functional morbidities, such as airway compromise, ocular surface exposure or such severe oculo-orbital disproportion that herniation of the globe occurs.

Bipartition distraction is a procedure combining frontofacial bipartition and monobloc distraction. Frontofacial advancement with a monobloc osteotomy can improve craniofacial aesthetics and function in syndromes featuring midface retrusion as described by Ortiz Monasterio and colleagues (1978) [5]. In 1979 van der Meulen described the median fasciotomy [6]. Tessier refined this technique as the classical facial bipartition, originally described for the treatment of hypertelorism and Apert syndrome [7]. The operation corrected hypertelorism and medially rotated the orbits. The bipartition also allowed an 'unbending' of the midface so that the central part of the face could be advanced to a greater degree than the lateral areas. Facial unbending has several potential functional advantages. The rotation and asymmetric advancement of the orbits permits a greater orbital volume increase without over advancing the lateral orbits and producing enophthalmos in the lateral aspect of the orbit. Facial unbending with distraction results in a greater advancement of the central part of the face and palate, which potentially leads to a greater enlargement of the upper airway volume [8].

Midface distraction offers significant advantages over techniques involving acute advancements with bone grafts [9–12]. Distraction osteogenesis allows large stable advancements [13, 14] and has also proved effective in the very young [15, 16]. Distraction may be achieved using either internal [17] or external devices [13, 18]. There is evidence that with internal distraction devices, the lateral aspect of the face advances farther than the central area of the face [13]. In an attempt to achieve preferential central advancement, the authors favour the RED (Rigid External Distraction) frame (KLS Martin) with centrally positioned threaded fixation plates plus wires, which apply pull in the region of the nasion, supraorbital ridge and pyriform margin [16]. The aim of combining bipartition with distraction using the RED device is to address the dysmorphology of the unique facies in Apert syndrome and also allow significant midface advancement.

8.2 Bipartition Distraction Technique

8.2.1 Presurgical Orthodontic Preparation

Presurgical orthodontic therapy is performed if needed, to create a midline diastema and diverge the roots of the maxillary central incisors, in order to facilitate the midline maxillary osteotomy [1]. It is indicated in patients in whom permanent central upper

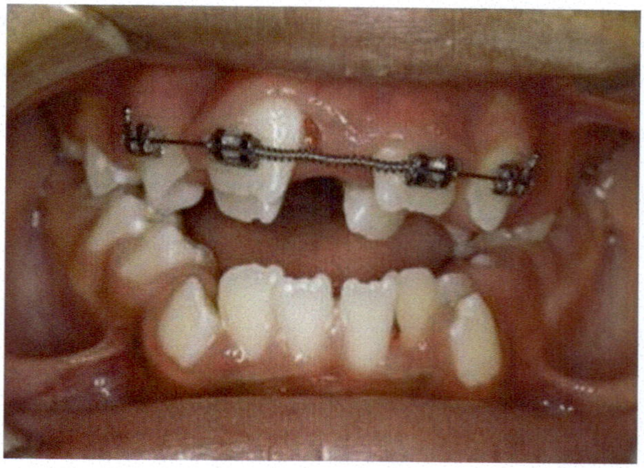

Fig. 8.1 Preoperative orthodontic treatment to create a midline diastema to facilitate a midline maxillary osteotomy

incisors have erupted and in which space between the incisor roots is insufficient to perform the midline maxillary osteotomy without damaging the periodontal membrane or teeth. Full arch or sectional fixed orthodontic appliances can be used (Fig. 8.1). All patients are seen by the dental team preoperatively to ensure optimal oral hygiene.

8.2.2 Surgical Technique

After induction of general anaesthesia, the endotracheal tube is secured with a circum-mandibular wire, and temporary lid occlusal sutures are performed. Coronal and upper sublabial incisions are made. A bifrontal craniotomy is performed (Fig. 8.2a). A V-shaped segment of bone is removed from the midline area of the frontal bone (Fig. 8.2b) to allow medial and upward rotation of the lateral orbits and to increase the amount of projection of the central facial skeleton compared to the lateral area. This manoeuver also increases the curvature of the frontal bone and widens the narrow upper dental arch. The bony interorbital distance is measured on table at the level of the medial canthi. In order to decide how much bone to remove, the ideal intercanthal distance is calculated preoperatively based on age and sex [19]. This value is overcorrected by 5 mm to aim for an interorbital distance of approximately 20–25 mm [20]. The two bipartition segments are wired together in the midline (Fig. 8.2c). The change in configuration of the supraorbital ridge means that the previously removed frontal bone segment often needs adjustment to provide a cosmetically acceptable fit before it is replaced.

After the two bipartitioned monobloc segments are mobilised and secured together, a pericranial graft is applied to the dura over the frontal lobes, to protect against CSF leaks. Three-hole threaded fixation plates (KLS Martin, Jacksonville, FL) are screwed onto the bone—one at the nasion, one on each side of the supraorbital bar in the midpupillary line and one on either side of the pyriform fossa [16]. Care is taken to site the pyriform margin plates so as to avoid damaging tooth roots. A central long fenestrated screw is inserted into the threaded fixation plates, and this

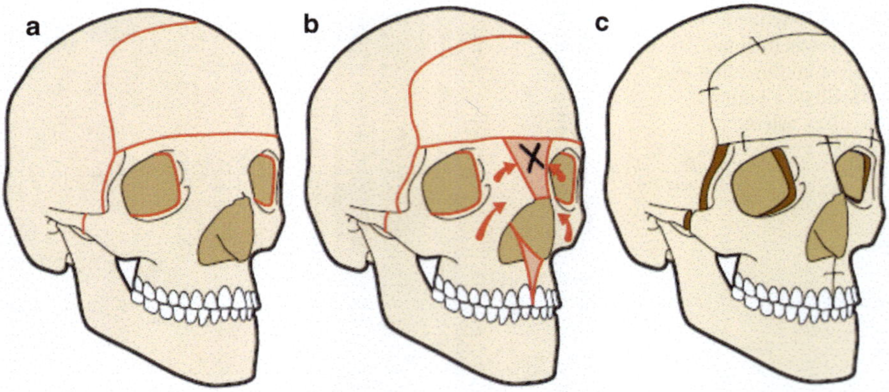

Fig. 8.2 A bifrontal craniotomy and monobloc osteotomies are first performed (**a**). A V-shaped segment of bone is excised from the midline area of the frontal bone, and the hard palate is split in the midline (**b**). This allows medial and upward rotation of the lateral orbits and also increases the amount of projection of the central facial skeleton, as compared to the lateral aspect. The two bipartition segments are wired together in the midline (**c**). The change in the configuration of the supraorbital ridge due to the bipartition means that the previously removed frontal bone segment often needs considerable adjustment to provide a cosmetically acceptable fit before it is replaced

is passed through the skin. Wires are later attached to this screw when the RED frame is applied. Lateral canthopexies are performed, and subperiosteal midface suspension sutures are inserted prior to closure of the coronal incision. The medial canthus is left attached to the bone.

The RED frame is applied parallel to the Frankfort plane. The wires attached to the fixation plates are attached and tightened onto two parallel bars, one at the level of the supraorbital rim and one at the level of the pyriform margin. These provide the vector of pull on the central midface. Two nasopharyngeal airways are inserted at the end of the procedure and sutured in place. A nasogastric tube is also inserted.

Device activation is started following a 7-day latency period. Activation proceeds at approximately 1.4 mm per day (0.7 mm twice a day). Initially, activation is performed by turning the screws at the back of the frame. Towards the end of the distraction period, final adjustments to the facial appearance are made by further tightening the maxillary and/or supraorbital wires at the front of the frame. The decision to stop distraction is based on clinical judgement. The main emphasis is on obtaining a satisfactory orbitozygomatic correction, rather than focussing on occlusal position, which can be later corrected with a Le Fort I osteotomy if necessary. The RED frame is removed after a 6-week consolidation period [1].

We chose an external distraction system (the RED frame) over an internal system in order to take complete advantage of the skeletal ‘unbending’ that the bipartition achieves. The internal systems apply their forces mainly to the malar regions to produce (particularly in the younger child) a bend of the face that worsens rather than reduces the existing concavity [13]. The RED frame with the wires attached at various sites allows differential pull on the central part of the face and permits fine adjustments during the advancement process. A proportion of the ‘unbending’ takes place initially at the time of osteotomies, but differential forward advancement also occurs at the points at which the distraction force is applied to the osteotomised segment (Figs. 8.3 and 8.4).

All patients undergo 3D CT scans preoperatively, immediately following removal of the frame and again at 6 months.

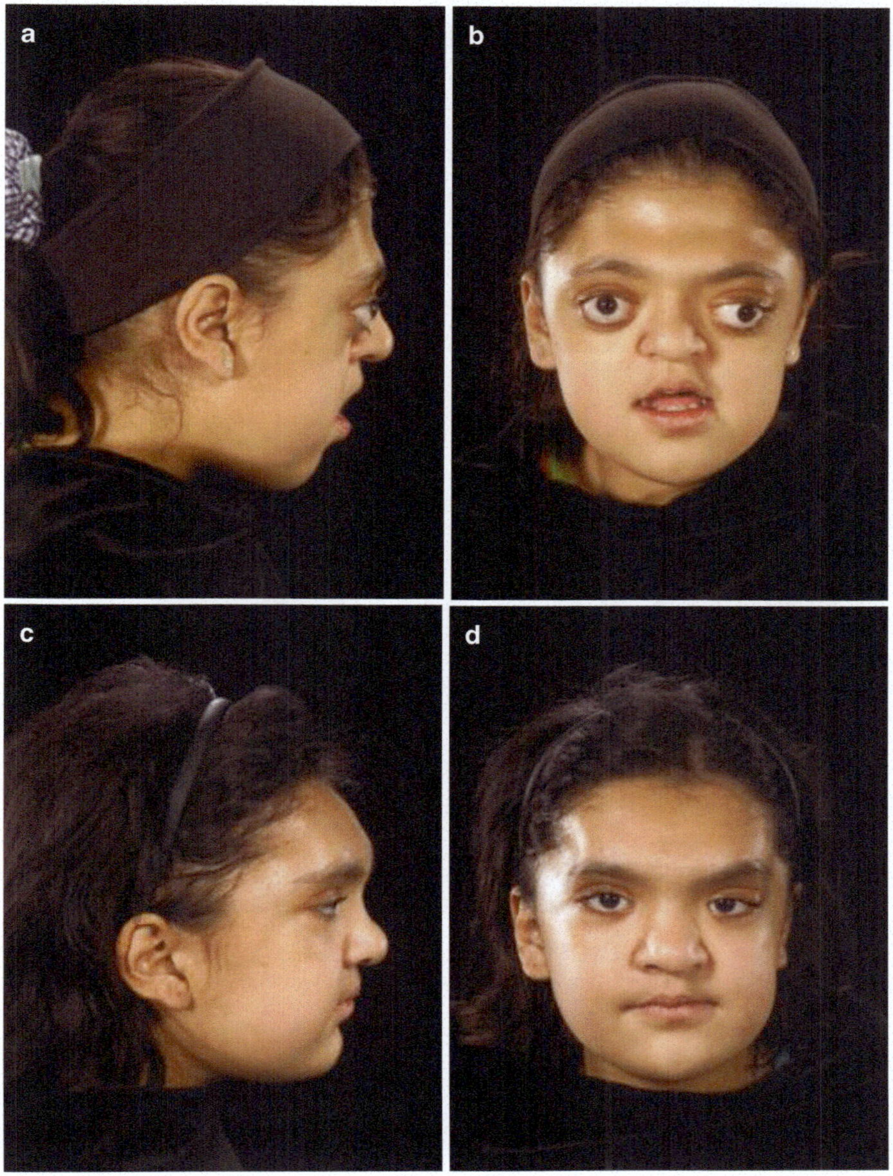

Fig. 8.3 (**a**, **b**) A female patient with Apert syndrome who underwent bipartition distraction at age 12 years. (**c**, **d**) Follow-up photographs are shown at about 14 months postoperative. Figure reproduced with permission from Greig et al. 2013

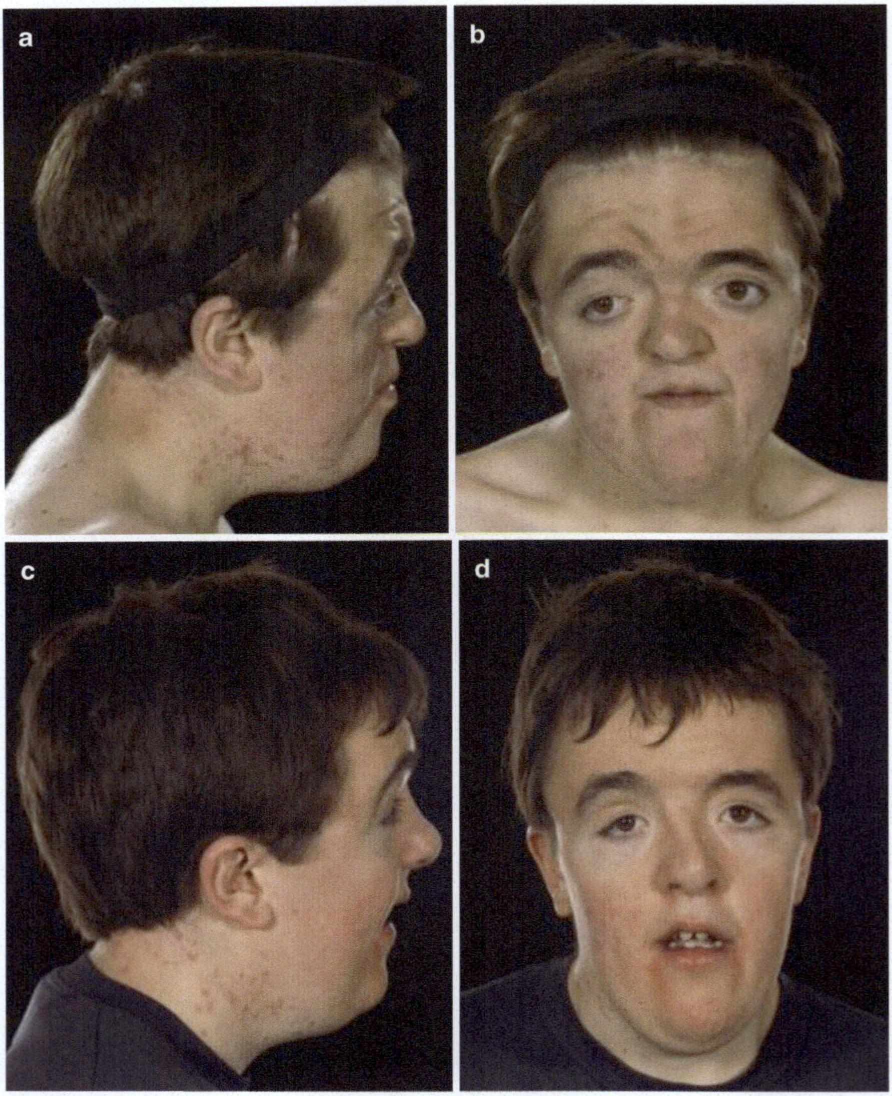

Fig. 8.4 (**a**, **b**) A male patient with Apert syndrome who underwent bipartition distraction at age 17 years. (**c**, **d**) Follow-up photographs are shown at 8 months postoperative. Figure reproduced with permission from Greig et al. 2013

8.3 Outcomes of Bipartition Distraction

A retrospective audit was performed of 20 patients (19 Apert, 1 Pfeiffer; age 1.6–21 years) who underwent bipartition distraction using the Rigid External Distraction (RED II) System (KLS Martin, Jacksonville, FL) from 2004 to 2010 [1]. There were ten females and ten males. There were two broad age groups: 17 patients of age 10–21 years (mean 15.2 years) and 3 patients of age 1.6–4 years (mean 2.6 years). The follow-up period ranged from 15 months to 7 years.

Indications for the procedure included upper airway obstruction [$n = 19$; 11 mild, 4 moderate, and 4 severe (five were on regular CPAP, three had an elective tracheostomy inserted at the time of surgery and removed at RED frame removal)], elevated intracranial pressure ($n = 3$) and the need for ocular surface protection ($n = 11$; five mild corneal exposure with punctate erosions needing lubricants, two moderate corneal exposure with evidence of old corneal scarring, four severe exposure with active ulceration and/or a history of globe herniation). Adolescent patients and patients without functional issues requested aesthetic improvement. Patients who had elective tracheostomies at the time of surgery had more than one indication for surgery with, for example, the need for ocular surface protection and/or elevated ICP.

Eleven of the 20 patients had presurgical orthodontic therapy using either full arch or sectional fixed appliances to open a space for the osteotomy. The remaining nine were too young or space already existed. The decision to open a space was surgeon-led.

The procedure produced functional and aesthetic benefits in all patients. Facial advancement improved corneal protection in all patients, relieving globe herniation in the most severely affected patients. Of the three patients who had evidence of elevated intracranial pressure, indicated by papilloedema on funduscopy and/or electrodiagnostic tests, papilloedema resolved postoperatively in all three patients. Another patient with an indwelling preoperative VP shunt developed elevated intracranial pressure postoperatively, diagnosed by deterioration in VEPs, and required a posterior vault expansion.

A subjective assessment was made of the severity of syndromic craniofacial dysostosis dysmorphology. Fourteen patients were graded as moderate and six as severe. Postoperative aesthetic appearance was graded: 14 had a mild appearance, 5 had a moderate appearance and 1 patient had a severe appearance. We found that 4 out of 20 patients (20%) had no change in their severity of appearance. Appearance was measured on a three-point scale (mild, moderate, severe), and it is recognised that this is not a sensitive evaluation. Examples of pre- and postoperative changes in appearance are shown (Figs. 8.3 and 8.4).

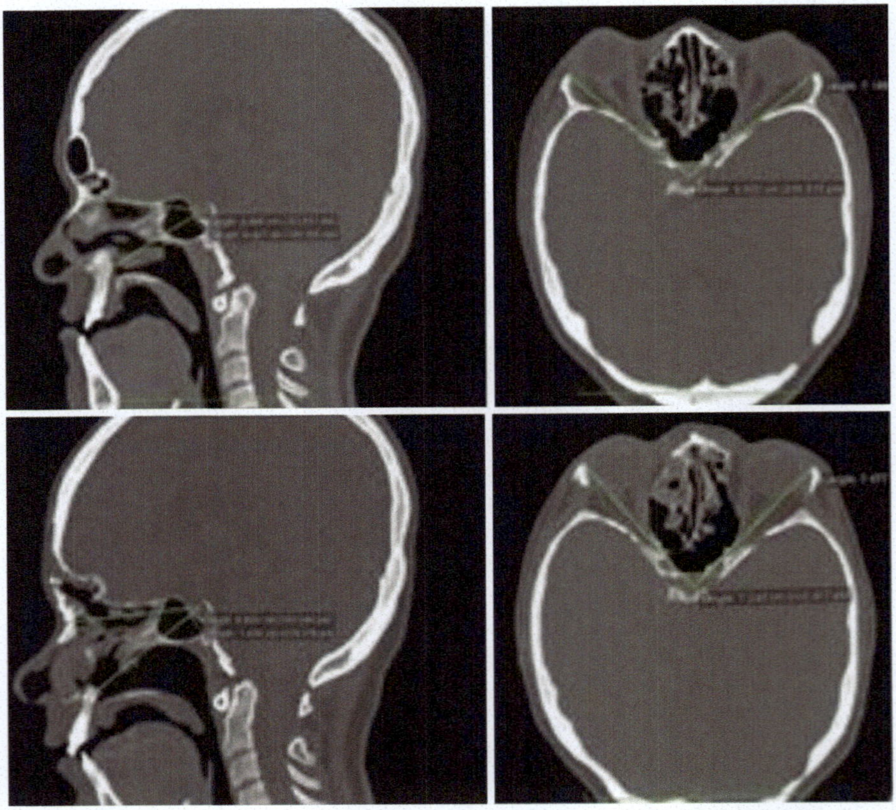

Fig. 8.5 Pre- and postoperative CT measurements were taken using OsiriX software of sella-nasion and sella-A point and compared with measurements between sella and the lateral orbital wall

Bipartition distraction produced a consistent differential central facial advancement. Mean central advancement at sella-nasion was 13.2 mm (SD 5.9 mm) and at sella-A point was 11.7 mm (SD 5.4 mm). Mean lateral advancement was 4.7 mm (SD 2.8 mm). The differential movements are shown (Figs. 8.5 and 8.6). The opportunity to perform distraction osteogenesis meant that the facial appearance could be 'fine-tuned' and adjusted until the facial aesthetic appearance was optimal. This is why the procedure was not performed as a single stage, even though some patients required relatively small advancements. Another reason was due to concerns about the safety of single-stage traditional or acute frontofacial advancement procedures as previously described [11].

Mean change in lateral interorbital distance was −5.4 mm (SD 4.6 mm). The mean change in bony interorbital distance was −4.4 mm (SD 2.8 mm). The mean reduction in lateral interorbital angle was 13.6° (SD 6.7°).

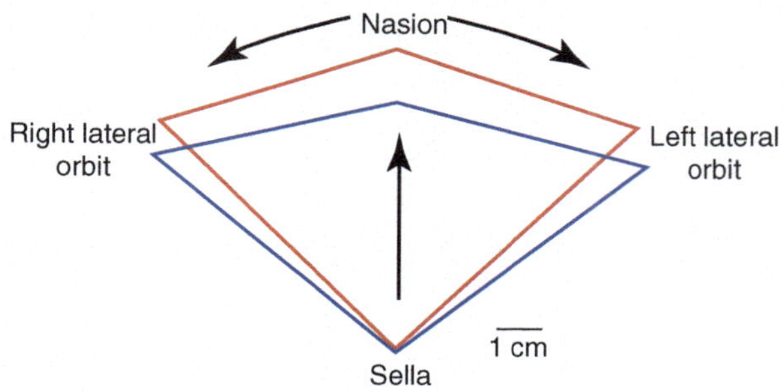

Fig. 8.6 CT scans demonstrating the differential advancement of the face after bipartition distraction, comparing average lateral and central movements for all patients. Central advancement was measured from sella to nasion (mean preop = 6.19 cm, mean postop = 7.52 cm), and lateral advancement was taken as the average measurements from the sella to the right lateral orbit (mean preop = 7.01 cm, mean postop = 7.49 cm) and from the sella to the left lateral orbit (mean preop = 6.93 cm, mean postop = 7.43 cm). Preoperative average measurements are shown in *blue*, and postoperative average measurements are shown in *red*. The *vertical arrow* shows the vector of anterior distraction. The *curved arrows* demonstrate that the face 'unbends' with this procedure. The figure is drawn to scale, and the scale bar represents 1 cm. Figure reproduced with permission from Greig et al. 2013

8.3.1 Postoperative Occlusal Issues

The operation results in a transverse expansion of the maxilla, which is not always symmetrical (because the two halves of the face may need to move by different amounts). Vertical mismatch between the two halves of the maxilla was not observed. The postoperative strategy is to allow the two halves of the maxilla to collapse spontaneously over a period of 3–6 months. Force was not applied to correct the maxillary width because of concern about moving the orbits apart. In addition, there is the risk of moving teeth into the osteotomy site where there is little bone. An older patient required active collapse of the maxilla, and a removable appliance was used to contract the maxillary width without moving the incisors into the osteotomy site. Definitive orthodontic treatment is undertaken after the bipartition either in preparation for orthognathic surgery or in isolation if the intermaxillary relationships are satisfactory. Two patients required an alveolar bone graft where there was insufficient bone to move the incisors together in the midline.

8.3.2 Complications

Complications observed during follow-up included the following: six temporary CSF leaks (four patients required a lumbar drain), five patients with late-onset postoperative seizures, five patients requiring RED frame repositioning, one palatal fistula, one velopharyngeal incompetence, five pin site infections, one retrofrontal abscess, three infections with sepsis, nine patients with increased strabismus, two patients with enophthalmos, one partial visual field loss and three patients requiring reintubation because of aspiration.

One major complication was a partial visual field loss in one eye. The patient aspirated and was reintubated and admitted to PICU from recovery. The patient developed a sluggish left pupil and left strabismus. There was no retrobulbar haemorrhage. We theorised that it could have been due to either rotation or traction on the optic nerve. Over-medialisation of the lateral orbital wall may have put pressure on the lateral rectus muscle belly.

CSF leaks can lead to intracranial infection if there is a communication between the nasopharynx and the intracranial compartment. Many of the initial monobloc distraction patients experienced this problem; therefore, a protocol was implemented. It included avoiding making the midline osteotomy posterior to the foramen caecum (thus avoiding tearing the dura over the crista galli), insetting a pericranial flap into the anterior cranial fossa floor defect and the application of TISSEEL fibrin sealant (Baxter, Deerfield, IL, USA) or DuraSeal (Covidien, Mansfield, MA, USA) to the pericranial flap in the cranial base prior to frontal reconstruction.

Frontofacial advancement is associated with a high complication rate, and complications can occur in between 10 and nearly 60% of patients [21]. Weighed against this are the enormous potential functional and aesthetic benefits of frontofacial distraction. Many of these operations, particularly in the younger age group, are undertaken for functional reasons and for prevention of the inevitable morbidity of phenotypically severe syndromic craniosynostosis. Mortality rates have varied between 0 and 4.5%. There has been a general decline in reported mortality rates with surgical experience, and the most recent series report mortalities of less than 1% [21]. The incidence of significant blood loss (greater than one blood volume) in patients undergoing monobloc osteotomy varied between 5.3 and 9.1%. CSF leaks following monobloc distraction are common (incidence 2–20%). Most of these leaks settle spontaneously. The incidence of frontal bone flap necrosis requiring debridement and a subsequent cranioplasty varied between 3 and 20% [21].

8.4 Geometric Morphometrics

Principal component analysis (PCA) allows the comparison of the shape of a postoperative skull of a patient with Apert syndrome to that of the preoperative skull and comparison to that of a normal skull [22]. Landmarks can be applied to 3D CT scans of the skull of a preoperative patient with Apert syndrome and warped to the mean of a skull which represents the mean of the normal population. Differences in surface distance can be shown by means of a colour map,

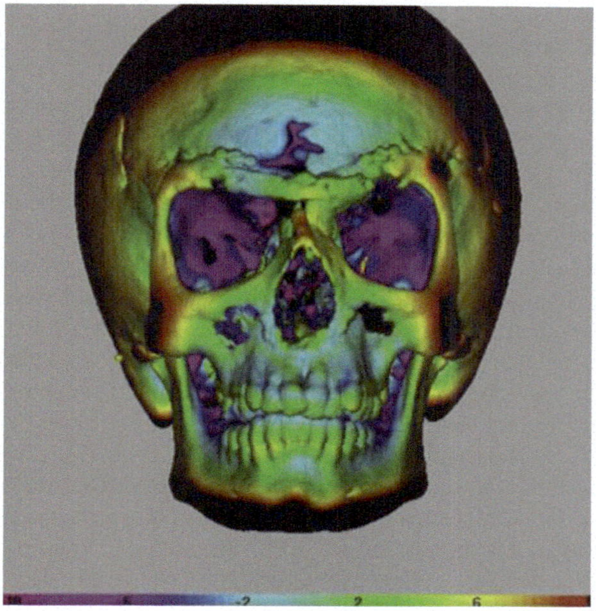

Fig. 8.7 Geometric morphometric colour map of postoperative versus expected normal 3D CT scan. Frontal view depicts positive and negative surface differences. *Light blue* and *green* areas show correspondence between the postoperative and normal scans. Figure reproduced with permission from Crombag et al. 2014

which superimposes the skulls over each other (Fig. 8.7). This technique allows preoperative and postoperative skulls to be compared with each other and also compared with a skull representing the mean of the normal population [22]. This tool has shown that facial bipartition distraction is effective in correcting the hypertelorism. The bipartition distraction procedure also corrects orbital position and midface hypoplasia and 'unbends' the face. However, the analysis has shown that it does not correct the shape of the orbits. Warping the skull from postoperative to normal shows that there is residual turribrachycephaly and deformity of the lateral orbital wall and zygoma (Fig. 8.7).

8.5 Alternative Surgical Approaches to Correct the Apert Face

Other groups have described their experience in treating the midface deformity in Apert syndrome using acute Le Fort III osteotomy [9, 23], Le Fort III midface distraction [13, 14, 24–29], dual Le Fort III minus I and Le Fort I midface distraction [30], monobloc distraction [24, 25, 31, 32] or facial bipartition [24, 25, 32, 33]. Posnick stated that 'A Le Fort III osteotomy is virtually never adequate for an ideal correction of the residual upper and midface deformity of Apert syndrome' and that when using the facial bipartition approach, a more normal arc of rotation of the midface complex is achieved with the midline split [25].

Another group has used Le Fort II midface distraction with simultaneous zygomatic repositioning to normalise the facial ratios in Apert syndrome patients [34]. The surgical aim was to vertically elongate and sagittally rotate the central midface, maintain globe position and improve the relationship between the inferior orbital rim and the anterior cornea. They performed morphometric analysis of 3D CT scans of four patients with Apert syndrome treated with Le Fort II distraction and zygomatic repositioning and compared them with five Apert patients treated with Le Fort III distraction, with five untreated patients with Crouzon syndrome and with six non-syndromic patients of comparable age [34]. Vertical and axial facial ratios were calculated. With Le Fort III midface distraction, the facial ratios of patients with Apert syndrome did not change with surgery and remained lower than the normal controls and the patients with Crouzon syndrome. With the Le Fort II segmental movement procedure, the central face advanced and lengthened more than the lateral orbit. Differential movement changed the preoperative abnormal facial ratios into ratios that were not significantly different from normal controls [34]. The Le Fort II distraction with simultaneous zygomatic repositioning also decreased the anterior open bite by rotating the palate clockwise. The procedure levelled the palpebral fissure by differentially moving the medial orbit and medial canthi to a position inferior to the lateral orbit and lateral canthi. It also reduced the prominent nasojugal folds and lengthened the nasal dorsum. The Le Fort II distraction with zygomatic repositioning the hypertelorism.

Pearls and Pitfalls

Pearls

Facial bipartition distraction:

- Corrects hypertelorism.
- Advances the midface.
- Unbends the face.
- Corrects the lateral canthal axis.
- Corrects upper facial asymmetry.
- Corrects the narrow upper dental arch.
- Good operation to improve function at any age and treats:
  - Upper airway obstruction
  - Elevated ICP
  - Globe exposure.
- Ideal timing for deformity correction is age 8–12 years, although osteotomies to correct occlusion may be required later.

Pitfalls

Facial bipartition distraction does not correct:

- Turricephaly
- Biparietal widening
- Midface height disproportion

It can have adverse effects on lower midface symmetry and occlusion.

Risks of surgery include infection, bleeding, CSF leaks, later-onset postoperative seizures, transverse expansion of the maxilla (with risks of palatal fistula, velopharyngeal incompetence or need for alveolar bone grafting), increased strabismus, overcorrection or under correction.

References

1. Greig AV, Britto JA, Abela C, et al. Correcting the typical Apert face: combining bipartition with monobloc distraction. Plast Reconstr Surg. 2013;131(2):219e–30e.
2. Forte AJ, Alonso N, Persing JA, Pfaff MJ, Brooks ED, Steinbacher DM. Analysis of midface retrusion in Crouzon and Apert syndromes. Plast Reconstr Surg. 2014;134(2):285–93.
3. Ponniah AJ, Witherow H, Richards R, Evans R, Hayward R, Dunaway D. Three-dimensional image analysis of facial skeletal changes after monobloc and bipartition distraction. Plast Reconstr Surg. 2008;122(1):225–31.
4. Kreiborg S, Cohen Jr MM. Ocular manifestations of Apert and Crouzon syndromes: qualitative and quantitative findings. J Craniofac Surg. 2010;21(5):1354–7.
5. Ortiz-Monasterio F, del Campo AF, Carrillo A. Advancement of the orbits and the midface in one piece, combined with frontal repositioning, for the correction of Crouzon's deformities. Plast Reconstr Surg. 1978;61(4):507–16.
6. van der Meulen JC. Medial faciotomy. Br J Plast Surg. 1979;32(4):339–42.
7. Tessier P. Apert syndrome: acrocephalosyndactyly type 1. In: Caronni EP, editor. Craniofacial surgery. Boston: Little Brown; 1985. p. 280–303.
8. Flores RL, Shetye PR, Zeitler D, et al. Airway changes following Le Fort III distraction osteogenesis for syndromic craniosynostosis: a clinical and cephalometric study. Plast Reconstr Surg. 2009;124(2):590–601.
9. Gosain AK, Santoro TD, Havlik RJ, Cohen SR, Holmes RE. Midface distraction following Le Fort III and monobloc osteotomies: problems and solutions. Plast Reconstr Surg. 2002;109(6):1797–808.
10. Denny AD, Kalantarian B, Hanson PR. Rotation advancement of the midface by distraction osteogenesis. Plast Reconstr Surg. 2003;111(6):1789–99; discussion 1800–1783.
11. Bradley JP, Gabbay JS, Taub PJ, et al. Monobloc advancement by distraction osteogenesis decreases morbidity and relapse. Plast Reconstr Surg. 2006;118(7):1585–97.
12. Hayward RJB, Dunaway D. The clinical management of craniosynostosis. Cambridge: Cambridge University Press; 2004.
13. Fearon JA. Halo distraction of the Le Fort III in syndromic craniosynostosis: a long-term assessment. Plast Reconstr Surg. 2005;115(6):1524–36.
14. Shetye PR, Kapadia H, Grayson BH, McCarthy JG. A 10-year study of skeletal stability and growth of the midface following Le Fort III advancement in syndromic craniosynostosis. Plast Reconstr Surg. 2010;126(3):973–81.

15. Polley JW, Figueroa AA, Charbel FT, Berkowitz R, Reisberg D, Cohen M. Monobloc craniomaxillofacial distraction osteogenesis in a newborn with severe craniofacial synostosis: a preliminary report. J Craniofac Surg. 1995;6(5):421–3.
16. Witherow H, Thiessen F, Evans R, Jones BM, Hayward R, Dunaway D. Relapse following frontofacial advancement using the rigid external distractor. J Craniofac Surg. 2008;19(1):113–20.
17. Arnaud E, Marchac D, Renier D. Quadruple internal distraction with early frontal-facial avancement for faciocraniodysostosis. Rev Stomatol Chir Maxillofac. 2004;105(1):13–8.
18. Polley JW, Figueroa AA. Management of severe maxillary deficiency in childhood and adolescence through distraction osteogenesis with an external, adjustable, rigid distraction device. J Craniofac Surg. 1997;8(3):181–5; discussion 186.
19. Hansman CF. Growth of interorbital distance and skull thickness as observed in roentgenographic measurements. Radiology. 1966;86(1):87–96.
20. Tessier P, Guiot G, Derome P. Orbital hypertelorism. II. Definite treatment of orbital hypertelorism (OR.H.) by craniofacial or by extracranial osteotomies. Scand J Plast Reconstr Surg. 1973;7(1):39–58.
21. Dunaway DJ, Britto JA, Abela C, Evans RD, Jeelani NU. Complications of frontofacial advancement. Childs Nerv Syst. 2012;28(9):1571–6.
22. Crombag GA, Verdoorn MH, Nikkhah D, Ponniah AJ, Ruff C, Dunaway D. Assessing the corrective effects of facial bipartition distraction in Apert syndrome using geometric morphometrics. J Plast Reconstr Aesthet Surg. 2014;67(6):e151–61.
23. McCarthy JG, Glasberg SB, Cutting CB, et al. Twenty-year experience with early surgery for craniosynostosis: II. The craniofacial synostosis syndromes and pansynostosis—results and unsolved problems. Plast Reconstr Surg. 1995;96(2):284–95; discussion 296–288.
24. Allam KA, Wan DC, Khwanngern K, et al. Treatment of apert syndrome: a long-term follow-up study. Plast Reconstr Surg. 2011;127(4):1601–11.
25. Posnick JC, Ruiz RL, Tiwana PS. Craniofacial dysostosis syndromes: stages of reconstruction. Oral Maxillofac Surg Clin North Am. 2004;16(4):475–91.
26. Meazzini MC, Allevia F, Mazzoleni F, et al. Long-term follow-up of syndromic craniosynostosis after Le Fort III halo distraction: a cephalometric and CT evaluation. J Plast Reconstr Aesthet Surg. 2012;65(4):464–72.
27. Marchac D, Renier D, Broumand S. Timing of treatment for craniosynostosis and faciocraniosynostosis: a 20-year experience. Br J Plast Surg. 1994;47(4):211–22.
28. Shetye PR, Davidson EH, Sorkin M, Grayson BH, McCarthy JG. Evaluation of three surgical techniques for advancement of the midface in growing children with syndromic craniosynostosis. Plast Reconstr Surg. 2010;126(3):982–94.
29. Oberoi S, Hoffman WY, Vargervik K. Craniofacial team management in Apert syndrome. Am J Orthod Dentofac Orthop. 2012;141(4 Suppl):S82–7.
30. Satoh K, Mitsukawa N, Hosaka Y. Dual midfacial distraction osteogenesis: Le Fort III minus I and Le Fort I for syndromic craniosynostosis. Plast Reconstr Surg. 2003;111(3):1019–28.
31. Witherow H, Dunaway D, Evans R, et al. Functional outcomes in monobloc advancement by distraction using the rigid external distractor device. Plast Reconstr Surg. 2008;121(4):1311–22.
32. Ko EW, Chen PK, Tai IC, Huang CS. Fronto-facial monobloc distraction in syndromic craniosynostosis. Three-dimensional evaluation of treatment outcome and facial growth. Int J Oral Maxillofac Surg. 2012;41(1):20–7.
33. Moreira Gonzalez A, Elahi M, Barakat K, Yavuzer R, Brinkmann B, Jackson IT. Hypertelorism: the importance of three-dimensional imaging and trends in the surgical correction by facial bipartition. Plast Reconstr Surg. 2005;115(6):1537–46.
34. Hopper RA, Kapadia H, Morton T. Normalizing facial ratios in apert syndrome patients with Le Fort II midface distraction and simultaneous zygomatic repositioning. Plast Reconstr Surg. 2013;132(1):129–40.

9 Midface Distraction: Orthodontic Considerations

Pradip R. Shetye and Barry H. Grayson

9.1 Introduction

Distraction osteogenesis has become an important clinical tool in craniofacial surgery. Initially applied to lengthening of the human mandible [1], the technique has subsequently been used to reconstruct all components of the craniofacial skeleton, including the maxilla, zygoma, and cranial vault. One of the most beneficial applications of distraction has been advancement of the midface in patients with cleft lip and palate, midface hypoplasia, and craniosynostosis syndromes.

Midface hypoplasia is a common finding in patients with syndromic craniosynostosis (Apert, Crouzon, and Pfeiffer syndromes). The midface hypoplasia is characterized by nasomaxillary and zygomatic hypoplasia, upper dental arch retrusion, and an anterior crossbite. There may also be associated exorbitism and increased intracranial pressure. The condition was traditionally treated using LeFort III or monobloc osteotomy with acute midface advancement, bone grafting, and rigid fixation. While this resulted in a decrease in corneal exposure and improvements in obstructive sleep apnea, dental relations, and dysmorphic facies, there were significant drawbacks to the LeFort III acute osteotomy with immediate advancement. Soft tissue resistance and deficiencies limited acute skeletal advancement. These were other problems: prolonged operative time, bleeding, infection prolonged surgical procedure (especially with monobloc advancement), extended hospital stays, and the need for bone graft harvest.

Distraction following LeFort III or monobloc osteotomy has become the preferred choice for midface advancement especially in the pediatric patient. The indications are discussed in more detail in Chapter 7. At our institution, LeFort III distraction is

---

P.R. Shetye, D.D.S., B.D.S., M.D.S. (✉) • B.H. Grayson, D.D.S.
Wyss Department of Plastic Surgery, NYU Langone Medical Center,
New York, NY 10016, USA
e-mail: pradipshetye@nyumc.org

J.G. McCarthy (ed.), *Craniofacial Distraction*,
DOI 10.1007/978-3-319-52564-8_9

undertaken for 4- to 7-year-old patients. The advantages of the distraction technique include elimination of the need for bone grafts and rigid fixation (thus avoiding secondary donor-site morbidity), possibility of larger advancement, reduced need for blood transfusion, and shorter hospital stays [2]. Computed tomography studies have demonstrated that new bone is generated at the site of the osteotomy [3]. Currently, midface distraction or monobloc can be achieved by using either an external halo device or paired internal (buried) devices. For larger advancement, our preference is to use a rigid external distraction (RED) device, as it provides better stabilization and control of the midface segment during the activation phase of distraction.

9.2 Preoperative Evaluation

As part of the planning for a midface distraction, the patient should undergo a comprehensive evaluation. Soft and hard tissue should both be examined in static and active positions. The occlusal cant, mandibular range of motion, and paths of opening and closing should be documented. The amount of corneal exposure and the relationship of the lateral and inferior orbital rims to the apex of the globe must be documented. Formal ophthalmologic and neurosurgical assessments are mandatory.

9.2.1 Diagnostic Records

The craniofacial skeletal relationship should be documented with a medical-grade or cone-beam computed tomography scan, 2- and 3-dimensional photographs, and dental study models. With current imaging software (such as Dolphin Imaging), a traditional lateral cephalogram, a panoramic radiograph, and a posteroanterior (PA) cephalogram can be generated from a computed tomography or cone-beam computed tomography. These records become important tools in evaluating craniofacial morphology and planning the placement of the distraction device and the occlusally bonded dental splint. These tools enable the clinician to calculate the appropriate distraction vector and plan the device placement. The dental study model is used to identify anticipated occlusal interferences and to construct the occlusally bonded dental splint, which is cemented to the dentition during the distraction process.

9.3 Predistraction Orthodontic Therapy

The patient preparing for LeFort III or monobloc distraction may need limited presurgical orthodontic treatment, depending on the occlusal findings. This may include maxillary expansion or leveling of the occlusal plane. The patient must also be seen by a pediatric dentist to confirm that he or she does not have any active decay. It is important to reinforce satisfactory oral hygiene during and after the distraction process.

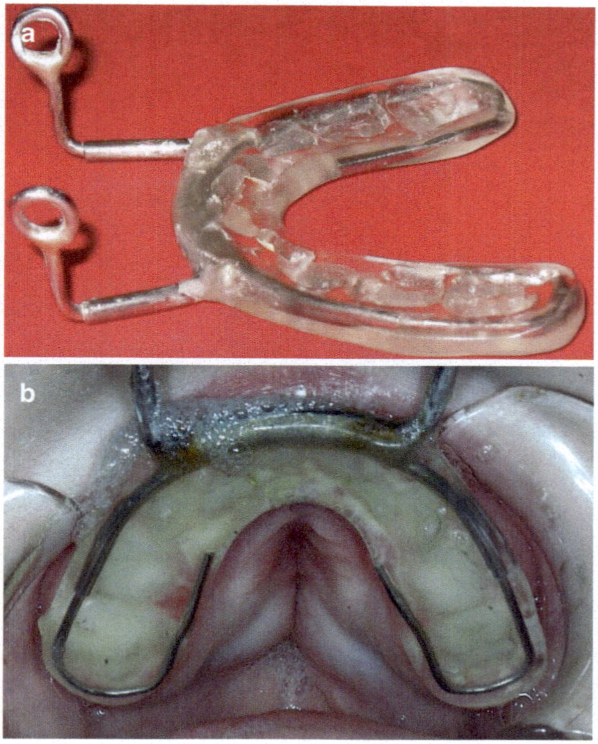

Fig. 9.1 Splint design (traditional) for LeFort III or monobloc distraction. (**a**) Splint construction using orthodontic headgear embedded in acrylic and fabricated on dental study model. (**b**) Splint cemented with glass inonomer cement on the maxillary dentition (applied in the operating room)

9.4 Splint Construction for LeFort III or Monobloc Distraction: Traditional

A traditional (or nonrigid) intraoral splint is constructed by incorporating an orthodontic headgear bow into the occlusal acrylic bite registration. The internal wire of the headgear bow (the thinner one) is closely adapted to the maxillary dentition, and the outer bow (the thicker one) is bent perpendicularly out and configured to construct outrigger hooks (Fig. 9.1). The height of the outrigger hooks will depend on the age of the patient and on the patient's planned vector of distraction. The inner wire is then embedded in self-curing acrylic dental resin to construct the dental splint. The dental splint is cemented in the operating room using light-cured glass ionomer cement. If the patient has multiple missing teeth, suspensory wires (026 gauge) are passed through drilled holes in the zygomas and the holes in the splint to

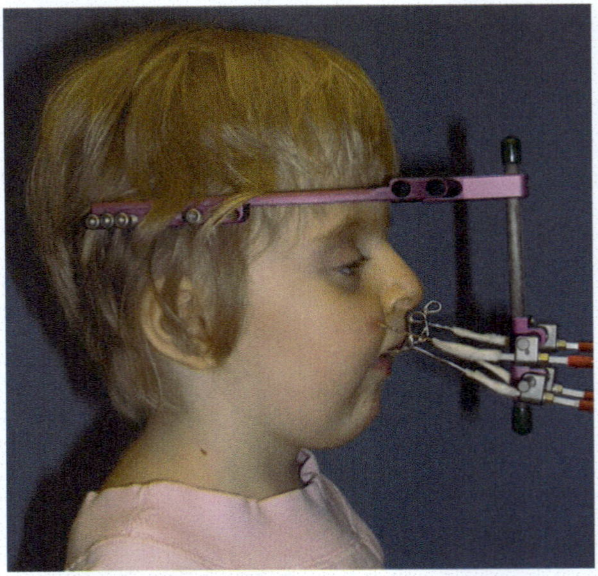

Fig. 9.2 Patient fitted with the external halo and attachments to the intraoral dental splint (traditional) and to the skeletal posts via 0.026-gauge stainless steel wires

reinforce it in the event that the cemented splint becomes detached from the dentition during the course of distraction. The dental splint is connected to the RED frame via .018 in. (026-gauge) stainless steel wires to the horizontal bar on the RED frame. The height of the vertical rod attachment can also be adjusted to achieve the desired height for the optimal distraction vector (Fig. 9.2).

9.5 Splint Construction for LeFort III or Monobloc Distraction: Rigid

This is a modified version of the distraction splint, and it has a rigid connection (instead of wire attachments) from the dental splint to the vertical rod of the RED device (Fig. 9.3). The design permits better control of the occlusal plane and, in turn, improves the position and the stability of the midface segment during the activation phase. The appliance consists of an intraoral component and an extraoral component that attaches to the RED device. The intraoral component consists of a wire mesh, which can be trimmed to adapt to the form of the maxillary arch form on the dental cast. Once adapted to the dental arch, it is embedded in self-curing acrylic dental resin to construct the dental splint. The attachment to the dental splint is adjustable in all three planes with the help of a driver. The horizontal extension from the dental splint is connected to the adjustable vertical rod, which, in turn, is attached to the vertical carbon rod of the RED device. The height of the vertical rod can also be adjusted to achieve the desired height for the optimal distraction vector (Fig. 9.4).

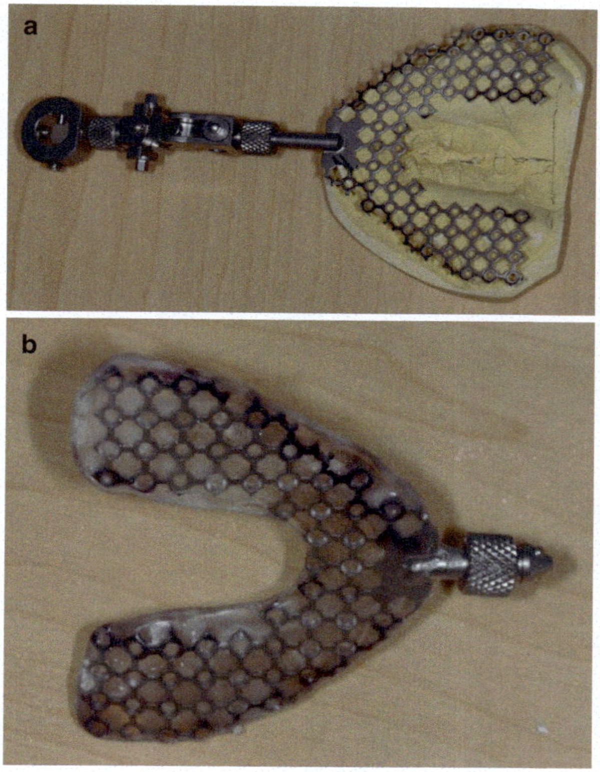

Fig. 9.3 Splint design (rigid) for LeFort III or monobloc distraction. (**a**) Splint construction using prefabricated wire mesh splint from KLS Martin®. (**b**) The intraoral splint is embedded in acrylic and fabricated on a dental study model

9.6 Orthodontic Therapy During Activation

9.6.1 Control of the Position of the Osteotomized LeFort III

To attain the desired occlusion and craniofacial form, it is essential to control the position of the osteotomized LeFort III/monobloc segment during distraction. In the traditional or acute LeFort III surgical advancement, the midface segment is acutely repositioned with the assistance of a prefabricated occlusal splint. The midface is buttressed in position with bone grafts and secured with rigid skeletal fixation plates. With precise preoperative planning, the procedure can be performed with a high degree of reliability. This stands in contrast to the LeFort III/monobloc distraction procedure, which has a certain degree of uncertainty with regard to the final position of the LeFort III midface segment. This is especially true when attempting to control the vertical position of the midface following completion of the

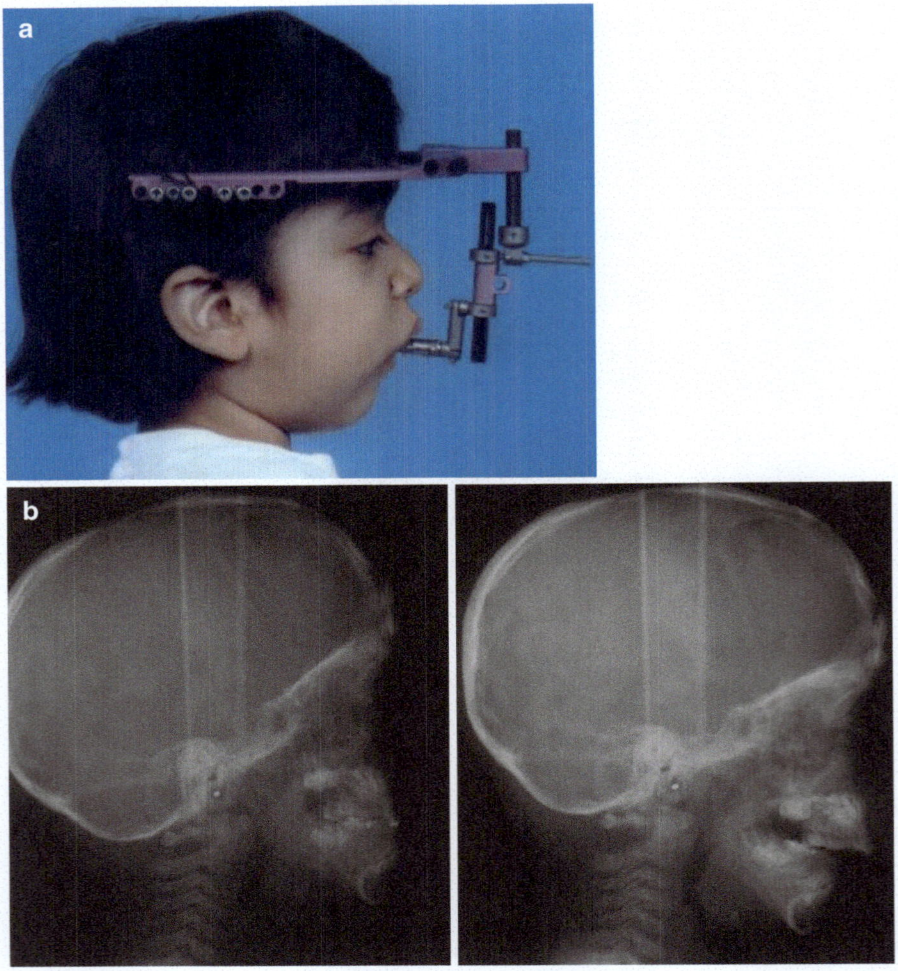

Fig. 9.4 (**a**) Patient fitted with the external halo and attachments to the rigid custom-fabricated dental splint. (**b**) Serial lateral cephalograms taken (*left*) pretreatment and (*right*) after device removal. Note the overcorrection accomplished with a positive dental overjet and control of the occlusal plane with rigid distraction splint

osteotomy. The final position of the midface following activation depends on the location and the direction (vector) of force application (relative to the maxillary occlusal plane).

The change in position of the osteotomized LeFort III segment during midface distraction can be predicted by controlling the *location* and *direction* of the force applied to the mobilized skeleton. The *center of resistance* of the mobilized *LeFort III /monobloc* segment is located slightly above the halfway point between the upper

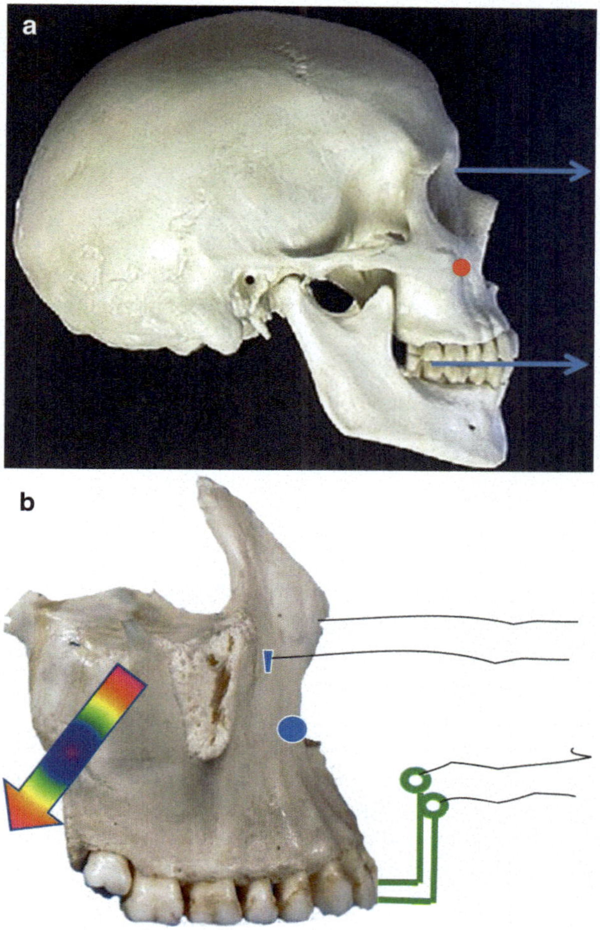

Fig. 9.5 (**a**) The center of resistance (*red dot*) of the mobilized LeFort III segment is located at a point 55% of the distance between the maxillary occlusal plane and the nasion. (**b**) The influence of the masseter muscle (*arrows*) causing posterior inferior descent on the position of the mobilized LeFort III segment when there is absence of a rigid splint (wire fixation)

incisor tip and the nasion [4]. The location of this point will vary according to the patient's age and degree of skeletal maturation. It can be measured at a point 55% of the distance between the maxillary occlusal plane and the nasion [4] (Fig. 9.5). If the distraction force is applied at this level, the LeFort III midface segment can be predicted to advance forward without adversely affecting the maxillary occlusal plane. The soft tissue envelope and the muscle attachments both exert influence on the actual location of the center of resistance. Having determined the center of resistance for the LeFort III segment, the surgeon can then apply appropriate forces to achieve a controlled change in the position of the midface during distraction osteogenesis.

Equally important is the fact that, if force is directed below the center of resistance, the LeFort III segment will rotate in a counterclockwise direction. This will result in an anterior openbite, as the maxillary incisors move superiorly and the molars move inferiorly. Conversely, if the line of force of distraction passes above the center of resistance and parallel to the maxillary occlusal plane, the bony segment will rotate in a clockwise direction, and this may cause excessive advancement of the zygomas and infraorbital rims.

Following the classic subcranial LeFort III or monobloc osteotomy and the mobilization of the osteotomized segment, absorbable sutures are used at the lateral orbital wall to return the mobilized segment to its native position relative to the cranium. An acrylic-and-wire splint (traditional) with outrigger hooks is then secured to the maxillary teeth with dental cement. If needed, distraction-fixation pillars (intraosseous screws) may be secured to the maxilla at the pyriform aperture. The RED device (KLS Martin) is secured to the cranium with pins. Two .018 in. 26-gauge stainless steel wires then connect the distraction posts and the oral splint to the distraction units on the crossarms of the RED device's vertical bar. Wires can also be passed from the pillars through the shin at the alar crease to the crossarm on the vertical bar of the halo device.

Patients undergoing midface distraction have a mean latency period of 5–7 days. The device is activated for 0.5 mm, twice per day, to complete the desired planned advancement. Activation of the device is concluded after sufficient maxillary advancement has been achieved, as judged by clinical (orbitozygomatic contour) and dental evaluations and through assessment of the lateral cephalometric findings. One of the objective criteria to conclude midface advancement during the activation phase is to bring the infraorbital rim just behind the plane of the cornea to avoid enophthalmos. At the end of distraction, especially in growing patients, at least 5–6 mm of positive overjet should be present. The device is left in position for an average consolidation period of 8 weeks. The RED devices and intraoral splints are removed in the operating room after the consolidation period. Lateral canthopexies are often performed during this procedure. There is no need for internal rigid fixation after removal of the distraction device.

9.7 Outcomes

9.7.1 Skeletal Changes

The effect of midface distraction on maxillary skeletal position and clinical appearance in patients with Crouzon, Pfeiffer, and Apert syndromes was studied at 1 year after distraction [5]. This retrospective longitudinal study examined the lateral cephalograms of patients who had undergone midface distraction with RED devices. The study demonstrated that, following distraction, the mean advancement was 17.16 mm at the upper incisal edge, 15.85 mm at point A, and 12.72 mm at the orbitale. The maxillary and mandibular skeletal discrepancies were significantly decreased, with the ANB angle changing from −5.87 to +13.17°. At the 1-year follow-up, the upper incisor edge, point A, and orbitale were all stable and did not exhibit any relapse. It is interesting to note that, post-distraction relapse, which can be observed following mandibular distraction, was not observed following midface distraction.

9.7.2 Comparison Between Traditional (Acute) and Distraction Midface Procedure

While traditional LeFort III or monobloc advancement and midface distraction osteogenesis are well described, there is a paucity of reports in the literature that compare the different techniques using a large series of patients.

A review of the clinical and cephalometric outcomes of midface advancement using the three different techniques for LeFort III midface advancement was reported by the NYU team [2]. The records of 212 syndromic craniosynostosis patients were reviewed from the period of 1973–2006. A total of 60 patients satisfied the inclusion criteria; the mean age of the sample at surgery was 6.2 years. In group 1 (1977–1987), fixation was performed using interosseous wiring and intermaxillary fixation; in group 2 (1987–1996), fixation was achieved using rigid-plate fixation; and in group 3 (2000–2005), the patients underwent midface distraction using the RED device. Cephalometric landmarks were identified and digitized at each of the time intervals (preoperative, postoperative, and 1 year postoperative).

The mean advancement measured at point A in group 1 was 9.7 mm; it was 10.6 mm in group 2 and 16.1 mm in group 3. There was no statistically significant difference in the amount of advancement between groups 1 and 2. However, when groups 1 and 2 were compared to group 3, there was a statistically significant difference ($P < .05$). No statistical significance was noted within or between the three groups at the 1-year follow-up, indicating relative stability of the advanced midface segment.

The clinical findings in this study also indicated that the distraction technique reduced operating time (mean below 6 h), blood loss (mean 678 mL), and length of hospital stay (mean 5.3 days). The improvements in these outcome metrics can be attributed to the less invasive nature of the distraction technique; the avoidance of bone graft harvest, intermaxillary fixation, plates, and screws; and the reduction of operating times (with attendant decreases in blood loss and hypothermia). The avoidance of bone grafts also decreases the risk of infection.

9.7.3 Soft Tissue Changes Following Distraction

The soft tissue profile changes following LeFort III (midface) distraction in growing patients with syndromic craniosynostosis were also studied [6]. The cohort consisted of 20 syndromic patients who underwent LeFort III distraction using a RED device. The mean age at surgery was 5.7 years (range: 3–12.5 years). Lateral cephalograms were obtained preoperatively (time 1), after distraction device removal (time 2), and 1 year after distraction (time 3). Profile landmarks (10 for skeletal or hard tissue and 11 for soft tissue) were identified and digitized at time points 1, 2, and 3. The *x* and *y* displacements of each landmark were studied to determine the ratio of changes in the soft tissue to changes in the hard tissue. The results showed that the ratio of horizontal changes in the soft tissue to those in the hard tissue was 0.73:1 for the nasal dorsum to the orbitale and 0.86:1 for the soft tissue tip of the nose to the anterior nasal spine. The same ratio at point A was 0.88:1. The horizontal ratio of the upper lip position to the labial surface of the maxillary incisor was 0.88:1. The ratio of nasal tip elevation to anterior nasal spine advancement was 0.27:1. The result of this study supported the hypothesis that a linear relationship exists between soft tissue changes and hard tissue (skeletal) changes in the horizontal direction for the midface landmarks following LeFort III distraction. However, the study showed a nonlinear relationship between soft tissue changes and hard tissue (skeletal) changes in the vertical direction.

9.7.4 Five-Year Follow-Up

Patients who underwent midface distraction were also followed 5 years post-distraction. Midface distraction stability that was observed at 1 year remained stable at 5-year follow-up. Orbitale point shows remodeling by moving posteriorly 0.58 mm, point A moved anteriorly by 2.08 mm, and upper incisor advanced by 1.93 mm. However, orbitale, point A, and upper incisor edge descended 3.23, 5.2, and 6.35 mm. This indicated that there was recordable vertical growth of the midface and minimal horizontal growth [7].

9.7.5 Airway Changes Following Distraction

Patients with syndromic craniosynostosis with severe upper respiratory tract obstruction can benefit significantly from midface distraction, as evidenced by improvement in the symptoms of obstructive sleep apnea and decannulation [8]. Midface distraction increases the angle of the velum in relation to the cranial base. The nasopharyngeal and velopharyngeal spaces, which are the areas most constricted in patients with advanced airway obstruction, are significantly expanded by LeFort III distraction. The ratio of bony advancement to anteroposterior airway expansion is approximately 1:0.5 in the nasopharynx and 1:0.25 in the velopharynx. Because of the proportionate expansion of the airspace in relation to bony sagittal advancement, a large midface advancement is required to produce a significant expansion of the compromised airspace. It was also observed that a constriction of the lateral airspace behind the velum is also relieved by midface advancement. Therefore, the volumetric increase of the airspace may be greater than what is suggested in the lateral cephalogram. Although LeFort III distraction can improve airway function, it must be emphasized that patients with syndromic craniosynostosis can have multiple anatomic sites of respiratory obstruction and dysfunction.

Pearls and Pitfalls

- Midface distraction, as compared to traditional advancement, achieves greater linear advancement with less morbidity.
- Vector control and prevention of counterclockwise rotation of the distracted segment must be part of preoperative planning.
- Activation in the growing child is not discontinued until there is overcorrection at the orbitozygomatic and maxillary occlusal plane.
- Device rigidity and force strength are absolute requirements.
- The distracted midface segment is stable at 1 and 5 years.

References

1. McCarthy JG, et al. Lengthening the human mandible by gradual distraction. Plast Reconstr Surg. 1992;89(1):1–8. Discussion 9–10
2. Shetye PR, et al. Evaluation of three surgical techniques for advancement of the midface in growing children with syndromic craniosynostosis. Plast Reconstr Surg. 2010;126(3):982–94.
3. Jensen JN, et al. Bone deposition/generation with LeFort III (midface) distraction. Plast Reconstr Surg. 2007;119(1):298–307.
4. Shetye PR, Giannoutsos E, Grayson BH, McCarthy JG. LeFort III distraction: part I. Controlling position and vectors of the midface segment. Plast Reconstr Surg. 2009;124(3):871–8.
5. Shetye PR, et al. Midterm follow-up of midface distraction for syndromic craniosynostosis: a clinical and cephalometric study. Plast Reconstr Surg. 2007;120(6):1621–32.
6. Shetye PR, et al. Soft-tissue profile changes following early Le Fort III distraction in growing children with syndromic craniosynostosis. Plast Reconstr Surg. 2013;132(4):945–54.
7. Patel PA, Shetye PR, Warren SM, Grayson BH, McCarthy JG. Five year follow-up of midface distraction in growing children with syndromic craniosynostosis. Plast Reconstr Surg. 2016. Accepted for publication.
8. Flores RL, Shetye PR, Zietler D, Berstein J, Wang E, Warren SM, Grayson BH, McCarthy JG. Assessment of airway changes following midface distraction for syndromic craniosynostosis: a clinical and cephalometric study. Plast Reconstr Surg. 2009;124(2):590–601.

Distraction of the Cranial Vault

10

Jordan W. Swanson and Jesse A. Taylor

10.1 Introduction

Building on the early clinical use of distraction osteogenesis by Codivilla and Ilizarov for orthopedic limb deformities [1, 2], and its maxillofacial application by McCarthy for lengthening the mandible [3], distraction was first applied to the cranial vault in 1997 by Do Amaral and colleagues who reported their experience distracting the fronto-orbital region in seven elementary school-aged children with Apert or Crouzon syndrome, with satisfactory results [4]. The following year, Lauritzen described two cases in which cranial springs were used to achieve gradual and effective expansion of the posterior vault and a monobloc segment, respectively [5]. In 1998, Hirabayashi reported the first distraction-mediated fronto-orbital advancement (FOA) in an infant with Apert syndrome [6]. In 2002, Imai and associates described refinement of a cranial distraction protocol in 20 patients with syndromic and nonsyndromic craniosynostosis [7].

Early use of DO in the cranial vault was not merely the employment of a new technology looking for novel applications. A growing literature evaluating outcomes of the first three decades of craniofacial surgery identified that a substantial number of patients who underwent fronto-orbital advancement required secondary surgical treatment for increased intracranial pressure or unsatisfactory

J.W. Swanson, M.D., M.Sc.
Division of Plastic Surgery, University of Southern California, Los Angeles, CA, USA

McGregor Integral Cleft and Plastic Surgery Program, Managua, Nicaragua
e-mail: jswans@gmail.com

J.A. Taylor, M.D. (✉)
The Perelman School of Medicine at the University of Pennsylvania, The Children's Hospital of Philadelphia, Colket Translational Research Building, 3501 Civic Center Blvd. 9th Floor, Philadelphia, PA 19104, USA
e-mail: Taylorj5@email.chop.edu

J.G. McCarthy (ed.), *Craniofacial Distraction*,
DOI 10.1007/978-3-319-52564-8_10

craniofacial morphology [6, 8, 9]. This was particularly true for patients with syndromic craniosynostosis [10, 11]. Some of these pioneers posited that by elevating and advancing the frontal and orbital bones off of and beyond the dura, subsequent resorption of the devascularized bone was potentially a contributing factor. This also potentially risked higher rates of dural injury and infection with revision surgery [6]. They suggested that cranial vault distraction might preserve frontal growth and might be accomplished in a shorter operating time, with decreased blood loss, and shorter hospitalization than with conventional techniques.

10.2 Benefits and Mechanisms of Cranial Vault Distraction

Distraction osteogenesis conveys several benefits as well as some drawbacks compared to conventional bony reconstruction [12]. As applied to the cranium, particularly for cranial expansion, the benefits appear to be borne out in several specific ways. Craniometric analysis shows that posterior vault expansion mediated by distraction can exceed conventional expansion volume by more than two-fold [13], and decreased relapse has been reported anecdotally [14]. The importance of gradual soft tissue expansion is crucial, because it is often the factor that limits the extent of expansion; furthermore, the consequence of a scalp incision breaking down under tension over exposed dura can be life threatening. In addition, an increasing body of evidence comparing conventional to distraction-mediated posterior vault expansion and fronto-orbital advancement show an improved perioperative morbidity profile [15, 16]. This may enable distraction to be safely applied in younger patients, facilitating earlier alleviation in cases of elevated intracranial pressure [17–21]. Two particular advantages of cranial vault distraction may be (1) preventing morbidity that could be life-threatening in severity and (2) enabling greater degrees of advancement and expansion to impart a more functionally beneficial outcome than would be achievable with conventional methods.

There are, however, several drawbacks of cranial vault distraction. The duration of the cranial distraction process, spanning weeks postoperatively rather than hours intraoperatively, requires family participation. Even with compliance, there is also the risk of mechanical device failure postoperatively. Device removal mandates a return to the operating room.

10.2.1 Mechanism of Ossification

In young children who undergo cranial vault expansion mediated by distraction devices, ossification is likely to result from a combination of osteogenesis from the bone edge and durally mediated ossification. To the degree that the cancellous component of cranial bone facilitates distraction osteogenesis, this is likely to play a greater role after the first year of age. To a degree, each of these forces may be substitutable. For instance, spring-mediated cranioplasty is likely to engender relatively greater dural ossification, because it is typically performed within the first 6 months of age, and most of the activation distance is achieved in the first few days postoperatively. In contrast, distraction osteogenesis is likely the primary mechanism of ossification in a monobloc frontofacial advancement in a 5-year-old patient. From a practical standpoint, the duality of distraction and dural osteogenesis may increase the risk of premature consolidation in a very young patient. Thus, a shorter latency period or faster rate of activation may be indicated in very young patients.

10.3 Device Selection

The three-dimensional architecture of the cranial vault introduces spatial and technical challenges in comparison to the vector of advancement of an extremity bone, or the uni- or bi-directional but uniplanar frontal movement of mandibular or midface advancement. This has implications for the patterns of osteotomy, completeness of osteotomy, and the orientation and vector of the distraction device. It also underscores the importance of device selection.

Internal metallic distraction devices are the mainstay of cranial vault distraction. Mounted footplates are secured to bone adjacent to an osteotomy. Alternatively, "Molina-type" distraction devices are attached with a single footplate. With rotatory movement, a piston is gradually extended to enable advancement in a pushing movement. Distraction devices with activation rods between 25 and 50 mm in length are utilized for cranial vault distraction. Ratcheting mechanisms prevent unwinding of the device between activation movements.

External "halo-type" devices are primarily utilized in conjunction with fronto-facial (monobloc) advancement (Chapter 7).

Absorbable devices for cranial distraction are currently in development, with the premise that they could avoid a second surgical procedure for device removal [22].

10.3.1 Springs

Developed by Lauritzen, a cranial expansion spring is a passive device applied under tension which, in trying to reattain its original form, can exert constant force on adjacent bone segments [23]. It is a segment of wire, approximately 1.5 mm in diameter, bent into a U shape. When the solitary ends are compressed together, they can exert a force of generally between 5 and 20 Newtons. Springs have been utilized in a variety of craniofacial applications including posterior vault distraction, anterior vault distraction, correction of Kleeblattschädel deformity, and fronto-facial advancement [24]. Springs can be either crafted by the surgeon preoperatively or purchased as part of a deployable system.

In contrast to conventional distraction devices, which are typically expanded at a constant rate throughout the activation phase, springs achieve much of their expansion in the first hours or days after placement. In the cranium, they achieve length by stretching adjacent open sutures. Given that they achieve their expansion quite rapidly after placement, it may be that dural ossification plays a greater mechanism in bone formation than intramembranous ossification from the osteotomized bony edges.

10.3.2 Magnetism

Magnetism has been utilized to mediate distraction in limb lengthening [25] and spinal growth rod movement to correct severe spinal curvature in children with scoliosis, using a magnet-driven controller [26]. In each application, an internal distraction device with a magnetic component is manipulated by way of transcutaneous interaction with an external magnetic controller in a clinic setting. This feature reduces the need for transcutaneous hardware, or return to the operating room for direct device advancement and manipulation, as is customary for scoliosis treatment. In the setting of cranial vault synostoses, magnetism has also been explored to mediate direct cranial expansion. In two rabbit studies, magnets were surgically affixed to osteotomized parietal bone segments, which were then oriented to polar opposite magnets on an external head frame [27, 28]. In a study comparing outcomes of magnet-mediated versus conventional surgical vault expansion, the study authors noted two differences between groups [28]. First, the cranial contours of the animals in the magnetic distraction group were rounded while those of the surgically repositioned group were more acutely angled. Second, the osteotomies in rabbits in the magnetic distraction group were essentially completely ossified, while in the surgically repositioned group, there were obvious gaps at the osteotomy sites filled with fibrous tissue. No known application of magnet-mediated cranial distraction has yet occurred in humans.

10.4 Posterior Vault Expansion

Since White's description of posterior vault distraction osteogenesis (PVDO) in 2009, a literature has developed describing its safety [13, 15, 29–36] and ability to convey robust cranial expansion [13, 29, 33]. Steinbacher and colleagues, in their initial series of eight patients, found the procedure to be effective and reliable with short-term follow-up [15]. A subsequent comparison of an early series of posterior vault distraction osteogenesis patients to patients with conventional posterior vault expansion showed a 15% decrease in blood loss and 40% decrease in hospital length of stay. However, other studies have shown more similar perioperative safety and morbidity profiles [37]. A craniometric analysis of 22 patients undergoing posterior vault distraction for syndromic craniosynostosis revealed an average distraction length of 27 mm, intracranial volume increase of 21.5%, and normalization of turribrachycephalic indices [29]. This reflects a considerable benefit over posterior cranial vault en bloc expansion, which is usually limited to at most 10 mm of expansion and is anecdotally associated with high rates of relapse [14]. From a technical standpoint, because the posterior bone plate does not need to be removed, the risky dissection over the torcula and high rate of posterior non-healing skeletal defects are avoided [38]. In a multicenter comparison of patients with syndromic craniosynostosis, those who underwent posterior vault distraction achieved an average 142 cm^3 of expansion versus an average of 66 cm^3 for fronto-orbital advancement, after controlling for growth [13]. The corrected mean volume difference per millimeter of advancement was 4.6 cm^3 for fronto-orbital advancement and 5.8 cm^3 for posterior vault distraction osteogenesis [13].

As far as patient selection, posterior vault distraction appears optimal for patients with syndromic synostosis, who typically exhibit bicoronal craniosynostosis and brachycephalic or turribrachycephalic cranial phenotype with constriction in the anteroposterior dimension. With synostosis of multiple cranial sutures, the likelihood of elevated ICP and associated developmental delay is higher. In the authors' opinion, this warrants early intervention for cranial expansion as soon as safe to do so. Posterior vault distraction expands the anteroposterior axis to normalize the cephalic index and achieve large distraction distances and associated volume expansion. The procedure can be performed safely at 3–4 months of age and appears to show durability of expansion. An additional advantage of early posterior vault distraction osteogenesis is that it preserves the growth of the anterior cranium for subsequent fronto-orbital advancement, which can be performed at an older age with potentially a more durable resulting contour [39, 40]. We have also recently noted that following posterior vault distraction but before any anterior cranial surgery, the degree of frontal bossing appears to improve, particularly in patients with Apert syndrome [29, 41].

It has been our institutional objective to treat syndromic synostosis patients with an algorithm that employs early posterior vault distraction osteogenesis. We found that the algorithm has been successful in delaying the timing of first fronto-orbital advancement in this patient cohort, compared to patients treated before the advent of posterior vault distraction osteogenesis [14]. This delay is likely to convey beneficial anterior growth as well as more optimal and durable result at the time of fronto-orbital advancement, if it is indeed indicated. Furthermore, the posterior vault distraction osteogenesis cohort showed a significant decrease in the number of fronto-orbital advancements performed in the first 5 years of life compared to the pre-PVDO group (0.6 v 1.5, $p = 0.0237$) and showed a trend toward decreased overall major craniofacial interventions (1.8 v 2.7, $p = 0.2087$) [14]. Subsequent craniofacial surgery and its timing are dictated by functional and aesthetic evaluation, and optimal patterns are emerging by syndrome type [14].

One unresolved question is the impact of posterior vault distraction osteogenesis on the skull base and foramen magnum. Cerebellar tonsillar herniation has long been associated with syndromic craniosynostosis, and Chiari malformations have been shown to be acquired defects, often exacerbated by ventriculoperitoneal shunting [42, 43]. The incidence of Chiari in Crouzon and severe Pfeiffer syndrome can be up to 70–100%. Fearon reasons that given this frequency, there is a high likelihood of needing decompression of the foramen magnum and enlargement of the lower posterior fossa but that such interventions are durable primarily after 1 year of age due to bony regrowth [42]. The Seattle team, on the other hand, has found that posterior vault expansion can be associated with spontaneous improvement of the Chiari herniation as well as resolution of the syrinx [44]. In our institutional experience, we have not seen considerable need for additional subsequent expansion of the lower posterior fossa or foramen magnum decompression (Fig. 10.1).

10.4.1 Surgical Technique

Posterior vault distraction is optimal for patients with syndromic or multisutural craniosynostosis, particularly as a primary vault expansion between 3 and 6 months of age, or shortly after presentation in older patients, and as a subsequent expansion for patients with suspicion for elevated ICP. Preoperative head computed tomography (CT) should be obtained. First, this can aid planning of osteotomies. Second, it can identify prominent emissary veins in the posterior fossa, the ligation of which could lead to venous thrombosis [45].

In a prone position with the head positioned on a Mayfield headrest, a stealth coronal incision is designed over the cranial vertex, acknowledging that it will likely be used for fronto-orbital advancement in the future. Dissection proceeds posteriorly and supra-pericranially and extends inferiorly past the occipital protuberance. The osteotomy is designed generally with the vertical limb to the cranial vertex and the horizontal limb to a position approximately 1 cm inferior to the

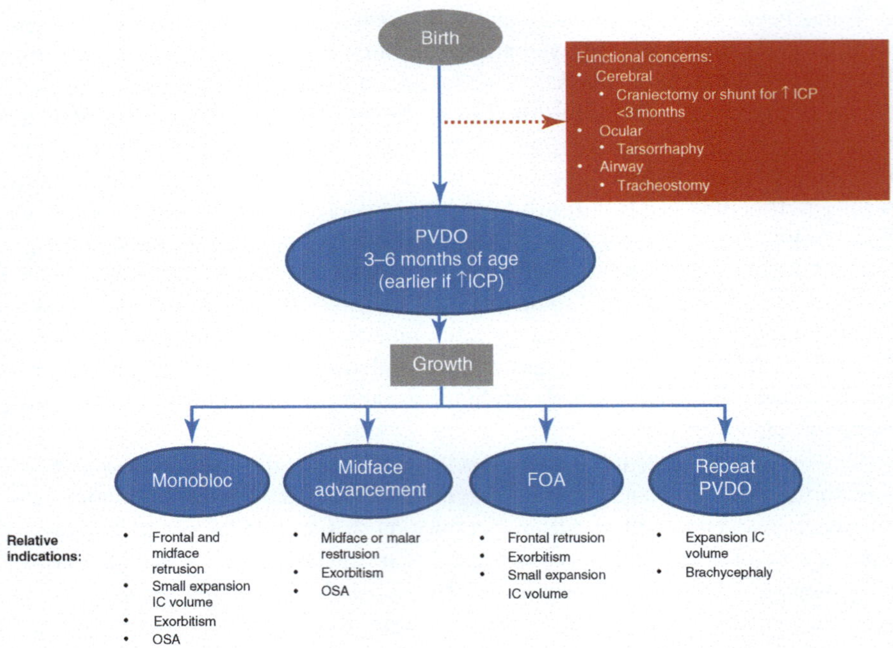

Fig. 10.1 Distraction of the Cranial Vault Algorithm

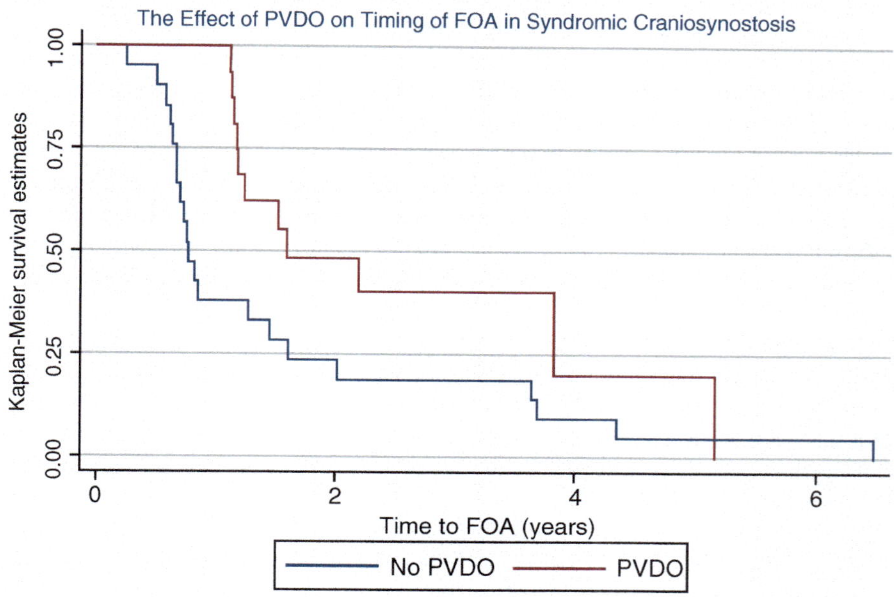

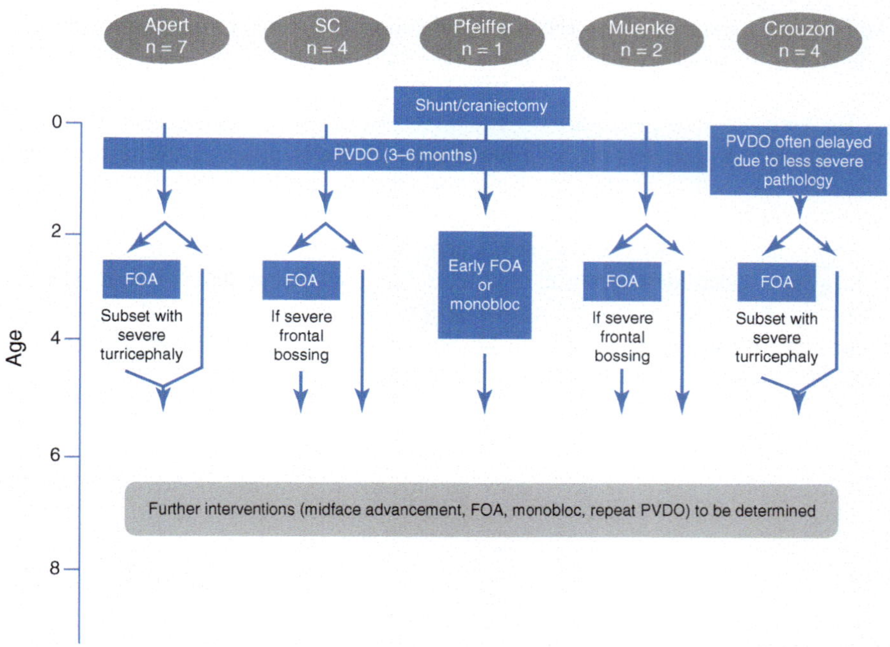

Fig. 10.1 (continued)

occipital protuberance. Interdigitating "teeth" can be employed in older patients; however, this is not necessary in infants given the degree of dural ossification. Osteotomies are marked, and the pericranium is stripped directly overlying the marks. The posterior craniotomy is performed taking care to avoid injury to the underlying dura. After completion of the osteotomy, further inferior dissection is performed along the posterior skull base, approximately 2–3 cm in distance. A series of vertical "barrel-stave" osteotomies are performed to enable six to eight inferiorly-based bone flaps to be "greenstick"—fractured and flexed with the distracted segment, so as to allow for greater volumetric expansion of the posterior cranial base.

Two linear distraction devices, generally 30–50 mm in length, are placed parietally on the cranium, generally at approximately the 2:00 and 10:00 clock positions in the coronal plane (Fig. 10.2). The device is oriented with the activating arm directed anteriorly. The device is placed to achieve a vector with the posterior portion canted downward slightly from the Frankfort horizontal, to decrease the turricephaly slightly. 4-0 PDS sutures are placed between the greenstick inferior bone flaps and the postero-inferior bone flap to prevent a step-off deformity. Each footplate is affixed with 4–8 blunt-tipped titanium screws, generally 3.5–5 mm in length. A piece of gelfoam is placed between the dura and internal table corresponding to the device footplates to prevent screw tips from tearing the dura during activation. If the lambdoid sutures are noted to be mobile, resorbable plates are placed spanning each suture so that the sutures do not flex during activation.

The anterior device arms are either able to exit the scalp through anterior apices of the stealth coronal incision or through separate stab incisions. Activating arms are attached and used to verify the distraction mechanism integrity, and the scalp is closed in layers.

Following a 2–5 day latency period, activation proceeds at a rate of 1 mm daily. Following a consolidation period of at least 2 months, the patient is returned to the operating room for removal of distraction devices under general anesthesia. Figure 10.3 illustrates a patient with Muenke syndrome and bicoronal craniosynostosis who underwent posterior cranial vault distraction.

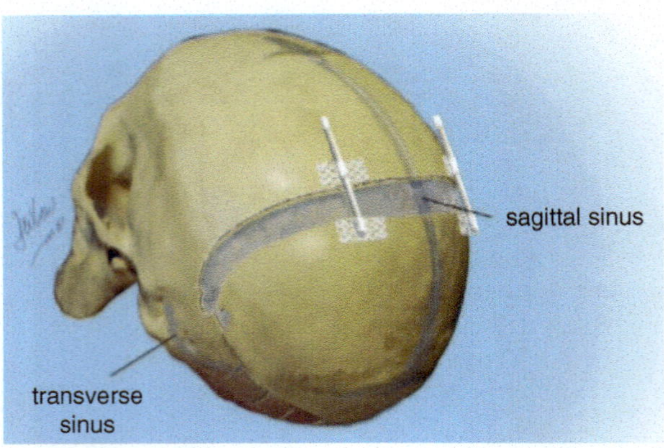

Fig. 10.2 Osteotomy design and distraction device placement for posterior vault distraction

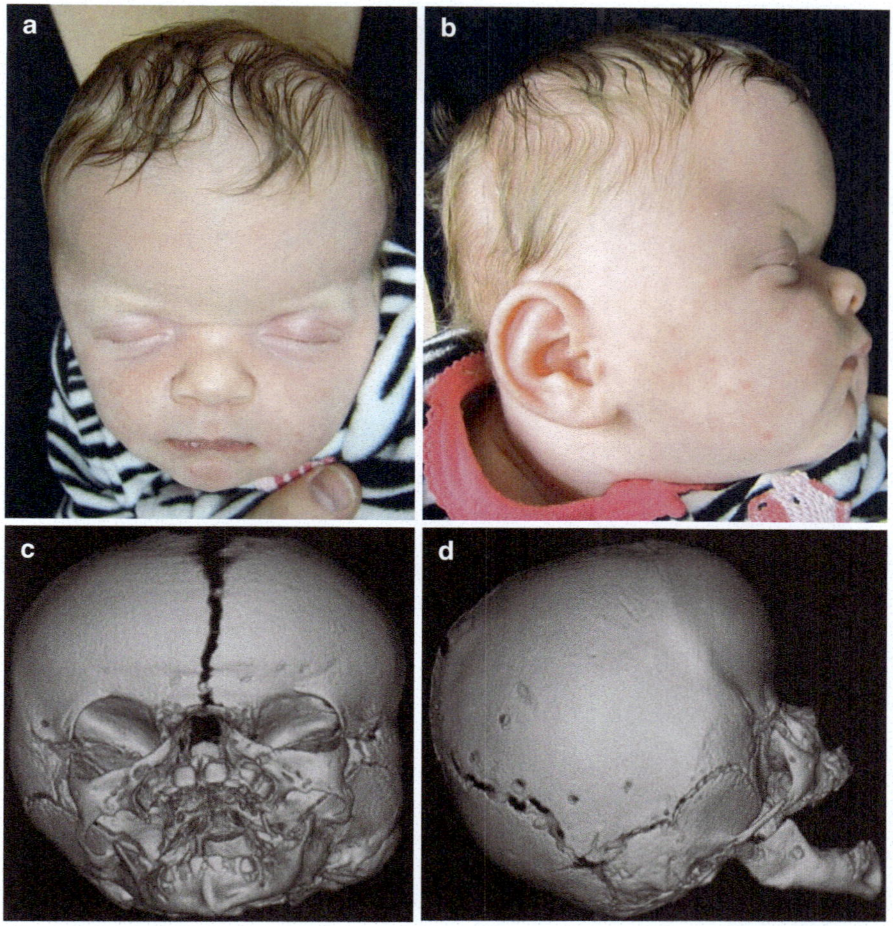

Fig. 10.3 Two-month-old male with Muenke syndrome (**a**, **b**). Preoperative CT images (**c**, **d**). Patient in consolidation phase of distraction (**e**, **f**) and post-distraction device removal CT scan (**g**, **h**). One year after posterior vault distraction osteogenesis without additional surgery (**i**, **j**)

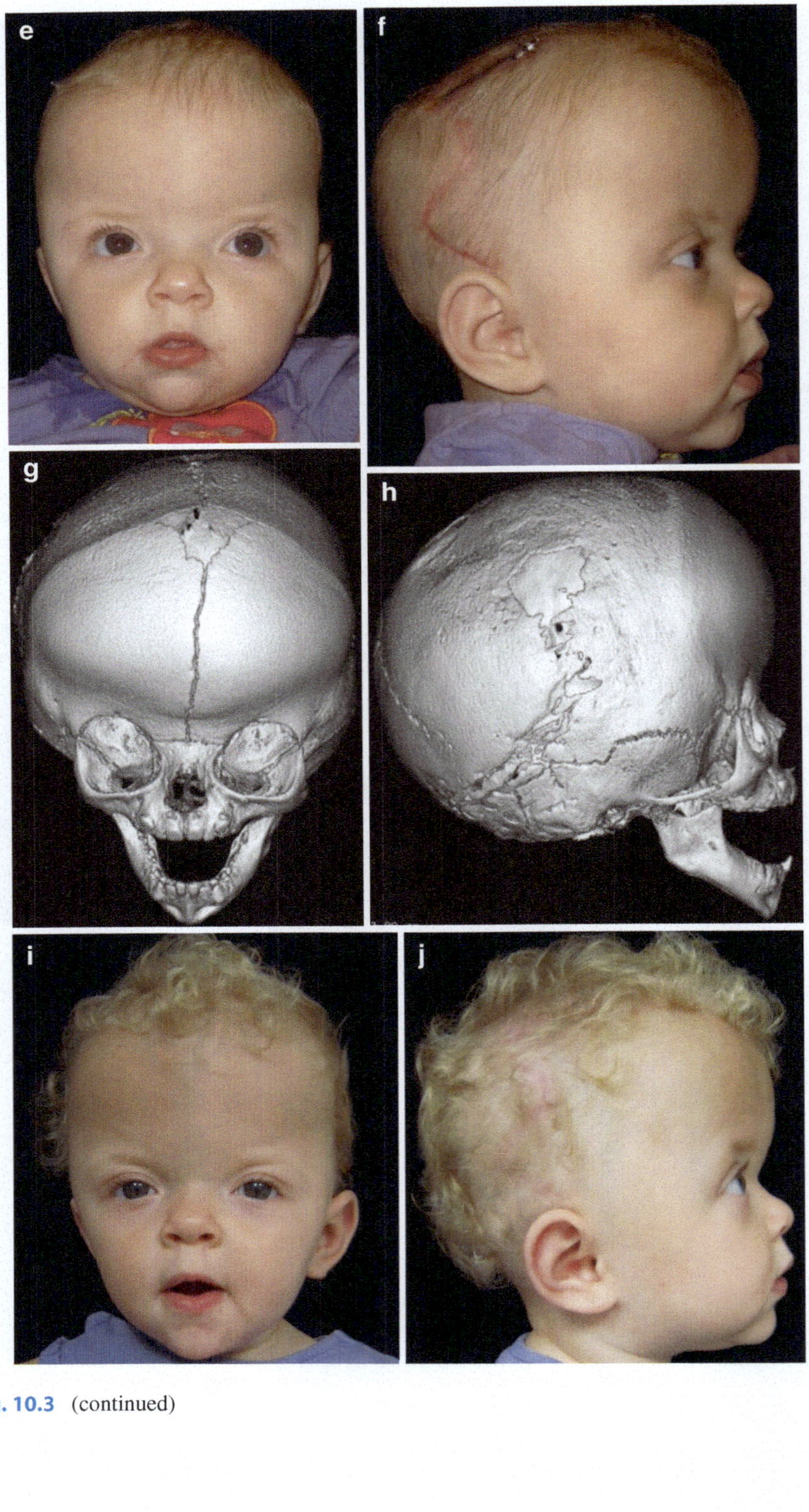

Fig. 10.3 (continued)

10.5 Middle Vault Expansion

While some groups have advocated middle vault expansion with semi-buried distraction devices, we have adopted spring-mediated middle vault expansion, both for its ease of use and consistency at achieving a satisfactory cranial morphology [5, 23, 24].

10.5.1 Surgical Technique

A sagittal strip craniectomy is performed via 3 cm transverse incisions slightly posterior to the anterior fontanelle and slightly anterior to the posterior fontanelle. A subgaleal tunnel is made between the two incisions anteriorly and posteriorly, and a 1.5 cm sagittal strip craniectomy is performed. Either two or three springs are placed transversely to the craniectomy, each ranging from 7 to 12 Newtons in force, with a higher force used posteriorly than anteriorly. Selection of spring force depends on (1) the age of the patient, (2) thickness of the bone, (3) degree of synostosis present, and (4) the extent of correction anticipated. The goal is to maximize force without tearing adjacent bone. The patient's strip craniectomy bone is morselized and then replaced deep to the springs as cranial bone graft to facilitate cranial bone regeneration deep to the springs. Springs are generally removed 3 months after the initial surgery in a one-hour outpatient procedure. Figure 10.4 illustrates a patient with sagittal craniosynostosis who underwent spring-mediated cranial vault remodeling.

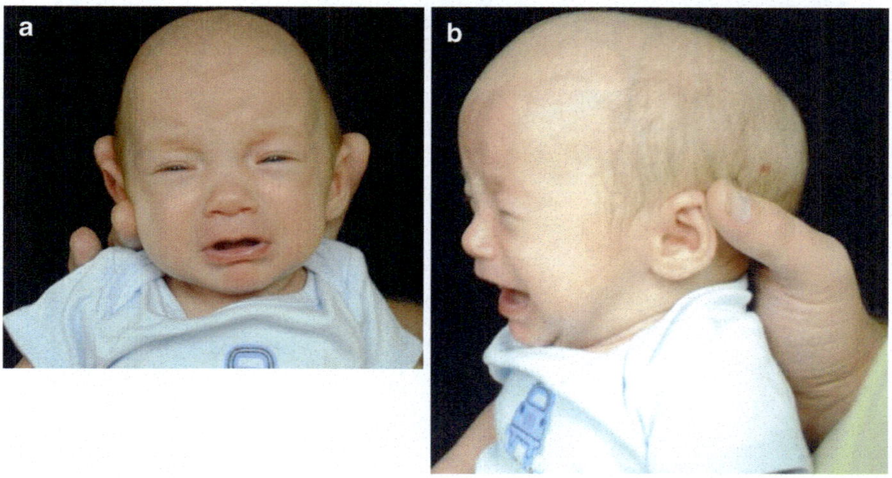

Fig. 10.4 Six-week-old with sagittal craniosynostosis (**a**, **b**). Preoperative CT scan (**c**, **d**). Postoperative plain lateral radiograph (**e**). One year postoperative appearance (**f–h**)

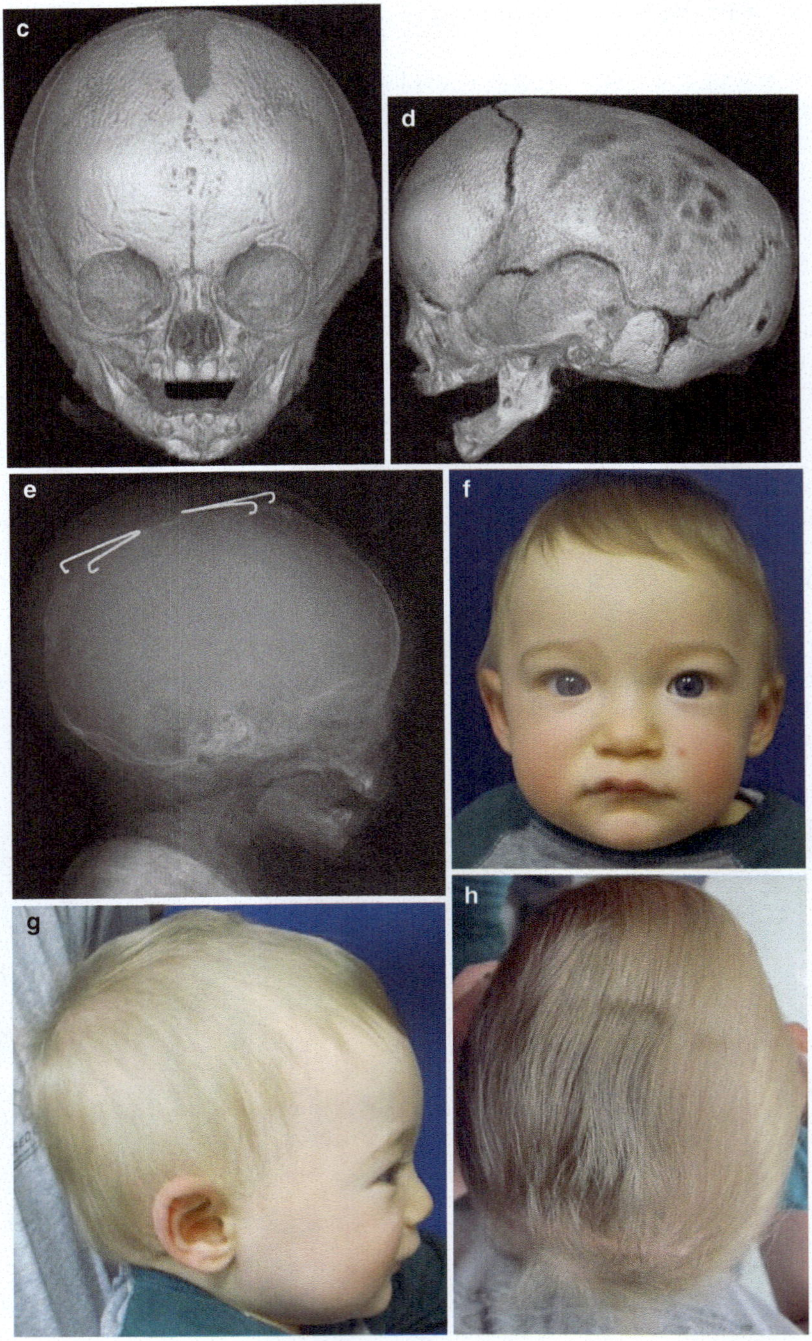

Fig. 10.4 (continued)

10.6 Anterior Vault Expansion

Anterior cranial abnormalities are more challenging, because they involve the constricted anterior cranial fossa and the orbits. Anterior cranial expansion has been reported for patients with syndromic synostosis in conjunction with occipital expansion [46, 47]. However, concerns over frontal distraction in syndromic patients include the inability to treat the turricephaly associated with the brachycephaly, long-term stability, and potential need for reoperation [38]. Anterior cranial vault distraction improves anterior cranial base dysmorphology to a greater extent than conventional surgery while concomitantly maintaining bone vascularity, both of which may provide for an enhanced growth trajectory and profile over time [48].

10.6.1 Unicoronal Craniosynostosis (UCS)

Unicoronal craniosynostosis (UCS) is the third most common of the single-suture synostoses and is characterized by ipsilateral supraorbital rim flattening, elevation and recession of the forehead, anterosuperior malposition of the sphenoid bone with a lateral and upwardly oriented greater wing of the sphenoid, deviation of the nasal root to the affected side, vertical orbital dystopia, temporal retrusion, and a hypoplastic cranial base [16]. Temporal hollowing is characteristic postoperatively and is attributed to a constricted temporal dimension along the anterior cranial fossa and orbit which is not corrected in a traditional advancement [49]. Furthermore, long-term aesthetic results have considerable shortcomings, and the rate of revision is not insignificant [50]. In particular, strabismus appears refractory to conventional fronto-orbital advancement [51].

Choi first described the application of unilateral distraction osteogenesis to patients with unicoronal craniosynostosis [52]. In order to correct the associated orbital deformity, a non-devascularizing technique was utilized which maintained the frontal and orbital components united en bloc. In subsequent comparison of the distraction patient cohort to a cohort which underwent conventional correction, the distraction group showed improved correction [48]. Using a similar technique to Choi, the authors found significant decreases in the duration of surgery (25% shorter), hospital stay (20% shorter), and trends toward decreased blood loss (57% less), and ICU stay (50% shorter), when compared to traditional fronto-orbital advancement [16, 53]. Significantly, we found that the rate of new-onset postoperative strabismus decreased from 60% in the conventional group to 0% following distraction [53]. Finally, the procedure could be performed at a much younger age group, on average 5 months, a time which may be particularly beneficial given the risk of elevated ICP.

10.6.2 Surgical Technique

Through a stealth coronal incision, subperiosteal elevation of the anterior cranial, forehead, and periorbital soft tissues is undertaken as with conventional fronto-orbital advancement and repositioning. A hemi-coronal suturectomy is performed with an ultrasonic scalpel following limited dural dissection (Fig. 10.5). Burr holes are then placed along anticipated osteotomies with one placed at the base of the fused coronal suture. Only the dura directly underlying a planned osteotomy is dissected, thus keeping the majority of the dura attached to the overlying frontal bone. The ultrasonic scalpel is used to perform all cuts typical of a unilateral fronto-orbital advancement extending to the medial third of the contralateral orbit; however, the bandeau is kept en bloc with the frontal bone. Bone cuts include a vertical "perforating" osteotomy contralateral to the affected side, at the inflection point of the deformity, from the contralateral orbit to the anterior fontanelle. Inferior orbital cuts are then made along the orbital roof, taking care to retract the brain and globe to prevent dural or periorbital injury. Additional radial osteotomies are made along the orbital roof to unfurl the horizontally shortened orbit.

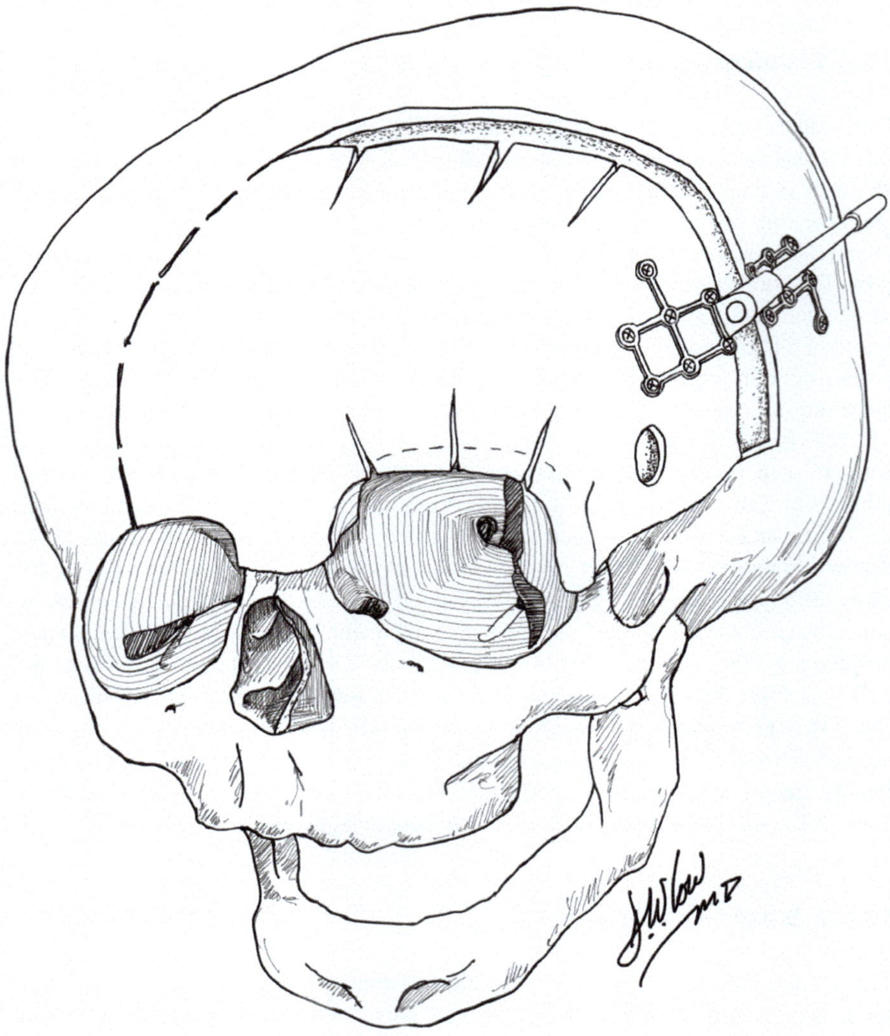

Fig. 10.5 Osteotomy design and burr hole placement for anterior vault distraction in unicoronal craniosynostosis

Accessed through the most caudal portion of the suturectomy at the level of the pterion, malleable retractors allow for careful osteotomy of the greater wing of the sphenoid and the lateral orbital wall.

A uniplanar cranial distraction device is rigidly fixated to the mid-parietal region with an anterior and slightly inferior vector to translocate the orbital rim to achieve slight overcorrection. The device is activated to ensure completeness of the osteotomy and returned to its original position. A drain is placed in the forehead and the scalp is closed in layers.

Activation is started on the second postoperative day at a rate of 1 mm per day. The endpoint of activation is slight overcorrection of the anterior frontal bone compared with the contralateral side. The subsequent consolidation phase ranges from 8 to 12 weeks. Figure 10.6 illustrates a patient who underwent distraction-mediated correction of unicoronal craniosynostosis.

10.6.3 Metopic Craniosynostosis

Metopic craniosynostosis is the second most common type of single-suture synostosis and it is the only subtype whose incidence is on the rise [54]. Early fusion of the metopic suture causes significant dysmorphology and hallmark characteristics including bilateral supraorbital retrusion, bilateral pterional constriction, trigonocephaly, and hypotelorism. Although fronto-orbital advancement and repositioning is generally the surgical treatment of choice, one of the central concerns in metopic synostosis is the timing of surgery, given the reduced head circumference and potentially attendant risk of cranial constriction. Distraction osteogenesis may offer improved durability of result, perhaps because of non-devascularizing osteotomies, when performed at a younger age.

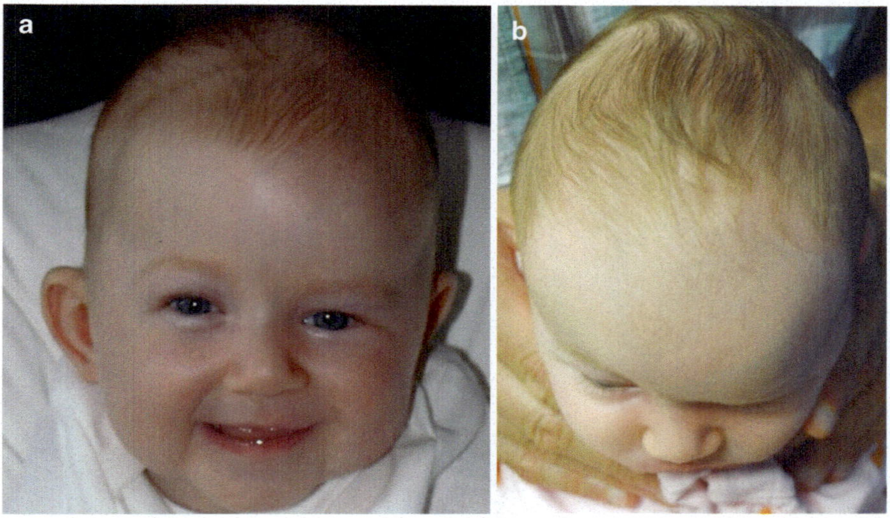

Fig. 10.6 Three-month-old female with right unicoronal craniosynostosis (**a**, **b**). Preoperative CT scan (**c**, **d**). Intraoperative view demonstrating osteotomies and position of distraction device (**e**). Close-up view demonstrating preoperative orbital dysmorphology and postoperative resolution (**f**, **g**). Two-year follow-up appearance (**h**, **i**)

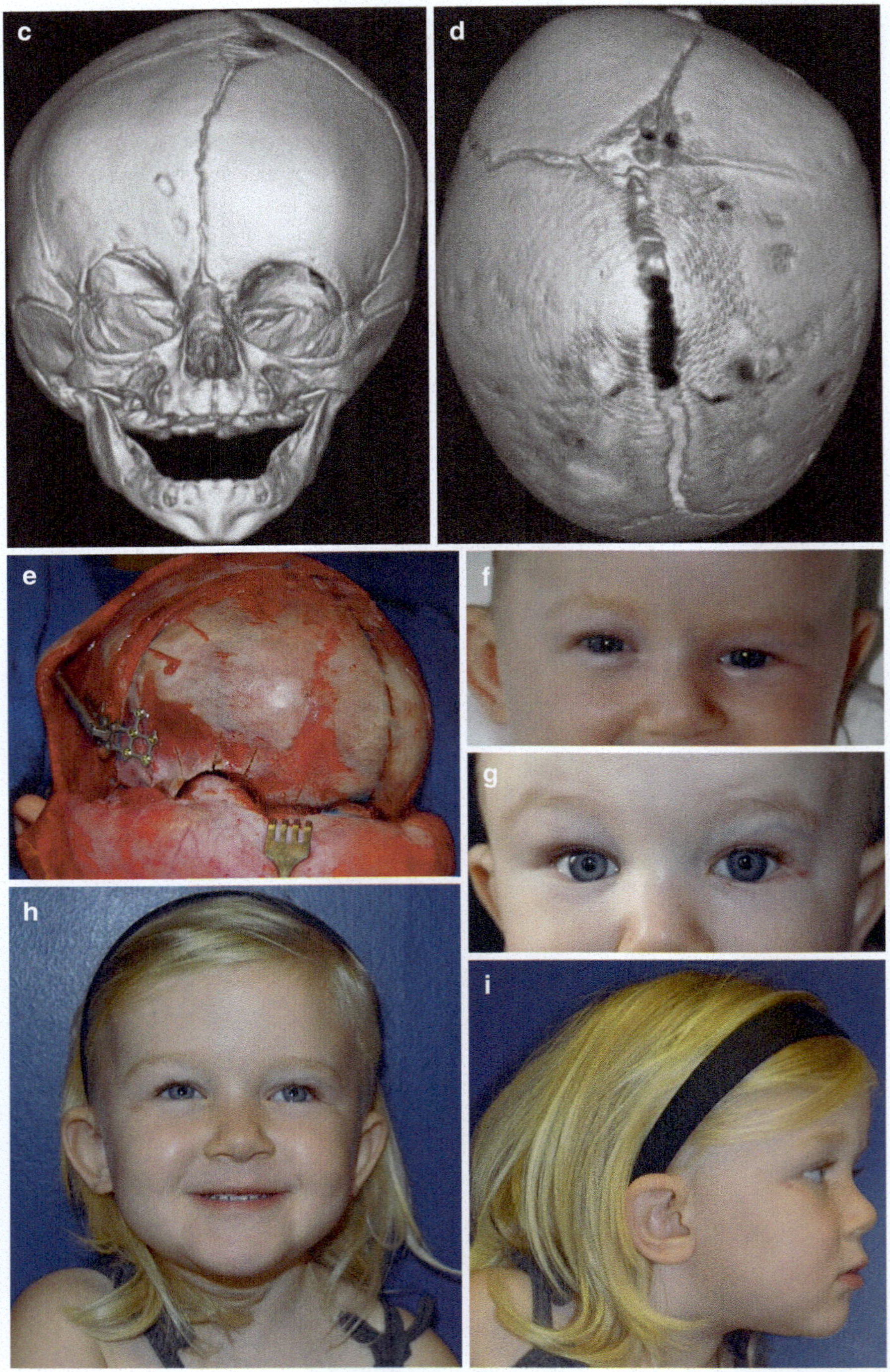

Fig. 10.6 (continued)

10.6.4 Surgical Technique

Through a coronal incision, subperiosteal elevation of the soft tissues of the forehead is undertaken as with conventional fronto-orbital advancement. A narrow, 5 mm, metopic suturectomy is performed with the Hudson brace and ultrasonic scalpel under direct visualization (Fig. 10.7). Following this, the ultrasonic

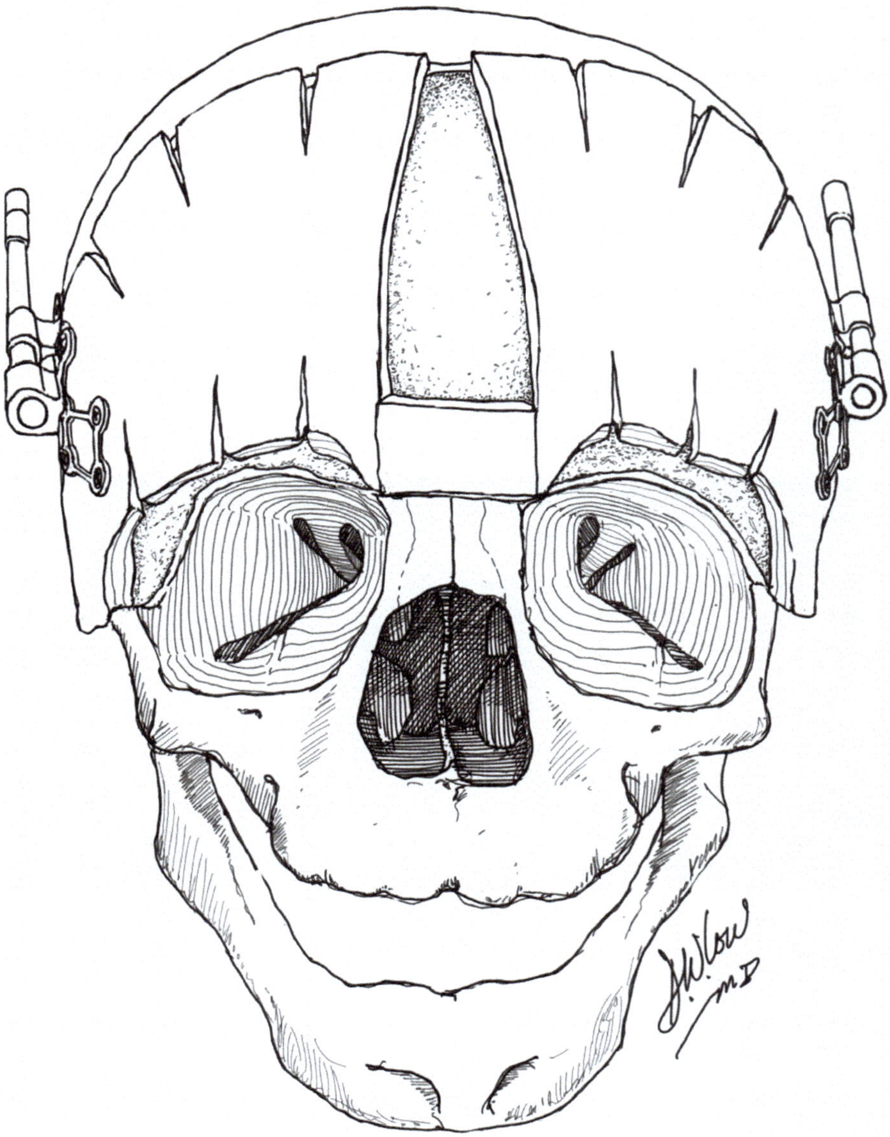

Fig. 10.7 Osteotomy and suturectomy design for bilateral anterior vault distraction in metopic craniosynostosis

scalpel is used to perform all cuts typical of a bilateral fronto-orbital advancement including coronally oriented osteotomies posterior to the coronal sutures at the transition between "normal" occiput and "abnormal" forehead. One key difference is that the frontal bandeau is not separated from the frontal bone as with fronto-orbital advancement and repositioning. Burr holes at the base of the coronal sutures in the pterional region permit limited dissection of the frontal and temporal lobes directly under the osteotomy sites to maintain bone vascularity. The sphenoid wing and orbital roof osteotomies are made via the pterional window. Additional radial osteotomies are made along the orbital roof and frontal bones to allow for gradual remodeling during distraction.

The dura in the region of the metopic suture is placed on stretch, and a 2 cm × 1 cm interpositional bone graft is placed at the nasofrontal junction and fixated with 3-0 PDS sutures to the nasal bones and bilateral frontal bones in a slightly advanced position. This allows for significant bilateral widening of the forehead on table. Uniplanar devices are rigidly fixated to the mid-parietal region in the forehead with an anteroposterior vector in order to translocate the forehead and orbital rims to their proper location. The scalp is then closed in layers. Activation is started on the second postoperative day at a rate of 1 mm per day. The endpoint of activation is slight overcorrection of the fronto-orbital deformity. Figure 10.8 illustrates a patient who has undergone distraction-mediated fronto-orbital remodeling for metopic craniosynostosis.

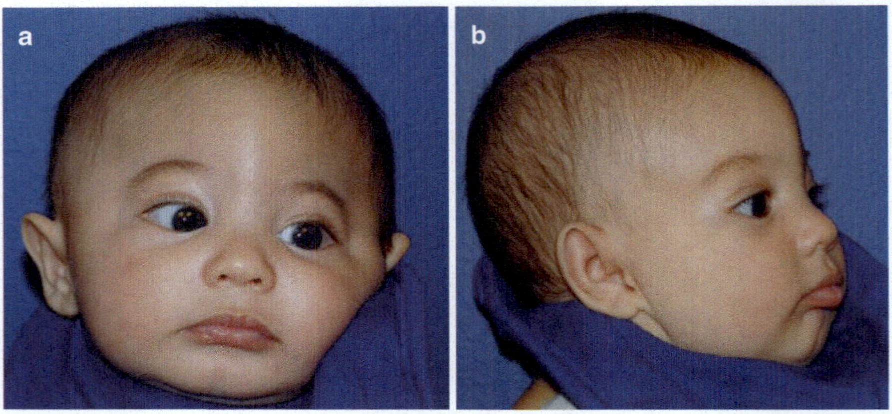

Fig. 10.8 Two-month-old male with metopic craniosynostosis (**a**, **b**). Preoperative CT scan (**c**, **d**). Postoperative CT scan demonstrating osteotomies and position of distraction devices (**e**, **f**). One-year follow-up photos (**g**–**i**)

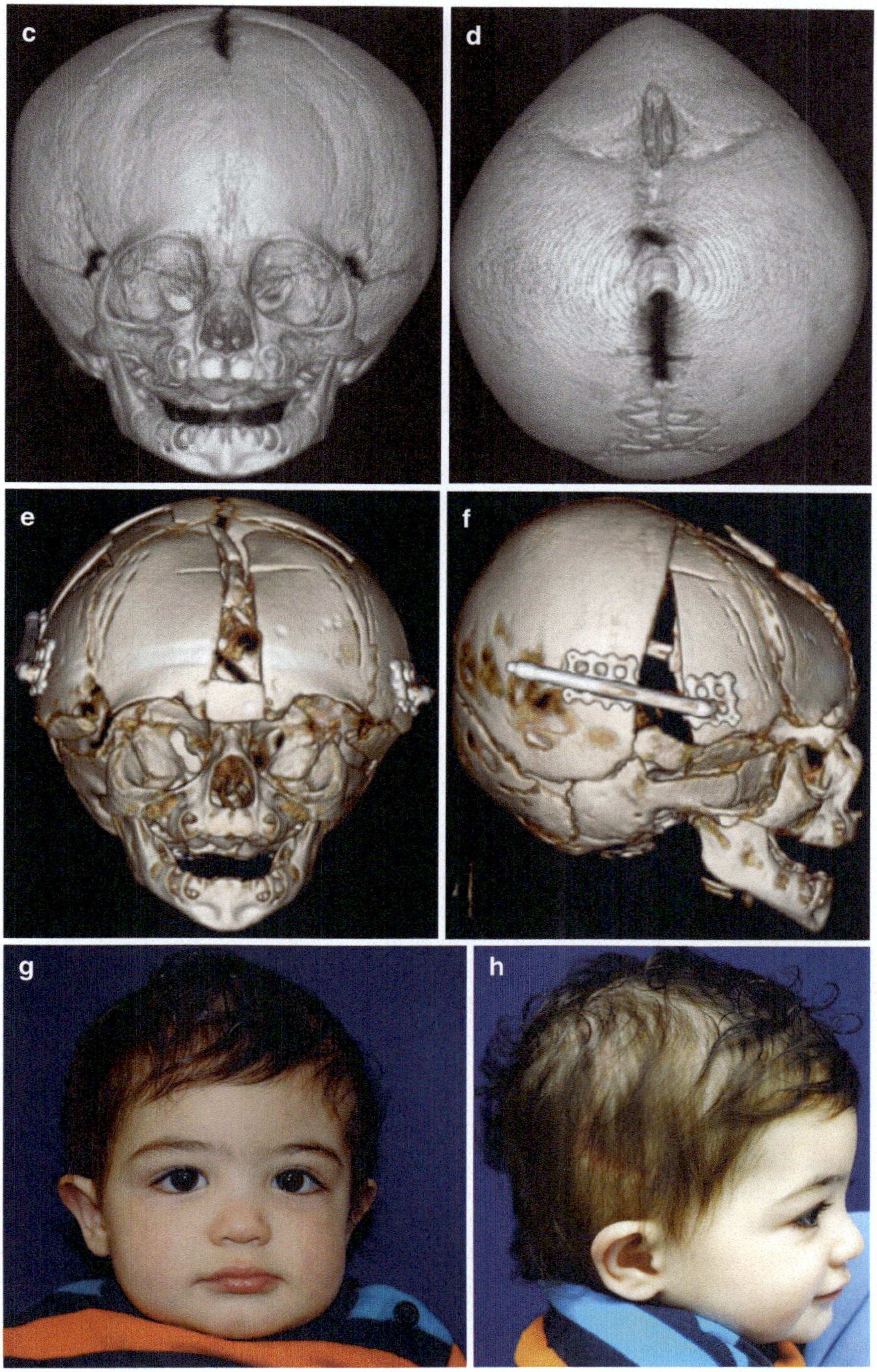

Fig. 10.8 (continued)

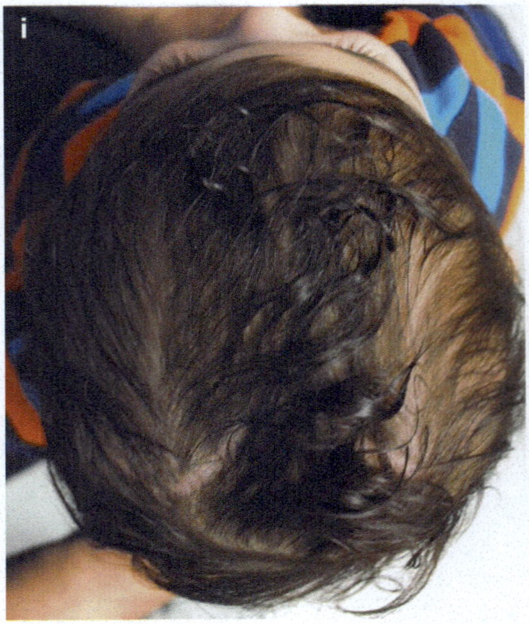

Fig. 10.8 (continued)

10.7 Total Cranial Vault Expansion

Patients with multi-suture synostosis, particularly those with cloverleaf or Kleeblattschädel deformity, present a significant challenge to the craniofacial surgeon. The severity of synostosis is associated with increased morbidity and mortality secondary to hydrocephalus, hindbrain herniation, and venous hypertension [1]; these factors ultimately drive neurodevelopmental impairment. Physical anomalies include a misshapen, trilobar skull, with a high "bossed" forehead, a bulging temporal region, and a flat posterior skull [55]. Multiple surgical procedures, including suturectomy, craniectomy, and subtotal calvariectomy, with adjunct ventriculoperitoneal shunting, have been described. In one study prior to widespread cranial vault distraction, staged correction was advocated due to the high morbidity of traditional early cranial vault remodeling [55].

Multi-vector distraction and spring-mediated cranial expansion in multi-suture craniosynostosis have been reported at 1 month and 6–9 months of age, respectively [56, 57]. We believe several principles underlie successful application of distraction in this challenging patient population. First, it enables a shorter operation, with an acceptable blood loss profile to facilitate consideration within the first 2 months of life. Second, it permits large, gradual expansion of the soft tissue envelope to enable large first-stage expansion. Third, with minimal devascularization, it may limit reduction of future growth compared to conventional cranioplasty.

Distraction-mediated surgical treatment is tailored to which sutures are involved. Suturectomies of involved sutures and liberation of involved fronto-orbital architecture are the baseline key tenants of treatment. Following osteotomies, distraction devices are placed perpendicular to the involved sutures so as to achieve expansion in multiple dimensions. Figure 10.9 illustrates a patient with bicoronal and sagittal craniosynostosis who underwent multi-vector distraction.

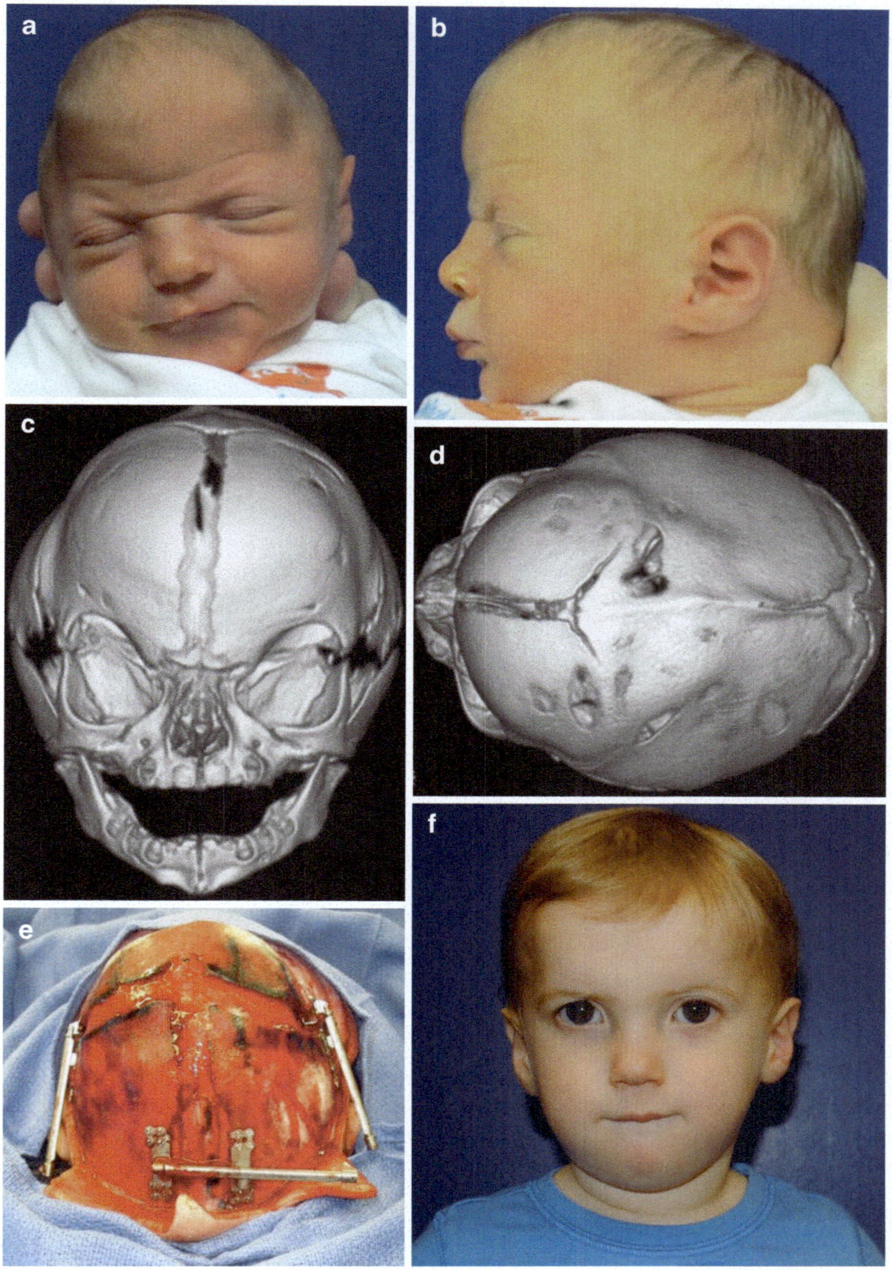

Fig. 10.9 Six-week-old male with bicoronal and sagittal craniosynostosis (**a**, **b**). Preoperative CT scan (**c**, **d**). Intraoperative photo demonstrating osteotomies and device placement (**e**). Eighteen-month postoperative appearance (**f–h**)

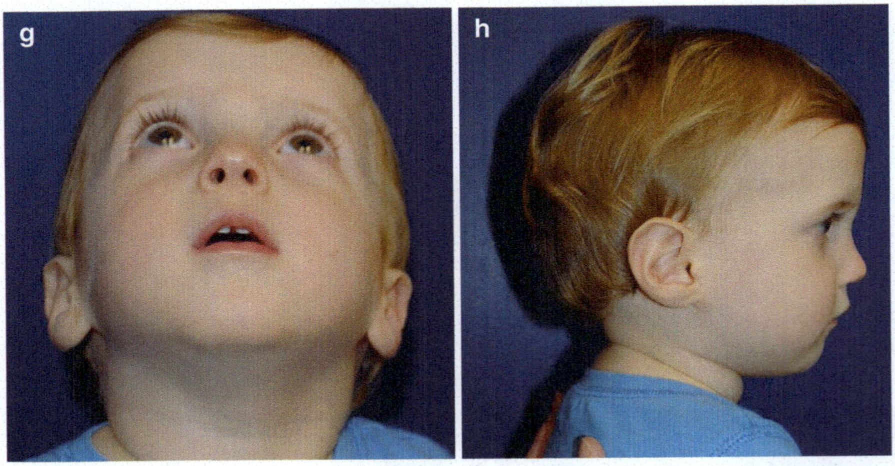

Fig. 10.9 (continued)

10.8 Complications

A structured literature review on posterior vault distraction by Grieves reported a 20–30% level of complications, similar to midface distraction advancements [58–60]. Dural injury and brain injury are possible, and they can be difficult to diagnose given the fact that the bone flaps remain in place, not allowing for inspection of the underlying dura [60]. Incomplete osteotomy can also be difficult to ascertain, as it can be difficult to feel the difference between a complete and incomplete osteotomy of the cranium in a young child. Device failure is common and may be due to screw thread failure, baseplate failure, failure at the interface of the bone and hardware, or external distractor arm failure [61].

Pearls and Pitfalls

- Cranial vault distraction offers a promising alternative to conventional cranial vault remodeling for treating craniosynostosis.
- Distraction enables an increased magnitude of cranial bone movement by utilizing gradual expansion of the scalp, and it has been shown to decrease operative morbidity, blood loss, and hospital length of stay compared to conventional expansion.
- Distraction may also allow for improved cranial growth trajectory and profile due to its non-devascularizing nature, although this remains untested.
- Nonetheless, cranial vault distraction involves a longer treatment process, often requiring family participation and an additional procedure for device removal.
- Posterior vault distraction has gained popularity as an initial intervention for syndromic craniosynostosis and can be performed safely at 3–6 months of age.

- Anterior vault distraction, for unicoronal or metopic synostosis, is more technically challenging due to pathologic involvement of the orbits and skull base.
- Future work will focus on development of improved distraction devices, the elimination of a second operation for device removal, and reduced length of treatment.

References

1. Codivilla A. On the means of lengthening, in the lower limbs, the muscles and tissues which are shortened through deformity. Am J Orthop Surg. 1905;2:353–69.
2. Ilizarov GA. The tension-stress effect on the genesis and growth of tissues. Part I. The influence of stability of fixation and soft tissue preservation. Clin Orthop. 1989;238:249–81.
3. McCarthy JG, Schreiber J, Karp N, et al. Lengthening the human mandible by gradual distraction. Plast Reconstr Surg. 1992;89:1–8.
4. do Amaral CM, Di Domizio G, Tiziani V, Galhardi F, Buzzo CL, Rinco T, Kharmandayan P, Bueno MA, Bolzani N, Sabbatini RM, Lopes LD, Lopes PF, Paiva B, Paiva RM, Turchiari LA. Gradual bone distraction in craniosynostosis. Preliminary results in seven cases. Scand J Plast Reconstr Surg Hand Surg. 1997;31(1):25–37.
5. Lauritzen C, Sugawara Y, Kocabalkan O, Olsson R. Spring mediated dynamic craniofacial reshaping. Case report. Scand J Plast Reconstr Surg Hand Surg. 1998;32(3):331–8.
6. Hirabayashi S, Sugawara Y, Sakurai A, Harii K, Park S. Frontoorbital advancement by gradual distraction. J Neurosurg. 1998;89:1058–61.
7. Imai K, Komune H, Toda C, Nomachi T, Enoki E, Sakamoto H, Kitano S, Hatoko M, Fujimoto T. Cranial remodeling to treat craniosynostosis by gradual distraction using a new device. J Neurosurg. 2002;96(4):654–9.
8. Wall SA, Goldin JH, Hockley AD, et al. Fronto-orbital re-operation in craniosynostosis. Br J Plast Surg. 1994;47:180–4.
9. Whitaker LA, Bartlett SP, Schut L, et al. Craniosynostosis: an analysis of the timing, treatment, and complications in 164 consecutive patients. Plast Reconstr Surg. 1987;80:195–206.
10. McCarthy JG, Glasberg SB, Cutting CB, et al. Twenty-year experience with early surgery for craniosynostosis: II. The craniofacial synostosis syndromes and pansynostosis—results and unsolved problems. Plast Reconstr Surg. 1995;96:284–95.
11. Williams JK, Cohen SR, Burstein FD, et al. A longitudinal, statistical study of reoperation rates in craniosynostosis. Plast Reconstr Surg. 1997;100:305–10.
12. McCarthy JG, editor. Distraction of the craniofacial skeleton. New York: Springer; 1999.
13. Derderian CA, Wink JD, McGrath JL, Collinsworth A, Bartlett SP, Taylor JA. Volumetric changes in cranial vault expansion: comparison of fronto-orbital advancement and posterior cranial vault distraction osteogenesis. Plast Reconstr Surg. 2015;135:1665–72.
14. Swanson JW, Samra F, Bauder A, Mitchell BT, Taylor JA, Bartlett SP. An algorithm for managing syndromic craniosynostosis utilizing posterior vault distraction osteogenesis. Plast Reconstr Surg. 2016;137(5):829e–41e.
15. Steinbacher DM, Skirpan J, Puchala J, Bartlett SP. Expansion of the posterior cranial vault using distraction osteogenesis. Plast Reconstr Surg. 2011;127:792–801.
16. Tahiri Y, Swanson JW, Taylor JA. Distraction osteogenesis versus conventional fronto-orbital advancement for the treatment of unilateral coronal synostosis: a comparison of peri-operative morbidity and short-term outcomes. J Craniofac Surg. 2015;26:1904–8.
17. Wall SA, Thomas GP, Johnson D, et al. The preoperative incidence of raised intracranial pressure in nonsyndromic sagittal craniosynostosis is underestimated in the literature. J Neurosurg Pediatr. 2014;14:674–81.

18. Renier D, Sainte-Rose C, Marchac D, Hirsch JF. Intracranial pressure in craniostenosis. J Neurosurg. 1982;57:370–7.
19. Speltz ML, Collett BR, Wallace ER, et al. Intellectual and academic functioning of school-age children with single-suture craniosynostosis. Pediatrics. 2015;135:e615–23.
20. Hashim PW, Patel A, Yang JF, et al. The effects of whole-vault cranioplasty versus strip craniectomy on long-term neuropsychological outcomes in sagittal craniosynostosis. Plast Reconstr Surg. 2014;134:491–501.
21. Spruijt B, Joosten KF, Driessen C, et al. Algorithm for the management of intracranial hypertension in children with syndromic craniosynostosis. Plast Reconstr Surg. 2015;136(2):331–40.
22. Cohen SR, Holmes RE, Amis P, Fichtner H. Internal craniofacial distraction with biodegradable devices: early stabilization and protected bone regeneration. J Craniofac Surg. 2000;11:354–66.
23. Lauritzen CG, Sugawara Y, Kocabalkan O, et al. Spring mediated dynamic craniofacial reshaping. Case report. Scand J Plast Reconstr Surg Hand Surg. 1998;32(3):331–8.
24. Lauritzen CG, Davis C, Ivarsson A, et al. The evolving role of springs in craniofacial surgery: the first 100 clinical cases. Plast Reconstr Surg. 2008;121:545–54.
25. Paley D. PRECICE intramedullary limb lengthening system. Expert Rev Med Devices. 2015;12(3):231–49.
26. Cheung KM, Cheung JP, Samartzis D, Mak KC, Wong YW, Cheung WY, Akbarnia BA, Luk KD. Magnetically controlled growing rods for severe spinal curvature in young children: a prospective case series. Lancet. 2012;379(9830):1967–74.
27. Rinehart G, Forget T, Zografakis J, Manepalli AN, Pittman T. Cranial vault expansion using transcutaneously activated magnetic implants. Pediatr Neurosurg. 1998;28(6):293–9.
28. Baird C, Fewings P, Manepalli A, Pittman T, Rinehart G. Cranial vault expansion: a comparison of magnetic coupled distraction to traditional surgical repositioning. Pediatr Neurosurg. 2000;33(1):2–6.
29. Goldstein JA, Paliga JT, Wink JD, et al. A craniometric analysis of posterior cranial vault distraction osteogenesis. Plast Reconstr Surg. 2013;131:1367.
30. Nowinski D, Di Rocco F, Renier D, et al. Posterior cranial vault expansion in the treatment of craniosynostosis. Comparison of current techniques. Childs Nerv Syst. 2012;28:1537–44.
31. Derderian CA, Bastidas N, Bartlett SP. Posterior cranial vault expansion using distraction osteogenesis. Childs Nerv Syst. 2012;28:1551–6.
32. Ylikontiola LP, Sándor GK, Salokorpi N, Serlo WS. Experience with craniosynostosis treatment using posterior cranial vault distraction osteogenesis. Ann Maxillofac Surg. 2012;2(1):4–7.
33. Serlo WS, Ylikontiola LP, Lähdesluoma N, et al. Posterior cranial vault distraction osteogenesis in craniosynostosis: estimated increases in intracranial volume. Childs Nerv Syst. 2011;27:627–33.
34. Thomas GP, Wall SA, Jayamohan J, et al. Lessons learned in posterior cranial vault distraction. J Craniofac Surg. 2014;25:1721–7.
35. Wiberg A, Magdum S, Richards PG, et al. Posterior calvarial distraction in craniosynostosis—an evolving technique. J Craniomaxillofac Surg. 2012;40:799–806.
36. Maurice SM, Gachiani JM. Posterior cranial vault distraction with resorbable distraction devices. J Craniofac Surg. 2014;25:1249–51.
37. Taylor JA, Derderian CA, Bartlett SP, Fiadjoe JE, Sussman EA, Stricker PA. Perioperative morbidity in posterior cranial vault expansion: distraction osteogenesis versus conventional osteotomy. Plast Reconstr Surg. 2012;129:674e–80e.
38. Hopper RA. New trends in cranio-orbital and midface distraction for craniofacial dysostoses. Curr Opin Otolaryngol. 2012;20:298–303.
39. Fearon JA. Evidence-based medicine: craniosynostosis. Plast Reconstr Surg. 2014;133:1261–75.
40. Fearon JA, Podner C. Apert syndrome: evaluation of a treatment algorithm. Plast Reconstr Surg. 2013;131:132–42.

41. Samra F, Swanson JW, Mitchell BT, Bauder AR, Taylor JA, Bartlett SP. Posterior vault distraction conveys anterior benefit in Apert syndrome. Boston: American Society of Plastic Surgeons; 2015.
42. Fearon JA. Chapter 35: Syndromic craniosynostosis. In: Neligan PC, editor. Plastic surgery, vol. 3: craniofacial, head and neck surgery, and pediatric plastic surgery. 3rd ed. London: Elsevier; 2013.
43. Francis PM, Beals S, Rekate HL, et al. Chronic tonsillar herniation and Crouzon's syndrome. Pediatr Neurosurg. 1992;18:202–6.
44. Levitt MR, Niazi TN, Hopper RA, et al. Resolution of syndromic craniosynos tosis-associated Chiari malformation type I without suboccipital decompression after posterior cranial vault release. J Neurosurg Pediatr. 2012;9:111–5.
45. Crocker M, Nesbitt A, Rich P, Bell B. Symptomatic venous sinus thrombosis following bone wax application to emissary veins. Br J Neurosurg. 2008;22:798–800.
46. Komuro Y, Hashizume K, Koizumi T, et al. Cranial expansion with distraction osteogenesis for multiple-suture synostosis in school-aged children. J Craniofac Surg. 2009;20:457–60.
47. Komuro Y, Shimizu A, Ueda A, et al. Whole cranial vault expansion by continual occipital and fronto-orbital distraction in syndromic craniosynosto- sis. J Craniofac Surg. 2011;22:269–72.
48. Choi JW, Ra YS, Hong SH, Kim H, Shin HW, Chung IW, et al. Use of distraction osteogenesis to change endocranial morphology in unilateral coronal craniosynostosis patients. Plast Reconstr Surg. 2010;126:995–1004.
49. Steinbacher DM, Wink J, Bartlett SP. Temporal hollowing following surgical correction of unicoronal synostosis. Plast Reconstr Surg. 2011;128:231–40.
50. Taylor JA, Paliga JT, Wes A, et al. A critical evaluation of long-term aesthetic outcomes of fronto-orbital advancement and cranial vault remodeling in the treatment of non-syndromic unicoronal craniosynostosis. Plast Reconstr Surg. 2015;135:220–31.
51. Samra F, Paliga JT, Tahiri Y, et al. The prevalence of strabismus in unilateral coronal synostosis. Plast Reconstr Surg. 2014;134(suppl 1):19–20.
52. Choi JW, Koh KS, Hong JP, Hong SH, Ra Y. One-piece frontoorbital advancement with distraction but without a supraorbital bar for coronal craniosynostosis. J Plast Reconstr Aesthet Surg. 2009;62:1166–73.
53. Taylor JA, Tahiri Y, Paliga JT, et al. A new approach for the treatment of unilateral coronal synostosis based on distraction osteogenesis. Plast Reconstr Surg. 2014;134:176e–8e.
54. Selber JM, Reid RR, Chike-Obi CJ, et al. The changing epidemiologic spectrum of single-suture synostoses. Plast Reconstr Surg. 2008;122:527–33.
55. Jarrahy R, Kawamoto HK, KEagle J, Dickinson B, Katchikian HV, Bradley JP. Three tenets for staged correction of Kleeblattschädel or cloverleaf skull deformity. Plast Reconstr Surg. 2009;123:310–8.
56. Mitchell BT, Swanson JW, Taylor JA. A new single-stage, distraction-mediated cranial vault expansion technique for the multisuture deformity. J Craniofac Surg. 2015;26(6):1923–5.
57. Tuncbilek G, Kaykcoglu A, Bozkurt G, Akalan N. Spring-mediated cranioplasty in patients with multiple-suture synostosis and cloverleaf skull deformity. J Craniofac Surg. 2012;23:374–7.
58. Meling TR, Høgevold H-E, Due-Tønnessen BJ, Skjelbred P. Comparison of perioperative morbidity after LeFort III and monobloc distraction osteogenesis. Br J Oral Maxillofac Surg. 2011;49:131–4.
59. Nout E, Wolvius EB, van Adrichem LNA, Ongkosuwito EM, van der Wal KGH. Complications in maxillary distraction using the RED II device: a retrospective analysis of 21 patients. Int J Oral Maxillofac Surg. 2006;35:897–902.
60. Greives MR, Ware BW, Tian AG, Taylor JA, Pollack IF, Losee JE. Complications in posterior cranial vault distraction. Ann Plast Surg. 2016;76(2):211–5.
61. White N, Evans M, Dover MS, Noons P, Solanki G, Nishikawa H. Posterior calvarial vault expansion using distraction osteogenesis. Childs Nerv Syst. 2009;25(2):231–6.

The manufacturer's authorised representative in the EU is Springer Nature Customer Service Centre GmbH, Europaplatz 3, 69115 Heidelberg, Germany. If you have any concerns regarding our products, please contact ProductSafety@springernature.com

Printed and bound by CPI Group (UK) Ltd, Croydon, CR0 4YY

25/09/2026

02222863-0003